COVID 19 – Monitoring with IoT Devices

Authored By

Ambika Nagaraj

St. Francis College
Koramangala, Bengaluru, Karnataka 560034
India

COVID 19 – Monitoring with IoT Devices

Author: Ambika Nagaraj

ISBN (Online): 978-981-5179-45-3

ISBN (Print): 978-981-5179-46-0

ISBN (Paperback): 978-981-5179-47-7

need for a court order if at any point you breach any terms of this License Agreement. In no event will any delay or failure by Bentham Science Publishers in enforcing your compliance with this License Agreement constitute a waiver of any of its rights.

3. You acknowledge that you have read this License Agreement, and agree to be bound by its terms and conditions. To the extent that any other terms and conditions presented on any website of Bentham Science Publishers conflict with, or are inconsistent with, the terms and conditions set out in this License Agreement, you acknowledge that the terms and conditions set out in this License Agreement shall prevail.

Bentham Science Publishers Pte. Ltd.
80 Robinson Road #02-00
Singapore 068898
Singapore
Email: subscriptions@benthamscience.net

BENTHAM SCIENCE

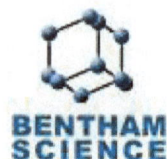

CONTENTS

FOREWORD I

Till December 2022, more than six hundred fifty-one million confirmed cases of COVID-19, whereas more than six million deaths were reported to WHO from all over the world. The SARS-CoV-2 virus and its variants spread mainly if there is close contact between people. In confined and enclosed places, short-range aerosol, airborne, droplet transmission happens at a conversational distance. It is recommended to avoid poor ventilation, and crowded indoor settings, and touching eyes, nose, or mouth after touching surfaces or objects. Anyone asymptomatic or pre-symptomatic carrying the virus can spread it. Singing, and breathing during the exercise can cause the virus to spread. Well-fitted three-layered masks, alcohol-based hand rubs, one-meter distance, cleaning hands, avoiding touching surfaces, and getting vaccinated can avoid SARS-COV-2 virus infection.

Monitoring public places, and hospitals, and understanding the overall situation in a country and the world is important to reduce the adverse impacts of Covid-19. Monitoring the situation, and venues without direct touch is possible through the Internet of Things (IoT) based solutions. The sensors, actuators, RFIDs, Near Field Communications, Unmanned Aerial Vehicles (UAVs) connected through the Wireless Sensor Network, and the Internet are the crucial elements in the monitoring of the COVID-19 situation.

Smart thermometers, Telehealth Consultations, wearables, robot assistance, and remote monitoring through the GPS-based ArogyaSetu are a few examples of IoT-enabled devices useful in COVID-19 monitoring. In particular, electronic sensors in the form of epidermal tattoos biomarkers cortisol, contact lenses for intraocular pressure, textiles face masks observe breathing patterns, airborne pathogens, inflammation markers, skin temperature, and metabolism monitoring, wristbands for the heartbeat and O_2 monitoring, and microneedle patches can help collect previously inaccessible physical and biochemical signals. Professor Steve Lindsay from Durham University developed the organic semiconducting (OSC) sensors that can detect fingerprints from body odor samples.

Author Dr. Ambika has good experience in the research field of WSN and academic experience. The content of the book is interesting and timely. Alone an IoT cannot bring insights and decisions based on the data collection, hence the author has elaborated machine learning techniques for the necessary actions based on the predictions. The predictions can help the government, social bodies, and individuals prepare themselves to handle the difficult situation of the pandemic. The content is highly relevant to extend the research in the health domain and to support the preparation of the policies in the governance of the country.

The pandemic created emotional and psychological impressions of low mood, tiredness, pessimism, poor sleep, and appetite, and feeling helpless, guilty, and hopeless, with a gradual reduction in work output. The IoT System monitoring the behavioral and allied patterns is equally important as that of social monitoring. The individual suffering from the infections needs to be monitored and counselled through the technological aspect. This will be an important input for all who would like to contribute and like to work in this direction.

Manoj Devare
Amity Institute of Information Technology
Amity University, Maharashtra
India

FOREWORD II

Covid sickness (COVID-19) is an irresistible illness brought about by the SARS-CoV-2 infection. The vast majority contaminated with the infection will encounter gentle to severe respiratory ailment and recuperate without requiring urgent treatment. In any case, some will turn out to be genuinely sick and require clinical consideration. More weak individuals and those with basic ailments like cardiovascular infection, diabetes, acute respiratory sickness, or disease are bound to foster difficult diseases. Anybody can get infected with COVID-19 and become genuinely sick or pass on at whatever stage in life. Observing and overseeing expected contaminated patients of COVID-19 is yet difficult with the most recent advancements. As a preventive measure, legitimate group checking, and the board frameworks are expected to be introduced in the open spots to restrict unexpected out brakes and confer further developed medical care. The quantity of new contaminations can be essentially diminished by taking on social distancing. In such scenarios, these smart IoT gadgets can become a very significant and important tool. The book introduces 5 chapters that discuss many interesting ideas that show how IoT devices are helping to tackle situations in the manufacturing and operational ecosystem of COVID-19.

Jyotir Moy Chatterjee
Department of Information Technology
Lord Buddha Education Foundation
Kathmandu-4600, Nepal

PREFACE

In patients with severe COVID-19, SARS-CoV-2 can cause not only antiviral immune responses to be activated but also uncontrolled inflammatory responses characterized by the significant release of pro-inflammatory cytokines. It can result in lymphopenia, lymphocyte dysfunction, and abnormalities in granulocytes and monocytes. Septic shock, severe multiple organ dysfunction, and infections by microorganisms may result from these immune abnormalities brought on by SARS-CoV-2. There is growing evidence that patients with viruses have resistant patterns closely linked to their disease progression. These patients exhibit lymphopenia, activation, and dysfunction of lymphocytes. They also have abnormalities in granulocytes and monocytes. They show elevated cytokines and increased immunoglobulin G (IgG) antibodies.

The well-defined scheme known as the Internet of Things (IoT) comprises digital, mechanical, and interconnected computing techniques. These devices can transmit data over a defined network without any human involvement. It is the network-compliant system of connected devices and operations, including; software, hardware, the network's connectivity, and any other necessary computer or electronic device that ultimately makes them responsive by supporting data altercation and collection. Utilizing an interconnected web made it possible for the healthcare system to be helpful for the proper monitoring of COVID-19 patients. The hospital readmission rate is reduced, and this technology improves patient satisfaction. The book is a description of how these devices aid in helping humanity.

Ambika Nagaraj
St. Francis College
Koramangala, Bengaluru, Karnataka 560034
India

CHAPTER 1

COVID -19

Abstract: Corona is a single-stranded RNA virus that has been around since the late 1960s when it was first discovered. The Nidovirales order includes the Corona viridae family of viruses. The crown-shaped spikes on the virus structure's outer surface inspire the name Corona. The virus has affected chickens and pigs, but there hasn't been a significant human-to-human transmission. The virus's mode of communication and other related information are continually updated every few weeks, increasing uncertainty. A Chinese study suggests that the COVID-19 pandemic had a significant psychological impact on more than half of the participants. One more ongoing review from Denmark revealed mental prosperity as adversely impacted. According to the American Psychiatric Association's survey, nearly half of Americans were anxious. The chapter details the disease, its symptoms and measures taken.

Keywords: Covid-19, SARS-CoV-2.

1.1. INTRODUCTION

The most recent infectious disease to rapidly spread across the globe is coronavirus disease 2019, also known as COVID-19 [1, 2]. The severe acute respiratory syndrome coronavirus 2 (SARS-CoV-2) [3] is the etiologic agent of COVID-19. The World Health Organization and the Public Health Emergency of International Concern declared the 2019–2020 pandemic due to the discovery of SARS-CoV-2 for the first time in Wuhan, China, in 2019. The disease began in Asia, but it has rapidly spread worldwide. It is the first coronavirus-related pandemic, according to the World Health Organization. Italy has risen to a prominent position in the international picture of infected patients due to the impressive growth in reported cases over time. Fig. (**1**) depicts the transmission of the disease. Fig. (**2**) represents SARS-CoV-2 virus depicting spike protein and mRNA core. Figs. (**3-5**) represent Integrative post-COVID symptoms model in non-hospitalized patients.

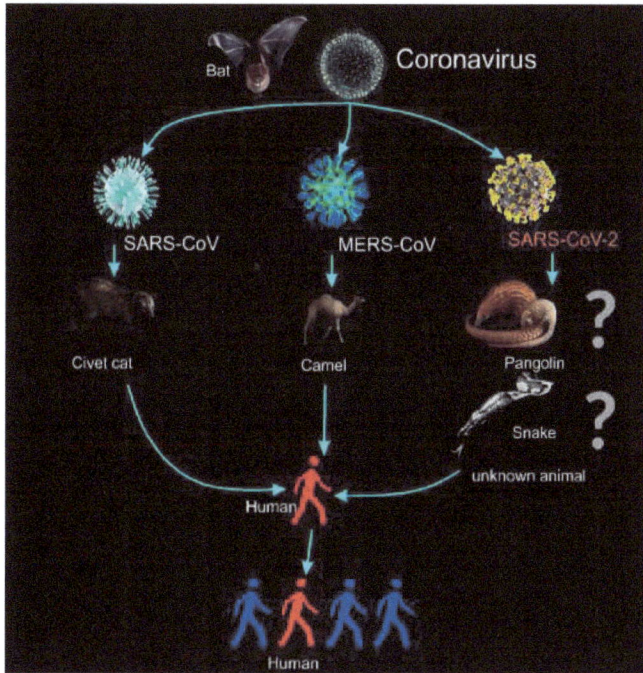

Fig. (1). Illustration for the transmission of coronaviruses [3].

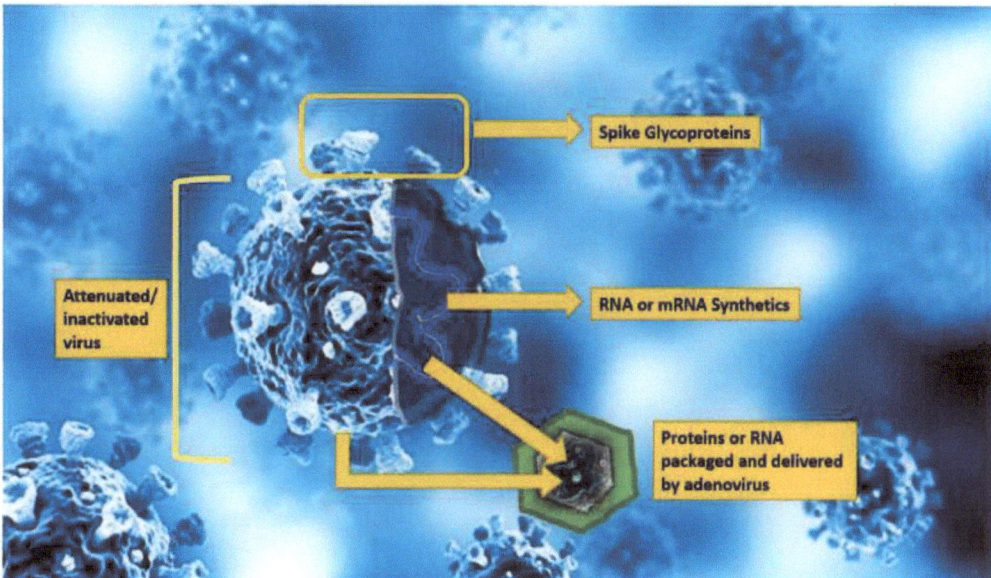

Fig. (2). Artist sketch of SARS-CoV-2 virus depicting spike protein and mRNA core [4].

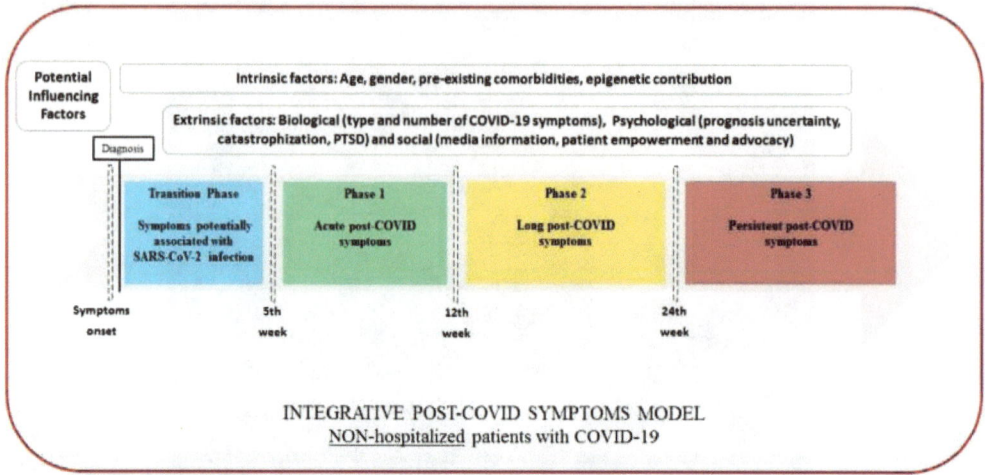

Fig. (3). Integrative post-COVID symptoms model in non-hospitalized patients showing transition phase (blue), and phases 1 (green), 2 (yellow), and 3 (red) of post-COVID symptoms. PTSD: post-traumatic stress disorder [5].

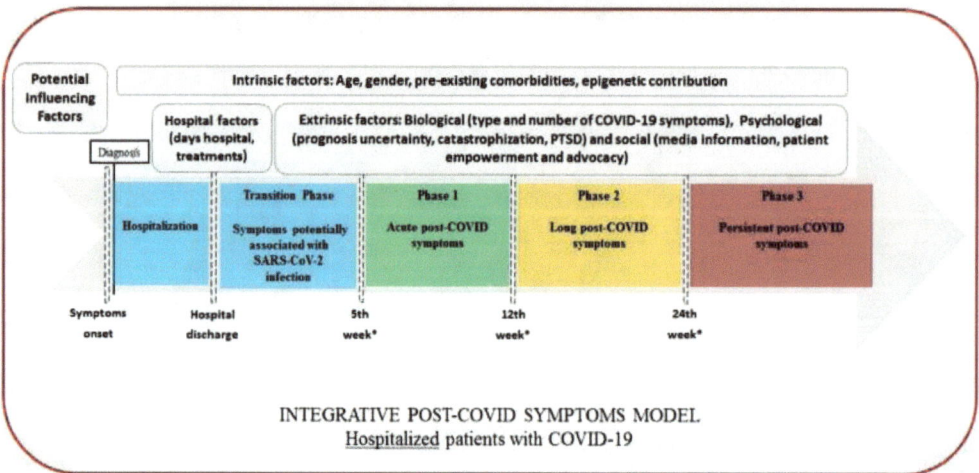

Fig. (4). Integrative post-COVID symptoms model in hospitalized patients showing transition phase (blue), and phases 1 (green), 2 (yellow), and 3 (red) of post-COVID symptoms. PTSD: post-traumatic stress disorder [5].

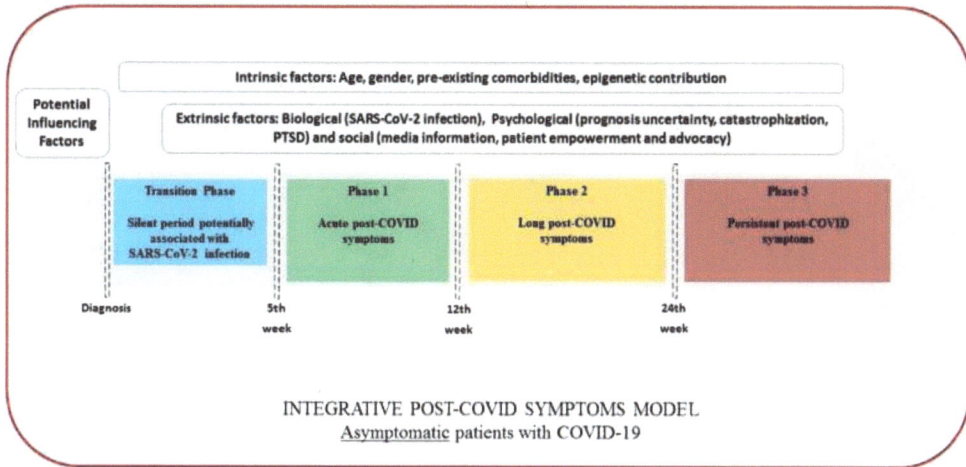

Fig. (5). Integrative post-COVID symptoms model in asymptomatic individuals showing transition phase (blue), and phases 1 (green), 2 (yellow), and 3 (red) of post-COVID symptoms. PTSD: post-traumatic stress disorder [5].

1.2. SYMPTOMS

Due to sustained human-to-human transmission, COVID-19 is rapidly spreading worldwide. At the beginning of the disease, pathogen concentrations are deficient, necessitating exact and sensitive detection techniques for prompt diagnosis and efficient surveillance. The correlation between the sensitivity of pathogen detection in clinical applications and pathogen enrichment methods based on sample preparation is significant. Additionally, the sensitivity of the COVID-19 diagnostic procedures remains low, necessitating the addition of electrophoresis and fluorescent dye labeling for detection.

The phase of change: Possible symptoms of acute COVID-19 infection: symptoms for four to five weeks;

Phase 1: Acute symptoms following COVID: symptoms between weeks 5 and 12;

Phase 2: Symptoms long after COVID: symptoms between weeks 12 and 24;

Phase 3: Consistent symptoms following COVID: symptoms that persist for over 24 weeks.

Long COVID syndrome [7], also known as a post-COVID-19 syndrome [8], first gained widespread recognition in social support groups and then spread to the scientific and medical communities. Because it affects COVID-19 survivors of all disease severity levels, including younger adults, children, and those who were not hospitalized, this illness is poorly understood. Female sex, more than five early symptoms, early dyspnoea, previous psychiatric disorders, and specific biomarkers may be associated risk factors. Fig. (**6**) represents a summary of multi-system clinical presentations of long COVID-19 syndrome.

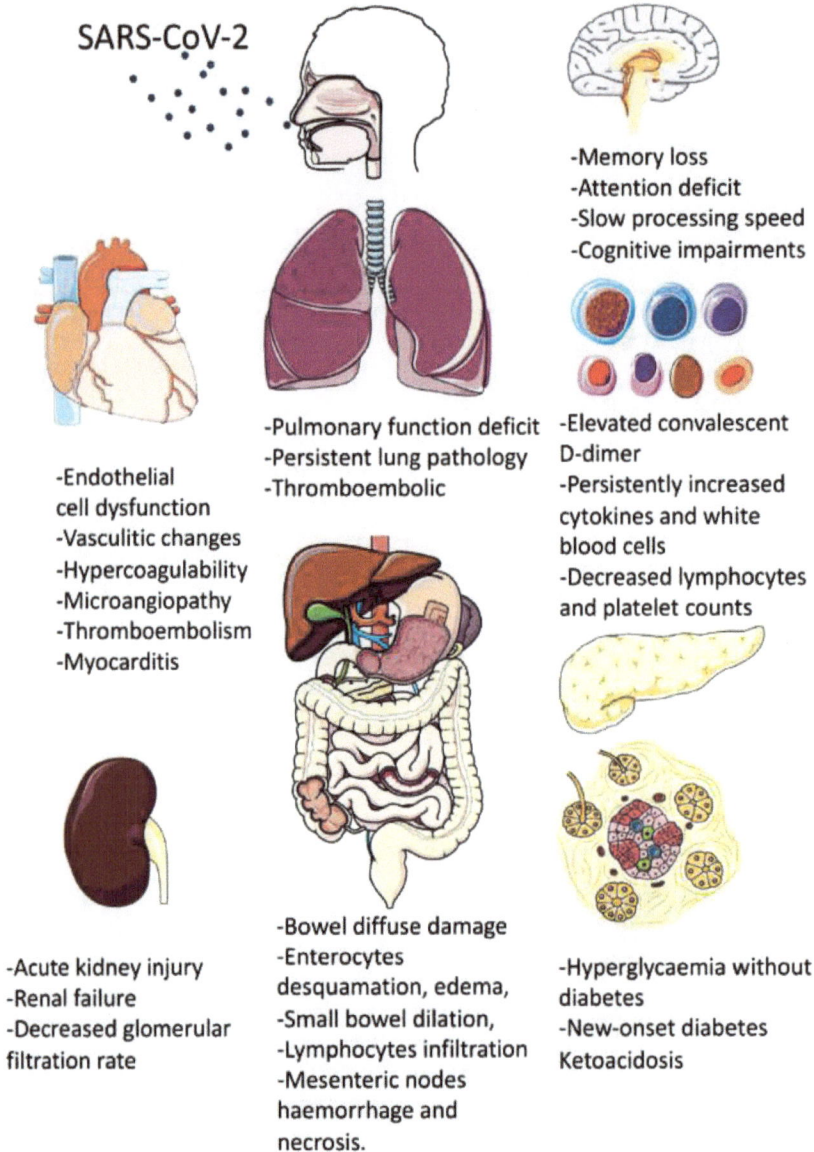

SARS-CoV-2

-Memory loss
-Attention deficit
-Slow processing speed
-Cognitive impairments

-Pulmonary function deficit
-Persistent lung pathology
-Thromboembolic

-Elevated convalescent D-dimer
-Persistently increased cytokines and white blood cells
-Decreased lymphocytes and platelet counts

-Endothelial cell dysfunction
-Vasculitic changes
-Hypercoagulability
-Microangiopathy
-Thromboembolism
-Myocarditis

-Acute kidney injury
-Renal failure
-Decreased glomerular filtration rate

-Bowel diffuse damage
-Enterocytes desquamation, edema,
-Small bowel dilation,
-Lymphocytes infiltration
-Mesenteric nodes haemorrhage and necrosis.

-Hyperglycaemia without diabetes
-New-onset diabetes Ketoacidosis

Fig. (6). Summary of multi-system clinical presentations of Long COVID-19 Syndrome [6].

An integrative review of the empirical and theoretical literature that has been published was carried out [9]. Post-COVID-19 syndrome, post-SARS-CoV-2, long COVID-19, long COVID-19 syndrome, and pathophysiology of post-COVID-19 were used in search of articles published as of August 30, 2021, in the PubMed, CINAHL, and Web of Science databases. There were a total of 27,929 articles found. It uses a constant comparison approach. It discovered patterns, variations, and relationships in the data through systematic categorization. Each group reviewed the data using an iterative compare-and-contrast strategy to integrate results from different articles.

It compares [10] a matched control group from the general population to individuals with covid-19 to determine the rates of organ-specific dysfunction after hospital discharge. It carried out an observational, retrospective, and matched cohort study on patients with covid-19 who were admitted to the hospital. It utilized the Emergency Clinic Episode Measurements Conceded Patient Consideration records for Britain up to August 31, 2020, and the General Practice Extraction Administration Information for Pandemic Preparation and Exploration up to September 30, 2020. For pandemic research and analysis, it extracts primary care records gathered from surgeries by NHS Digital. These records include information on over 56 million people registered at NHS England general practice surgeries and are updated every two weeks. A subset of approximately 35,000 clinical codes has been included in the extract for potential use in the pandemic-related analysis. For deaths occurring up until September 30, 2020, and registered by October 7, 2020, death registrations from the Office for National Statistics were linked. It matched patients to controls for potential confounding factors in the relationship between outcomes and covid-19 hospital admission. Age, sex, ethnicity, region, and poverty were all included in the list of personal characteristics. The diagnoses were identified as comorbidities from the hospital and primary care diagnoses. It calculated rate ratios from the rates of death, readmission, and multiorgan dysfunction per 1000 person-years for patients and controls after hospital discharge. 53 795 of the 86 955 people hospitalized for covid-19 at the end of the study had been released alive.

1.3. MEASURES

1.3.1. Demographic Information

Demographic factors associated with COVID-19 vaccination among adults over the age of 18 were reported in all studies. Age, gender, education, and ethnicity were the demographics that it evaluated the most frequently. Having children, being employed, being religious, and smoking status were among the less regularly used constructs. In most studies, the intention to receive the COVID-19 vaccine was significantly correlated with age, gender, and education. After the coronavirus outbreak in March, April, May, and September 2020, eight studies showed that older men and women were more likely to get vaccinated than younger people and women. According to a survey that was carried out in the United States, older populations were more willing to vaccinate than younger ones because the risk of mortality elicits a more significant proportion of willing participants than morbidity alone. Fig. (**7**) represents a conceptual framework for the hypothesized predictors of intention to receive COVID-19 vaccines based on the modified health belief model.

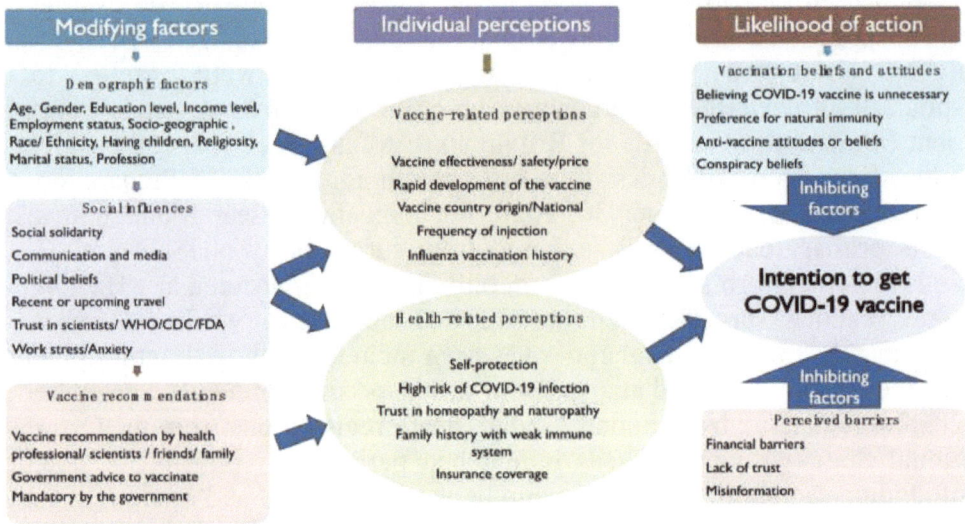

Fig. (7). Conceptual framework for the hypothesized predictors of intention to receive COVID-19 vaccines based on the modified health belief model (HBM) [11].

The study [12] followed Helsinki's international ethical guidelines. The study's participation was entirely voluntary and completely free. All of the questionnaires and any requested personal identification information were anonymous. There were three sections to the questionnaire. It included gender, age, autonomous region and place of residence, and professional situation in the first. The second section took anthropometric variables like height, weight, and Body Mass Index. It took food and nutrition variables like following the Mediterranean Diet, eating more, and participating in food preparation. The third and final section gathered data on physical activity-related variables like the type of exercise, dedicated time, and information research needed to perform the exercise. It used the Google questionnaire platform and social media platforms like WhatsApp, Instagram, Twitter, and Facebook for dissemination. There were a total of 1073 responses to the questionnaire, but it discarded eight of them due to differences in age, weight, or height.

Another study [13] followed PRISMA guidelines in the systematic review and mini meta-analysis. Its goal is to determine how often medical students are anxious during this pandemic. The following data were extracted using a pre-designed data extraction form - country, sample size, anxiety prevalence, the proportion of females, average age, anxiety assessment instruments, response rate, and sampling strategies. Nine criteria were used to assess quality, each receiving a zero or one score. After screening the titles and abstracts for compliance with the inclusion criteria, it eliminated 1338 of the initial 1361 potential records. Fig. (**8**) provides graphical abstract.

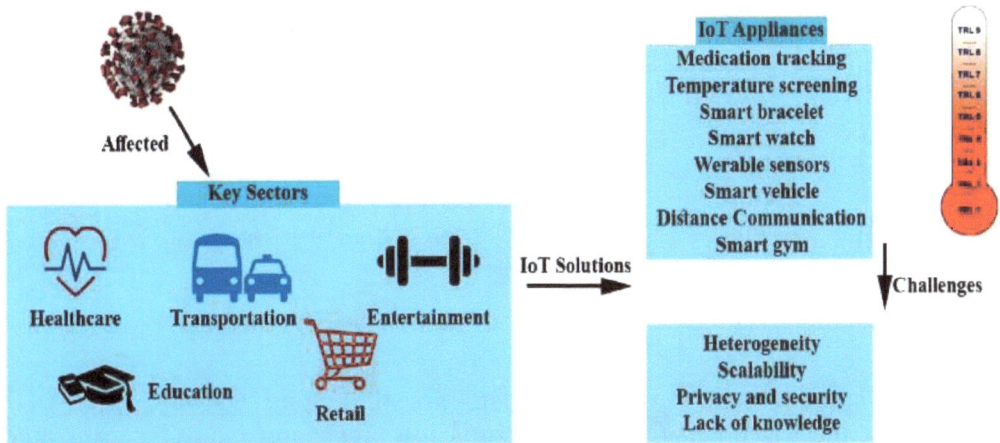

Fig. (8). Graphical Abstract [14].

The purpose of this study [15] is to discuss the questionnaire development process. A structured questionnaire was used to collect the primary data for this study. In addition to the demographic data, the survey had three significant sections. The demographic information section has four main questions: gender, age, education level, and participants' occupation. The following team, part 1, consists of questions about the field participants' current employment and the kinds of IoT service experiences they have had. On a five-point level of agreement Likert scale, the participants were asked to rate their responses to share their perceptions. The 12 advantages gained from using IoT services during COVID-19 are listed in Part 2 of the questionnaire. The survey used twelve related statements. The third section of the survey asks respondents about 12 difficulties they encountered when utilizing IoT services during COVID-19. During May and June of 2021, a structured online questionnaire was used to collect the data for this study. The sampling strategy was convenient sampling, in which IoT users from various fields were conveniently identified. It utilized IBM Statistical Package for Social Science (SPSS) version 28 for this study's data analysis. Cronbach alpha values and corrected item-total correlation were used to evaluate each construct's consistency and reliability. Fig. (**9**) represents COVID-19's Impact on IoT Research and Development.

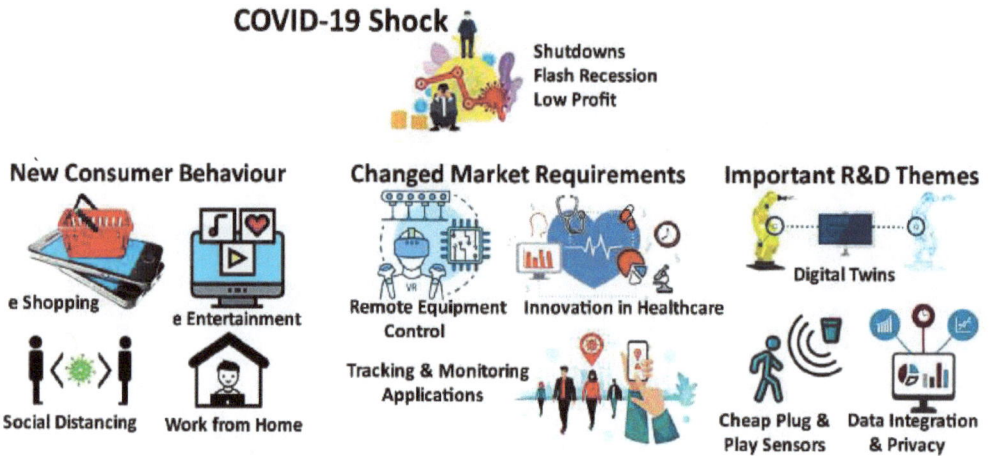

Fig. (9). COVID-19's Impact on IoT Research and Development [16].

The five layers of the proposed system are the cloud (Devare, 2019), the application, the fog layer, the data transmission layer, and the IoT sensor layer. Machine learning and deep learning algorithms are used in the Fog layer's system architecture to diagnose patients' diseases and generate and send users diagnostic and emergency alerts. The architecture's wearable IoT layer gathers data from various medical, location, body, environmental, and meteorological sensors [17]. The data transmission layer sends the collected data to the Fog layer for real-time processing and diagnosis of the patient's health. An alert signal is sent to the patient's mobile phone for prompt prevention once the patient's health condition has been diagnosed. This layer divides the patient's health status into healthy and unhealthy classes—the cloud layer of the architecture stores the analysis's findings. The Cloud layer [18, 19] sends alerts to healthy individuals about infected areas. There are 5644 rows and 111 features in the COVID-19 dataset. One hundred images from the primary database are used in the experiments.

The work [20] aims to investigate how the Internet of Things (IoT) can help prevent COVID-19. The combination of human services tools, clinical treatment framework, Web design, software, and services make up the IoT approach's operating principle. The IoT framework allows it to collect data, monitor reports, comprehend databases, test images, conduct investigations, and so on. Online methods have been utilized to collect data. We used a practical research design for this study. In total, 150 online questionnaires were distributed in the Indian city of Chennai, Tamilnadu. The part-time job in the critical care division is clinical examination.

Using the Application's Peripheral Interface, the IoT-health monitoring process [21] looks into physiological metrics and COVID-19 symptoms [22] communicated to the health center. The API is regarded as the infection level measurement database. When self-quarantined individuals exhibit COVID-19 symptoms, the IoT sensor calculates the geographical details, assisting in the notification of relatives. There are three levels of the developed system: Layers for IoT, cloud [23], and mobile. Each layer serves a specific purpose in successfully monitoring COVID-19 patients and making use of recordings. The wearable IoT, responsible for collecting patient data, is the first layer. The cloud layer establishes fundamental security measures before accepting the data from the cloud-based microcontroller. By ensuring data ownership and credibility, the cloud system's (Devare, 2019) data are received by the web front layer. Mel-frequency Cepstral Coefficients (MFCC) feature extraction is used to process the collected signal data. The derived features based on the MFCC are fed into the neural network that recognizes the patient's health status. Using the COVID-19 Open Research Dataset, it used a MATLAB implementation tool to create the analyzed system. It gathers information regarding the health of patients. The dataset examines 4700 scholarly articles. Fig. (**10**) represents IoT with cloud involvement for the COVID-19 situation. Fig. (**11**) shows three-layer design of COVID-19-patient health-monitoring framework .

1.3.2. Depressive Symptoms

Since its inception in Wuhan, China, in December 2019, the coronavirus disease 2019 (COVID-19) [24 - 26] has affected more than 200 nations. As of December 2020, the World Health Organization (WHO) reported 75 million confirmed cases of COVID-19 and 1.6 million deaths worldwide. Effective public response to this health crisis has relied heavily on social isolation.

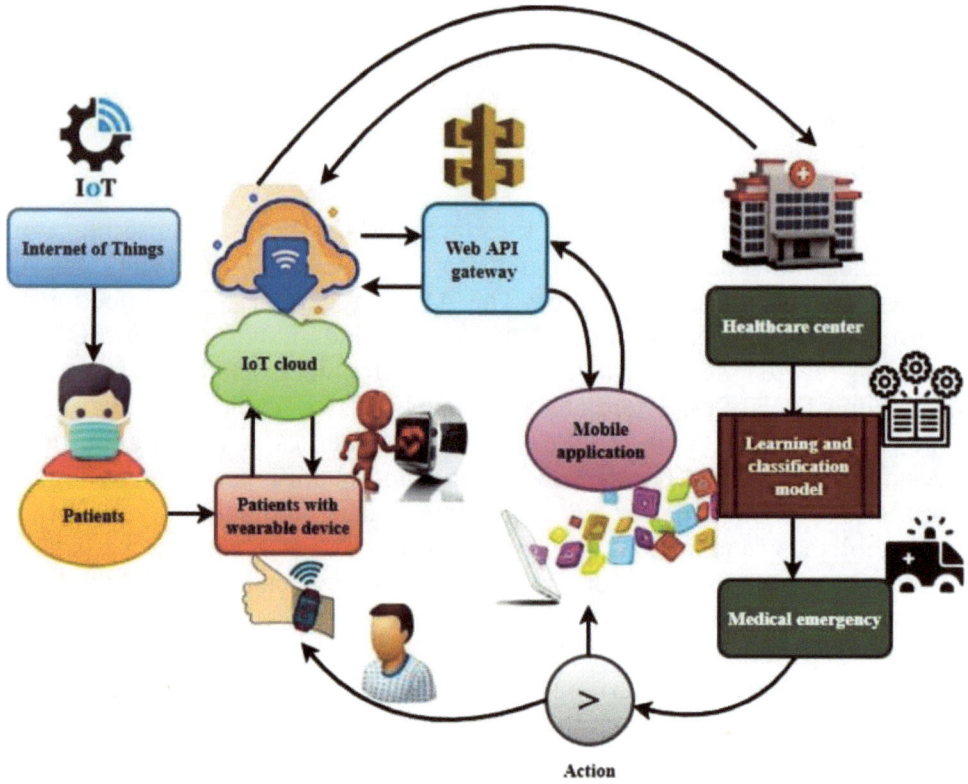

Fig. (10). IoT with cloud involvement for the COVID-19 situation [21].

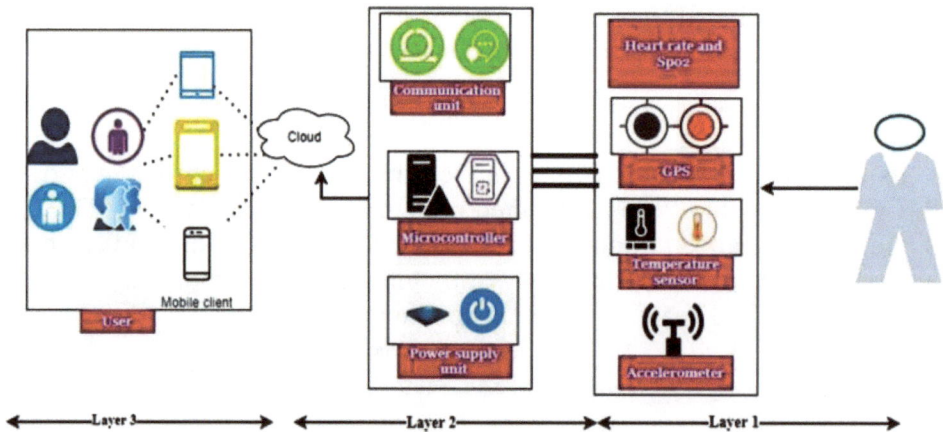

Fig. (11). Three-layer design of COVID-19-patient health-monitoring framework [21].

This study [27] demonstrated that frontline public health workers play a crucial role in protecting public mental health by highlighting the depressive symptoms experienced by individuals subjected to mandatory social isolation during the COVID-19 pandemic. From February 28 to March 6, 2020, a cross-sectional online survey was conducted in Shenzhen, China, to gather information from individuals in a mandatory home or centralized social isolation. Their depressive symptoms, as well as their perceptions of the tone of media coverage, the quality of people-centered public health services, and the risk of COVID-19 infection, were evaluated. After controlling for several variables, including demographics, the duration and location of mandatory social isolation, family infection status and isolation status, time spent on COVID-related news, and online social support, three rounds of stepwise multiple regression were used to examine the moderating effects. Fig. (**12**) illustrates direct and first-order indirect effects of various COVID-19 mitigation policies on the National well-being system components.

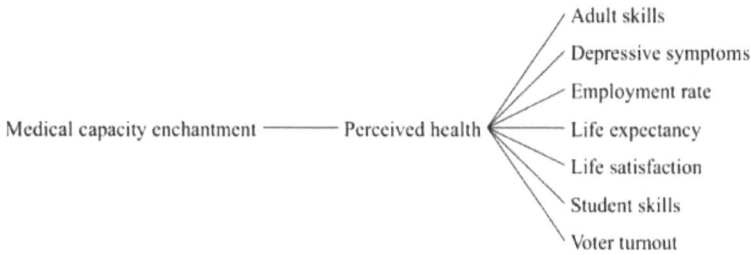

(a)

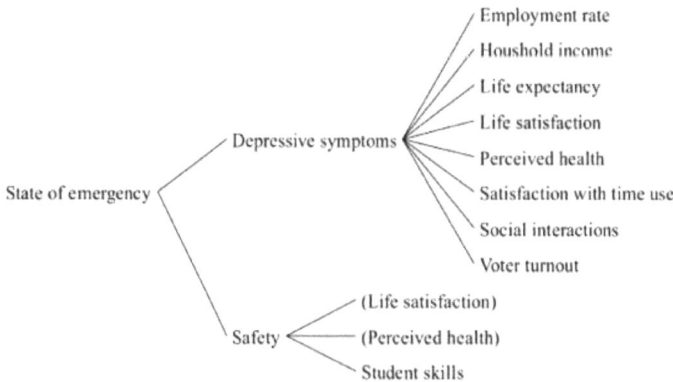

(b)

Fig. (12). Direct and first-order indirect effects of various COVID-19 mitigation policies on the of the National Well-being System components [28].

iResponse [29], a technology-driven framework for coordinated and autonomous pandemic management, enables data-driven planning and decision-making, pandemic-related monitoring and policy enforcement, and resource planning and provisioning. There are five modules in the framework: Data Analytics and Decision Making, Resource Planner, Monitoring and Break-the-Chain, Cure Development and Treatment, and Data Storage and Management Data from IoT-based sensors, social media, electronic health records, hospital occupancy data, Wi-Fi, GPS, travel itinerary, testing labs, intelligent devices, and other sources are used to collect it. This information is handled. Both in-house and cloud-based data are used to store the data. These server farms are heterogeneous, which implies they are fit for putting away different information, for example, organized, unstructured, multi-media, spatial, and EHRs. It can train several machine learning and deep learning algorithms on data that data centers provide. In addition, these trained models can carry out specific actions with real-time data. Data visualization capabilities are used to display the obtained results both statically and interactively. The work's modeling and analysis were carried out on the R statistical platform. Fig. (**13**) represents the same.

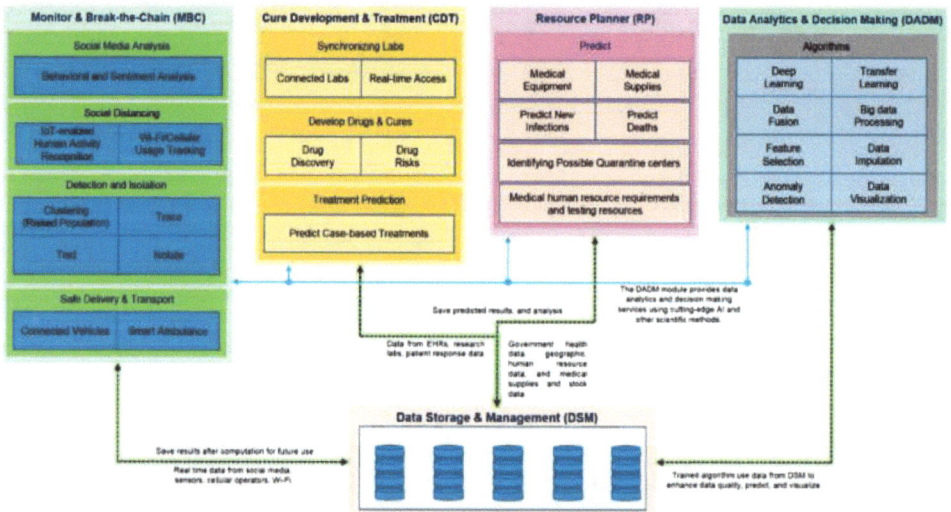

Fig. (13). iResponse framework [29].

Psychiatric outpatients who gave their consent to the study's [30] purpose and data collection participated for four weeks. The "active data" obtained from responses to self-reported questionnaires and the "passive data" gathered from multimodal sensors on smartphones comprise the collected data. Given that the mental health survey was based on behavior over the previous two weeks, the period for collecting data was set at two weeks. The app reads and stores data that are continuously generated by smartphone sensors. All sensor data are saved without the participant's intervention or command. The application can get to the sensor and store the sensor's data in the background. It can obtain facial Expression Features and Landmarks from facial images. A model for converting facial images into facial landmarks and expression features is included in the application. For each questionnaire, the application sends a notification to the participant's smartphone at the specified time, allowing the participant to respond. IRIS is a database with a distributed architecture that supports the collection, storage, processing, distributed processing, analysis, visualization, and sharing of big data. It can process large-scale time-series data quickly. According to a predetermined table, the smartphone stores the received data as a CSV file. Two hundred and nine psychiatric outpatients were recruited for the study. It collected all participants' data for four weeks following the procedure. Fig. (**14**) represents the same.

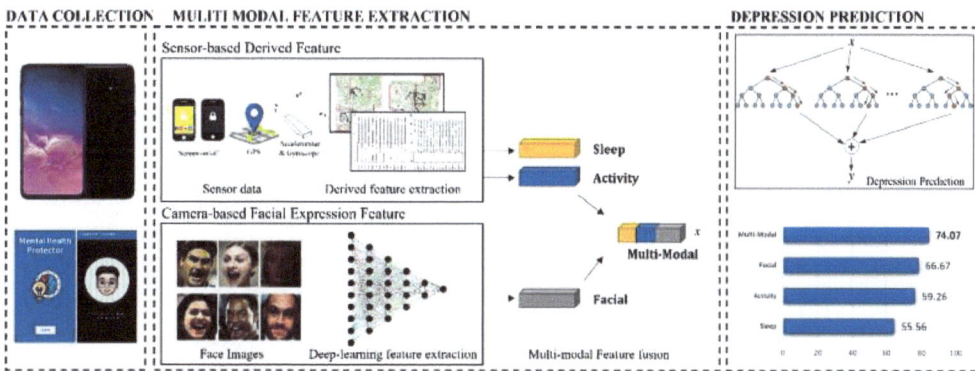

Fig. (14). Overview of the Smartphone-Based Depressed Mood Prediction System [30].

1.3.3. Emotional Health

Mental disorders significantly increase the global disease burden on their own. The estimates of the worldwide burden of disease made by the WHO in 2005 demonstrate the relative importance of various health issues worldwide. In all developing regions, non-communicable conditions rapidly become the most common cause of illness. By employing an integrated measure of disease burden—the disability-adjusted life-year, which is the sum of years lived with disability and years lost to death—the Global Burden of Disease report has revealed the extent to which mental disorders contribute. According to the report, neuropsychiatric conditions account for a quarter of all disability-adjusted life years and a third of those attributed to non-communicable diseases. However, the size of this contribution varies from country to country and income level to income level. Mental disorders are the neuropsychiatric conditions that contribute the most to disability-adjusted life years.

In the design of our EmotIoT algorithm [31], which uses IoT devices to collect and analyze user data during various activities, the recommendation includes six stages for developing an IoT system. The first step is to establish the user's characteristics, to be analyzed, including activities, frequency, and location, as well as the context in which it will use the system. It establishes the emotional parameters that the system will take into account during the analysis. The sensors and devices used to collect the data identified in Stage 1 must be determined during the Device Requirements Study stage. Investigations are done on requirements like cost, sensing frequency, usability, accessibility, and bandwidth. The IoT system's logical processes and architecture are designed during the Logic and Architecture Design stage. For smart devices, it uses Bluetooth LE to communicate with our system and collect user survey data. Through HTTP, the system obtains stored user data from the database. The IoT smart gateway keeps an eye on data processing, reducing the number of calls to the cloud. EmotIoT gathers both self-reported and IoT user data and the user's emotions. The recommendations for new games will be based on these data. A questionnaire collects users' data, opinions about the games, and feelings while participants must answer while playing. The collected data are analyzed in the data analysis stage to determine how relationships with games affect users' emotions. At the data prediction stage, the user must select the predictive models that will be used to examine the connections between user data and the system's specific performance. In the IoT Framework stage, it plans the calculation that permits the IoT framework to prescribe or adjust to accomplish client objectives. Fig. (**15**) represents the same.

The proposed system [32] could be beneficial for monitoring health at the patient level, regionally, during epidemic disease outbreaks, or in the current COVID-19 attack. The proposed system's multi-node architecture may store the subject's social facial image and GPS location and perform the initial screening at various locations. The FCMN architecture consists of several connected 1-to-N FCSN nodes spread across the globe. For the initial screening, encrypted data from each FCSN node is sent in real-time to a cloud database server connected to the internet, including body temperature, facial image, and GPS location. Real-time monitoring of health record trends for specific geographical regions, epidemic diseases, or particular patients could also be accomplished using the remote monitoring system for the assigned health worker or government authorities. It uses the facial image match algorithm. It can also track a subject or patient's travel track, and the patient's health information and GPS coordinates can be stored in a cloud database with the date and time of the records while maintaining adequate privacy protection for the data. It could keep the subject's health information in the N-FCSN systems and send the encrypted version to a cloud database server with a wireless connection. Fig. (**16**) represents the same.

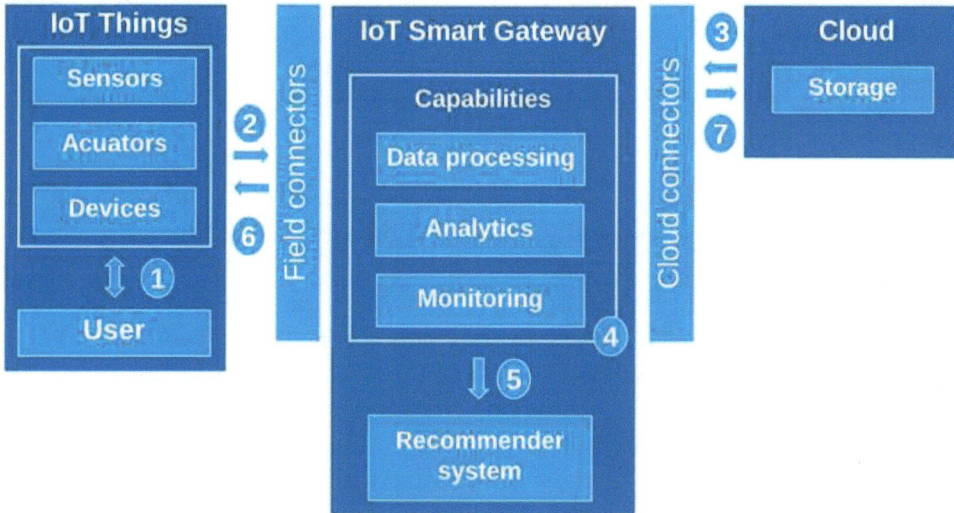

Fig. (15). Proposed Architecture [31].

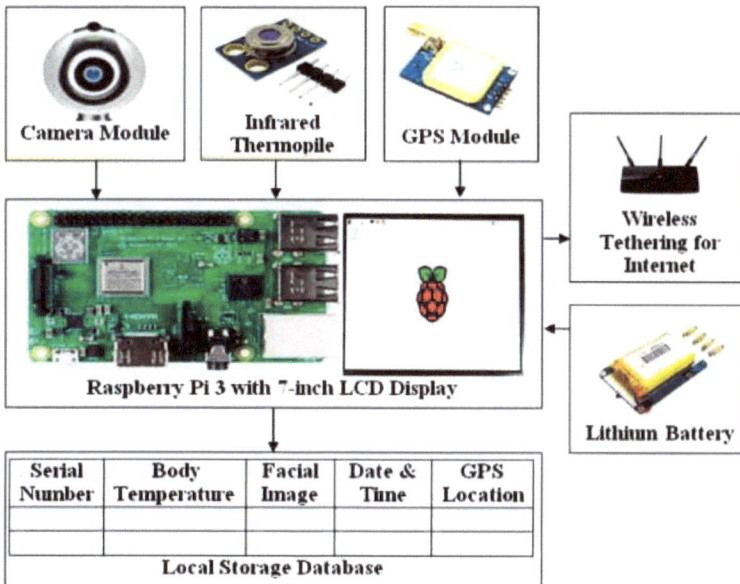

Fig. (16). Hardware Architecture [32].

1.4. POTENTIAL IMPACT

Since December 2019, when Covid illness episodes were first revealed in Wuhan, China, a rising number of cases have been accounted for in all nations on all landmasses aside from Antarctica. Staying inside, avoiding social contact, washing one's hands, travel restrictions, lockdowns, and other measures have all been implemented by nations worldwide to prevent the disease from spreading. Some of these measures, like lockdowns, are severe, affect everyday life in unusual ways, and have significant financial effects.

Models based on machine learning have been used to find patterns in health conditions and diseases. Typically, historical datasets of healthcare records and other patient data are used to train machine learning models. The diagnosis and treatment of chronic diseases like cancer were made possible by recent advances in machine learning technology in developing nations' healthcare systems. Classifying intricate data patterns with machine learning algorithms is very easy. As a result, medical applications that require sophisticated proteomics and genomics analyses use machine learning algorithms. Several issues with disease detection and diagnosis rely heavily on machine learning algorithms.

The combination of clinical devices and software applications that provide a wide range of medical care services connected to IT frameworks for medical services is referred to as the Internet of Medical Things (IoMT) or medical care IoT. The medical services industry has recognized IoMT innovations' extraordinary capabilities due to their proficiency in gathering, analyzing, and transmitting health information. Telemedicine is the practice of working with remote patient observation using IoMT advancements. It lets doctors evaluate, diagnose, and treat patients without knowing them.

1.4.1. Using Machine Learning

The present and future states of the data can be forecasted or predicted based on the type of data prediction and analytical techniques used. Various modeling, statistical, data mining, artificial intelligence, and machine learning techniques are utilized when analyzing past or current data to predict future trends. Defining the task, gathering relevant data from various sources, analyzing the data, statistical analysis, data modeling, deploying the collected data using multiple methods, and monitoring the model are the different stages of this kind of analysis and prediction. This kind of predictive analysis is frequently used in various use case scenarios like predicting market sales, customer needs, healthcare status, collection analysis, and fraud detection.

1.4.2. Using IoT Devices

An amalgamation of medical devices and software applications that provide extensive healthcare services and are connected to healthcare IT systems is known as the healthcare IoT. The Internet of Things can be used to monitor patients remotely, track medication orders, and use wearables to send health information to healthcare providers. The healthcare industry has recognized IoMT technologies' transformative potential due to their data collection, analysis, and transmission efficiency. Battery-operated Internet of Things buttons have been installed in several Vancouver hospitals to maintain high cleaning standards and reduce the number of hospital-acquired infections. Wanda QuickTouch is the name of these buttons, which were made to be quickly put into use in any facility, no matter how big it is, to notify management of any sanitation or maintenance issues that could harm public safety.

1.5. OVERVIEW OF THE BOOK

The respiratory disease is COVID-19. Clinicians might utilize chest imaging to analyze individuals with Coronavirus side effects while anticipating RTPCR results or when RT-PCR results are pessimistic and the individual has Coronavirus side effects. Most patients with the coronavirus disease 2019 (COVID-19) outbreak in China present with influenza-like illness or mild pneumonia, with severe or critical pneumonia occurring in 19 percent of cases. The primary signs and symptoms are fever, cough, fatigue, and myalgia. It appears that COVID-19 ILI expression is not specific. It cannot suspect a claim without any indication of exposure based on any particular symptom. IoT devices play a significant role in detecting the disease. The Internet of objects is a system of detectors accumulating information from remote environments. They build E-health administration. It provides sick details to the health workers. The patient vitals and area can be shipped at standard intermissions to therapeutic structures for surveillance. The writing commences by introducing the COVID, its symptoms, methodologies considered to collect data, followed by its investigation.

A supervised learning algorithm builds a model from a known set of input data—the learning set—and an available set of responses to the output—to make reasonable predictions about how the new input data will react. Use supervised learning if you already have data for the production you want to predict. The second chapter talks about different supervised algorithms used in the analysis.

A machine learning method called semi-supervised learning (SSL) trains a predictive model with a large amount of unlabeled data and a small amount of labeled data. In contrast to unsupervised learning, SSL can be applied to a wide range of issues, including classification, regression, clustering, and association. In contrast to supervised learning, the method uses a small amount of labeled data and a large amount of unlabeled data, which cuts down on time spent on data preparation and saves money on manual annotation. The third chapter semi-supervised algorithms in literature.

An algorithm that uses untagged data to learn patterns is known as unsupervised learning. The expectation is that it will compel the machine to construct a concise representation of its world and generate imaginative content through mimicry, a primary mode of human learning. Clustering, association, and dimensionality reduction are the three direct purposes of using them. The fourth chapter details the unsupervised algorithms designed.

The COVID-19 pandemic provided IoT-inspired frameworks and solutions with a much-needed sanity check. Authorities successfully managed the coronavirus's spread thanks to IoT solutions like contact tracing and remote health monitoring. The fifth chapter explains IoT usage in detecting COVID cases.

CONCLUSION

Coronaviruses are RNA viruses with a single strand that can infect not only humans but also a wide range of animals. These infections were first concentrated by Tyrell and Bynoe in 1966, who refined them from patients with the regular virus. These viruses were dubbed coronaviruses because of their spherical virions, shell, and surface projections that resemble a solar corona. Corona means crown in Latin, and there are four subfamilies of coronaviruses that have been identified thus far: alpha, beta, gamma, and delta. Gamma and delta coronaviruses came from pigs and birds. At the same time, alpha and beta coronaviruses came from mammals, particularly bats. These viruses have genomes ranging from 26 to 32 kilobytes in size. Among the seven other subtypes of these viruses, the beta-coronaviruses have the potential to cause severe illness and death. Infections caused by alpha-coronaviruses can be mildly symptomatic or even asymptomatic. The SARS-CoV virus and the beta-coronavirus SARSCoV-2 are related. The chapter details the disease in different stages.

REFERENCES

[1]   S. Zaim, J.H. Chong, V. Sankaranarayanan, and A. Harky, "COVID-19 and multiorgan response", *Curr. Probl. Cardiol.,* vol. 45, no. 8, p. 100618, 2020.
[http://dx.doi.org/10.1016/j.cpcardiol.2020.100618] [PMID: 32439197]

[2]   C. Covid, R. Team, C. Covid, R. Team, S. Bialek, V. Bowen, N. Chow, A. Curns, R. Gierke, A. Hall, and M. Hughes, "Geographic differences in COVID-19 cases, deaths, and incidence - United States,

February 12-April 7, 2020", *MMWR Morb. Mortal. Wkly. Rep.,* vol. 69, no. 15, pp. 465-471, 2020.
[http://dx.doi.org/10.15585/mmwr.mm6915e4] [PMID: 32298250]

[3]   T. Nguyen, D. Duong Bang, and A. Wolff, "2019 Novel coronavirus disease (COVID-19): Paving the
road for rapid detection and point-of-care diagnostics", *Micromachines.,* vol. 11, no. 3, p. 306, 2020.
[http://dx.doi.org/10.3390/mi11030306] [PMID: 32183357]

[4]   M. Ting, and J.B. Suzuki, "SARS-CoV-2: Overview and its impact on oral health", *Biomedicines.,* vol.
9, no. 11, p. 1690, 2021.
[http://dx.doi.org/10.3390/biomedicines9111690] [PMID: 34829919]

[5]   C. Fernández-de-las-Peñas, D. Palacios-Ceña, V. Gómez-Mayordomo, M.L. Cuadrado, and L.L.
Florencio, "Defining post-COVID symptoms (post-acute COVID, long COVID, persistent post-
COVID): An integrative classification", *Int. J. Environ. Res. Public Health.,* vol. 18, no. 5, p. 2621,
2021.
[http://dx.doi.org/10.3390/ijerph18052621] [PMID: 33807869]

[6]   Z. Yan, M. Yang, and C.L. Lai, "Long COVID-19 syndrome: A comprehensive review of its effect on
various organ systems and recommendation on rehabilitation plans", *Biomedicines.,* vol. 9, no. 8, p.
966, 2021.
[http://dx.doi.org/10.3390/biomedicines9080966] [PMID: 34440170]

[7]   S.J. Yong, "Long COVID or post-COVID-19 syndrome: Putative pathophysiology, risk factors, and
treatments", *Infect. Dis.,* vol. 53, no. 10, pp. 737-754, 2021.
[http://dx.doi.org/10.1080/23744235.2021.1924397] [PMID: 34024217]

[8]   A. Nalbandian, K. Sehgal, A. Gupta, M.V. Madhavan, C. McGroder, J.S. Stevens, J.R. Cook, A.S.
Nordvig, D. Shalev, T.S. Sehrawat, N. Ahluwalia, B. Bikdeli, D. Dietz, C. Der-Nigoghossian, N.
Liyanage-Don, G.F. Rosner, E.J. Bernstein, S. Mohan, A.A. Beckley, D.S. Seres, T.K. Choueiri, N.
Uriel, J.C. Ausiello, D. Accili, D.E. Freedberg, M. Baldwin, A. Schwartz, D. Brodie, C.K. Garcia,
M.S.V. Elkind, J.M. Connors, J.P. Bilezikian, D.W. Landry, and E.Y. Wan, "Post-acute COVID-19
syndrome", *Nat. Med.,* vol. 27, no. 4, pp. 601-615, 2021.
[http://dx.doi.org/10.1038/s41591-021-01283-z] [PMID: 33753937]

[9]   J.D. Pierce, Q. Shen, S.A. Cintron, and J.B. Hiebert, "Post-COVID-19 Syndrome", *Nurs. Res.,* vol. 71,
no. 2, pp. 164-174, 2022.
[http://dx.doi.org/10.1097/NNR.0000000000000565] [PMID: 34653099]

[10]   D. Ayoubkhani, K. Khunti, V. Nafilyan, T. Maddox, B. Humberstone, I. Diamond, and A. Banerjee,
"Post-covid syndrome in individuals admitted to hospital with covid-19: Retrospective cohort study",
BMJ., vol. 372, p. 693, 2021.
[http://dx.doi.org/10.1136/bmj.n693] [PMID: 33789877]

[11]   B.A. AlShurman, A.F. Khan, C. Mac, M. Majeed, and Z.A. Butt, "What demographic, social, and
contextual factors influence the intention to use COVID-19 vaccines: A scoping review", *Int. J.
Environ. Res. Public Health.,* vol. 18, no. 17, p. 9342, 2021.
[http://dx.doi.org/10.3390/ijerph18179342] [PMID: 34501932]

[12]   E. Sánchez-Sánchez, G. Ramírez-Vargas, Y. Avellaneda-López, J.I. Orellana-Pecino, E. García-Marín,
and J. Díaz-Jimenez, "Eating habits and physical activity of the spanish population during the COVID-
19 pandemic period", *Nutrients.,* vol. 12, no. 9, p. 2826, 2020.
[http://dx.doi.org/10.3390/nu12092826] [PMID: 32942695]

[13]   I. Lasheras, P. Gracia-García, D. Lipnicki, J. Bueno-Notivol, R. López-Antón, C. de la Cámara, A.
Lobo, and J. Santabárbara, "Prevalence of anxiety in medical students during the COVID-19
pandemic: A rapid systematic review with meta-analysis", *Int. J. Environ. Res. Public Health.,* vol. 17,
no. 18, p. 6603, 2020.
[http://dx.doi.org/10.3390/ijerph17186603] [PMID: 32927871]

[14]   M. Yousif, C. Hewage, and L. Nawaf, "IoT Technologies during and Beyond COVID-19: A
comprehensive review", *Future Internet.,* vol. 13, no. 5, p. 105, 2021.

[http://dx.doi.org/10.3390/fi13050105]

[15]   N. Sultana, and M. Tamanna, "Exploring the benefits and challenges of internet of things (IoT) during Covid-19: A case study of Bangladesh", *Discover Internet of Things.*, vol. 1, no. 1, pp. 1-12, 2021. [http://dx.doi.org/10.1007/s43926-021-00020-9]

[16]   M. Umair, M.A. Cheema, O. Cheema, H. Li, and H. Lu, "Impact of covid-19 on iot adoption in healthcare, smart homes, smart buildings, smart cities, transportation and industrial IoT", *Sensors.*, vol. 21, no. 11, p. 3838, 2021. [http://dx.doi.org/10.3390/s21113838] [PMID: 34206120]

[17]   B. Geethanjali, and B. Muralidhara, A wireless sensor system to monitor banana growth based on the temperature. *Information and Communication Technology for Sustainable Development.* vol. 933. Springer: Singapore, 2020, pp. 271-278. [http://dx.doi.org/10.1007/978-981-13-7166-0_26]

[18]   M.H. Devare, Cloud computing and innovations. *Applying Integration Techniques and Methods in Distributed Systems and Technologies.* IGI Global: US, 2019, pp. 1-33. [http://dx.doi.org/10.4018/978-1-5225-8295-3.ch001]

[19]   M.H. Devare, Challenges and opportunities in high performance cloud computing. *Handbook of Research on the IoT, Cloud Computing, and Wireless Network Optimization.* IGI Global: US, 2019, pp. 85-114. [http://dx.doi.org/10.4018/978-1-5225-7335-7.ch005]

[20]   J. Prabhu, P.J. Kumar, S.S. Manivannan, S. Rajendran, K.R. Kumar, S. Susi, and R. Jothikumar, "IoT role in prevention of COVID-19 and health care workforces behavioural intention in India-an empirical examination", *Int. J. Pervas. Comput. Commun.*, vol. 16, no. 4, pp. 331-340, 2020. [http://dx.doi.org/10.1108/IJPCC-06-2020-0056]

[21]   M.M. Jaber, T. Alameri, M.H. Ali, A. Alsyouf, M. Al-Bsheish, B.K. Aldhmadi, S.Y. Ali, S.K. Abd, S.M. Ali, W. Albaker, and M. Jarrar, "Remotely monitoring COVID-19 patient health condition using metaheuristics convolute networks from IoT-based wearable device health data", *Sensors.*, vol. 22, no. 3, p. 1205, 2022. [http://dx.doi.org/10.3390/s22031205] [PMID: 35161951]

[22]   N.E.S.S.J. Islam, K.S.N. Fabiano, L. Treanor, M. Absi, Z. Hallgrimson, M. Leeflang, L. Hooft, and C. van der Pol, "Thoracic imaging tests for the diagnosis of COVID-19", *Cochrane Database Syst. Rev.*, vol. 30, p. CD013639, 2021. [http://dx.doi.org/10.1002/14651858.CD013639.pub2] [PMID: 32997361]

[23]   M.H. Devare, Convergence of manufacturing cloud and industrial IoT. *Applying Integration Techniques and Methods in Distributed Systems and Technologies.* IGI Global: US, 2019, pp. 49-78. [http://dx.doi.org/10.4018/978-1-5225-8295-3.ch003]

[24]   A. Abd-Alrazaq, M. Alajlani, D. Alhuwail, A. Erbad, A. Giannicchi, Z. Shah, M. Hamdi, and M. Househ, "Blockchain technologies to mitigate COVID-19 challenges: A scoping review", *Comput. Methods Programs Biomed. Update.*, vol. 1, p. 100001, 2021. [http://dx.doi.org/10.1016/j.cmpbup.2020.100001] [PMID: 34337586]

[25]   N. Ambika, Aiding IoT and cloud to control COVID-19: A systematic approach. *Pervasive Healthcare.* Springer: Cham, 2022, pp. 349-365. [http://dx.doi.org/10.1007/978-3-030-77746-3_21]

[26]   A.A. Al-Atawi, F. Khan, and C.G. Kim, "Application and challenges of iot healthcare system in COVID-19", *Sensors.*, vol. 22, no. 19, p. 7304, 2022. [http://dx.doi.org/10.3390/s22197304] [PMID: 36236404]

[27]   B. Cao, D. Wang, Y. Wang, B.J. Hall, N. Wu, M. Wu, Q. Ma, J.D. Tucker, and X. Lv, "Moderating effect of people-oriented public health services on depression among people under mandatory social isolation during the COVID-19 pandemic: A cross-sectional study in China", *BMC Public Health.*, vol. 21, no. 1, p. 1374, 2021.

[http://dx.doi.org/10.1186/s12889-021-11457-6] [PMID: 34247618]

[28]   N. Strelkovskii, E. Rovenskaya, L. Ilmola-Sheppard, R. Bartmann, Y. Rein-Sapir, and E. Feitelson, "Implications of COVID-19 mitigation policies for national well-being: A systems perspective", *Sustainability.,* vol. 14, no. 1, p. 433, 2021.
[http://dx.doi.org/10.3390/su14010433]

[29]   F. Alam, A. Almaghthawi, I. Katib, A. Albeshri, and R. Mehmood, "iResponse: An AI and IoT-enabled framework for autonomous COVID-19 pandemic management", *Sustainability.,* vol. 13, no. 7, p. 3797, 2021.
[http://dx.doi.org/10.3390/su13073797]

[30]   J. Hong, J. Kim, S. Kim, J. Oh, D. Lee, S. Lee, J. Uh, J. Yoon, and Y. Choi, "Depressive symptoms feature-based machine learning approach to predicting depression using smartphone", *Healthcare,* vol. 10, no. 7, p. 1189, 2022.
[http://dx.doi.org/10.3390/healthcare10071189] [PMID: 35885716]

[31]   J. Navarro-Alamán, R. Lacuesta, I. García-Magariño, and J. Lloret, "EmotIoT: An IoT system to improve users' wellbeing", *Appl. Sci.,* vol. 12, no. 12, p. 5804, 2022.
[http://dx.doi.org/10.3390/app12125804]

[32]   V. Khullar, H.P. Singh, Y. Miro, D. Anand, H.G. Mohamed, D. Gupta, N. Kumar, and N. Goyal, "IoT fog-enabled multi-node centralized ecosystem for real time screening and monitoring of health information", *Appl. Sci.,* vol. 12, no. 19, p. 9845, 2022.
[http://dx.doi.org/10.3390/app12199845]

CHAPTER 2

Supervised Learning Algorithms

Abstract: Numerous domains now employ learning algorithms. It has distinct performance metrics appropriate for them.. Based on a predetermined set of paired input-output training samples, a machine learning paradigm known as "Supervised Learning" is used to gather information about a system's input-output relationship. An input-output training sample is also known as supervised or labeled training data because the output is regarded as the input data or supervision label. Supervised learning aims to build an artificial system that can learn the mapping between input and output and predict the system's output, given new information. The learned mapping results in the classification of the input data if the output takes a limited set of discrete values representing the input's class labels. Regression of the information occurs if the output takes continuous values. The chapter details the various algorithms, technologies used and their applications.

Keywords: Known Label, Regression, Supervised Algorithms.

2.1. INTRODUCTION

Numerous supervised learning methods [2] have found applications in processing multimedia content and supervised learning accounts for a significant amount of machine learning research. In supervised learning, a mapping between a set of input variables X and an output variable Y is learned and used to predict outputs for data that has not been seen. The availability of annotated training data is the defining characteristic of supervised learning. The name evoked the concept of a "supervisor" who directs the learning system regarding the labels to associate with training examples. In classification problems, these labels are typically class labels. From these training data, supervised learning algorithms generate models that can be used to classify other unlabeled data. Fig. (1) represents contrastive learning pipeline for self-supervised training.

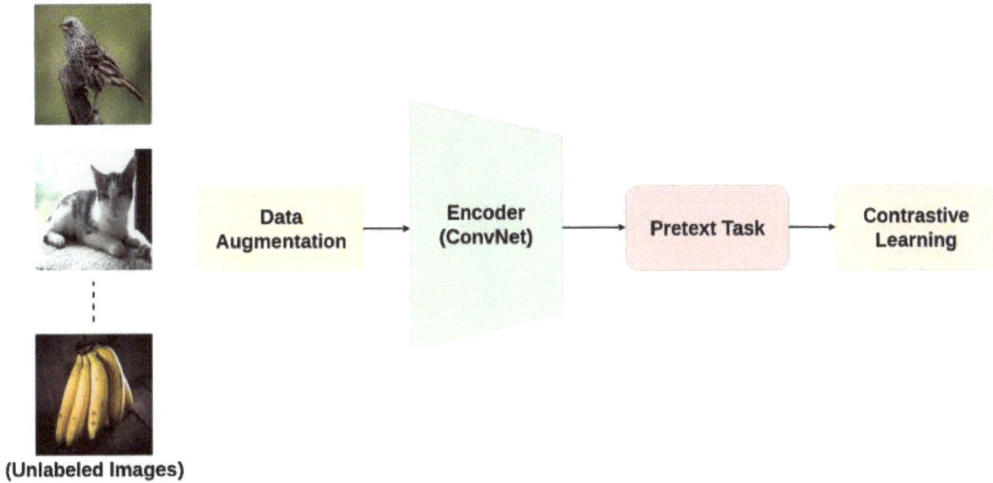

Fig. (1). Contrastive learning pipeline for self-supervised training [1].

The five main components of the proposed system model [3] are as follows: pre-processing, balancing, feature extraction, classification, and validation of the data are all included. The three-sigma rule, normalization, and interpolation of missing values are used to pre-process electricity data. The next model uses the pre-processed data for data balancing. The data are balanced using the Adasyn algorithm. Thirdly, the essential features are extracted from time series data using a VGG-16, and fourthly, the critical parts are given to FA-XGBoost for classification. A high-resolution accurate, intelligent meter data set provided by China's State Grid Corporation serves as the basis for testing the proposed system. 1032 are the input dimensions or features. The collection of data lasted for three years. Forty-two thousand three hundred seventy-two customers' electricity consumption data are included. The recently released data reveals the undisputed fact that 9% of all customers are victims of electricity theft. Fig. (**2**) depicts the same.

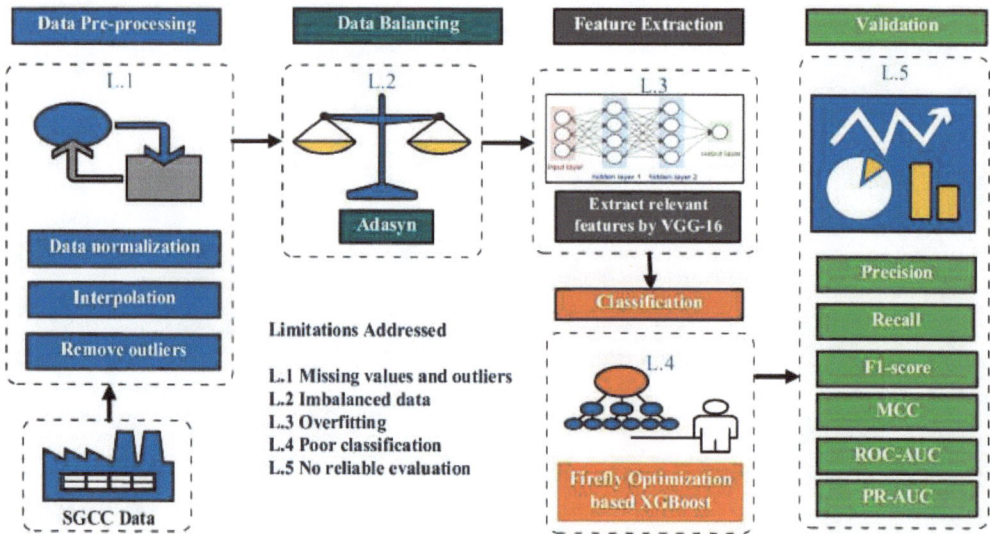

Fig. (2). Proposed model [3].

2.2. SUPERVISED LEARNING ALGORITHMS

2.2.1. Support Vector Machine

A computer algorithm known as a support vector machine (SVM) uses examples to teach itself how to label objects. By looking at many scanned images of handwritten zeroes, ones, and other digits, SVM can learn to recognize them. Additionally, SVMs have been successfully utilized in many biological applications. The automatic classification of microarray gene expression profiles is a common biomedical application for support vector machines. It can determine a diagnosis or prognosis by analyzing the gene expression profile derived from a tumor sample or peripheral fluid.

The speech recognition process [4] is improved by utilizing a hybrid Support Vector Machine (SVM) and Dynamic Time Warping (DTW) algorithm to contribute to the proposed framework. It is a smartphone-dependent system for speech recognition to execute a single command based on matching against the user command and the recorded speech templates. The proposed solution is a machine learning-based system for controlling smart devices through speech commands with an accuracy of 97 percent. To train the system to recognize these commands using the smartphone's microphone and voice command matching, each user should record these commands for various home appliances. Then, only a smartphone is used to send orders. A machine learning model is used to match the voice commands of elderly, sick, or disabled individuals using an expandable dictionary of predefined user commands. An SVM library and MATLAB running on a laptop PC (2.2 GHz, 8 GB RAM) were utilized in the work. Fig. (**3**) portrays the same.

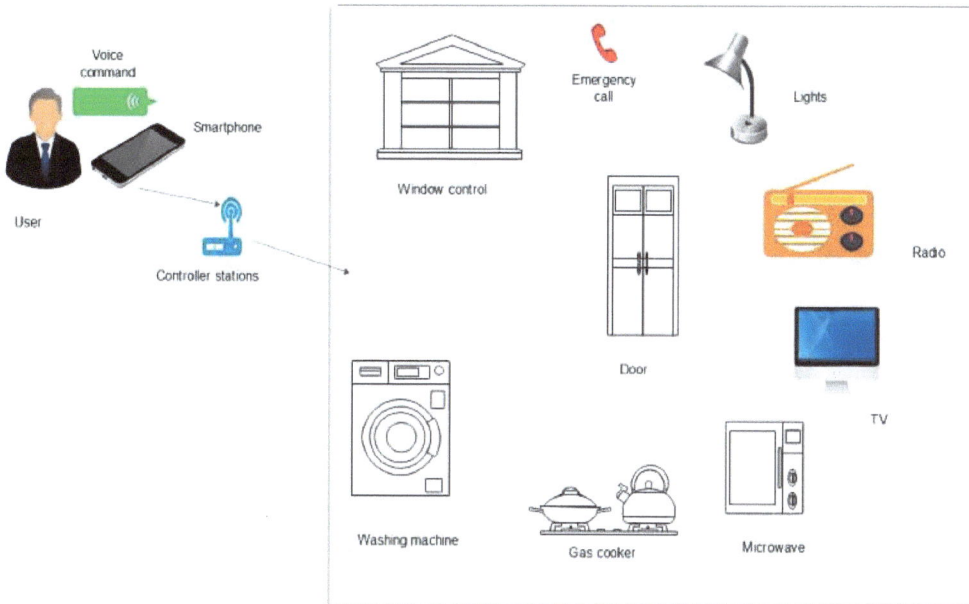

Fig. (3). proposed system [4].

The work [5] involves pre-processing the signal and extracting features from it. These features are specific, signal-specific characteristics of heart sounds that are suitable for classification. At Imam Ghaem Hospital in Mashhad, Iran, the system collects PCG data from 116 newborns between the ages of one and twenty. When there is environmental noise, it records at sampling frequencies of more than 8 kHz. The next step is determining the timing intervals between the signal's S1 and S2 components after de-noising. The feature extraction stage extracts features from the PCG signals that can represent properties deemed helpful for the diagnosis. Following the detection of cardiac cycles, it is essential to determine which process possesses the most significant number of symptoms of heart disease. Identifying the most informative cycle can be extremely useful for assessing cardiac function. Fig. (**4**) represents the same.

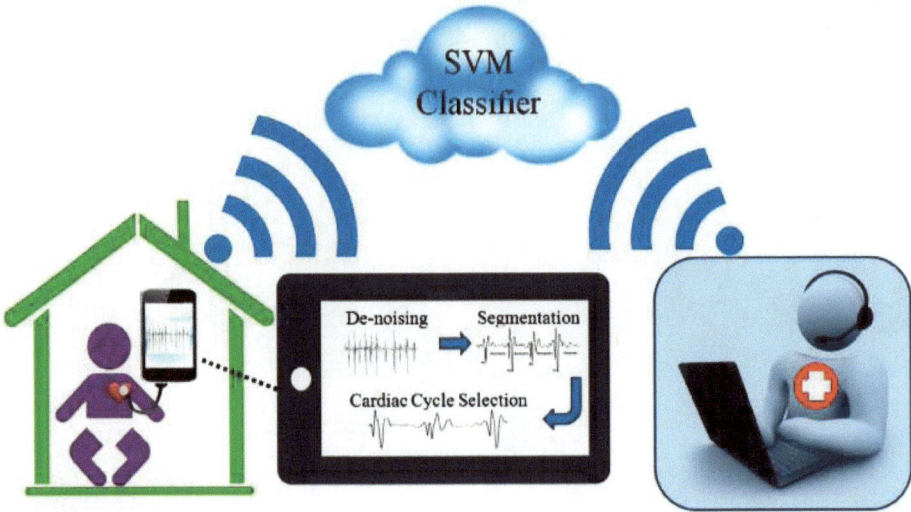

Fig. (4). SVM classifier [5].

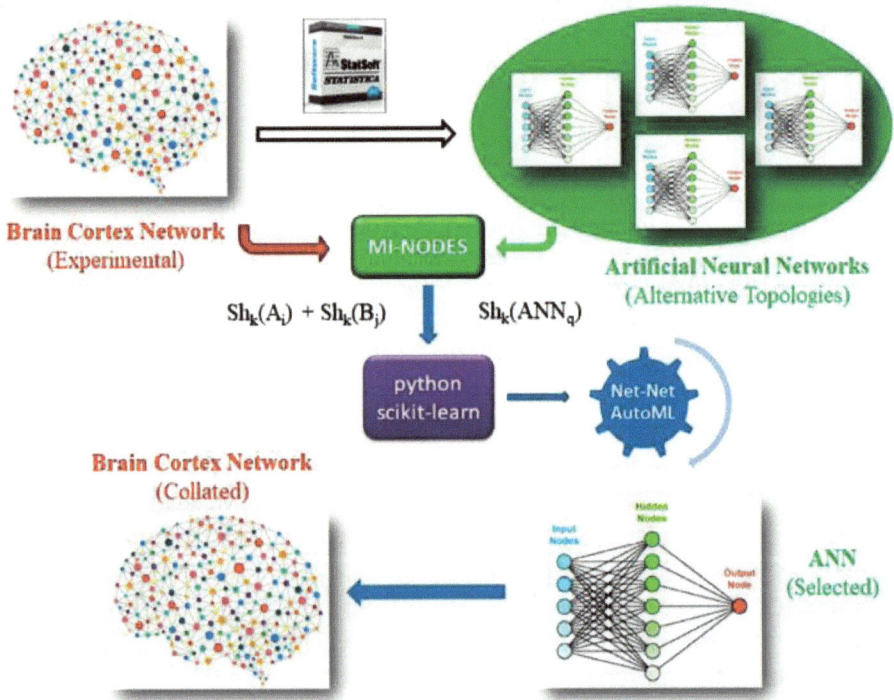

Fig. (5). Proposed flow [6].

2.2.2. Artificial Neural Network

A computational system composed of highly interconnected processing elements known as neurons that process information in response to external stimuli is referred to as a generic artificial neural network [7]. An artificial neuron is a simplified representation that uses mathematical equations to mimic the behavior of biological neurons in terms of threshold firing and signal integration. Testing and learning are the two distinct modes in which an artificial network operates. The web shows a set of examples during learning. The output is "guessed" at the beginning of the training process by the network. Layers are typically used to organize neural networks. A collection of processing units, also known as neurons, make up each layer of a layered network. Each component receives and processes information in an input-output fashion. Fig. (**5**) portrays the proposed work.

The study [8] is a novel, searchable, secure algorithm that lets users encrypt on their own and upload it to the distributed ledger. Using the blockchain users API, users can search for keywords anonymously. The user can revoke the policy and request a new key if they lose the key. It shields you from attacks that use active collusion. The selection of attributes and features is the basis for access control. Access is granted to a user who meets the criteria based on the required details; otherwise, access is denied. The administration, the patient, the doctor, and the lab technician are the four main participants in the framework. There are setup, initialization, update, and search steps in the enhanced homomorphic encryption that has been proposed. The algorithm's configuration is provided in the setup step, where initialization provisions set the parameters. In the binary version, the concept of displacement is put into action with the help of a probability function. The new location of each member in each dimension of the problem might change or stay the same. It depends on the value of this probability function. The system will track the user's actions and interactions with the system. The work provides a secure, searchable, and blockchain-based access control system. Homomorphic encryption is used for keyword searching, storing, retrieving, and sharing personal healthcare data. The initial experiment included 3050 rounds. Fig. (**6**) portrays the same.

It can find three kinds of tumors in MRI images using the proposed neural model [9]- meningioma, glioma, and pituitary tumors over sagittal, coronal, and axial views without input images preprocessed to remove parts of the skull or vertebrae in advance. The strategy of classifying and segmenting brain tumors is the objective. A dataset of T1-CE MRI images from 233 patients, including standard views of meningiomas, gliomas, and pituitary tumors, was used to train and test the proposed neural model. The study is a tumor segmentation CNN architecture with multiple paths. The CNN architecture classifies each pixel using one of four possible output labels as it processes an MRI image (slice) pixel by pixel, covering the entire image. 0 is the healthy area, 1 is a tumor in the meninges, 2 is a glioma, and 3 is a tumor in the pituitary. Three convolutional pathways with three scale kernels are used to process each window and extract the features. Two convolutional stages with ReLU rectification and a 3 3 max-pooling kernel with a stride value of 2 make up each pathway. There are 128, 96, and 64 feature maps in the large, medium, and minor courses, respectively. From 2005 to 2010, it took 2D slices from 233 patients at Nanfang Hospital in Guangzhou and General Hospital at Tianjing Medical University in China. Meningiomas (708 pieces), gliomas (1426 slices), and pituitary tumors (930 portions) are included in the dataset's standard views. Fig. (**7**) depicts the same.

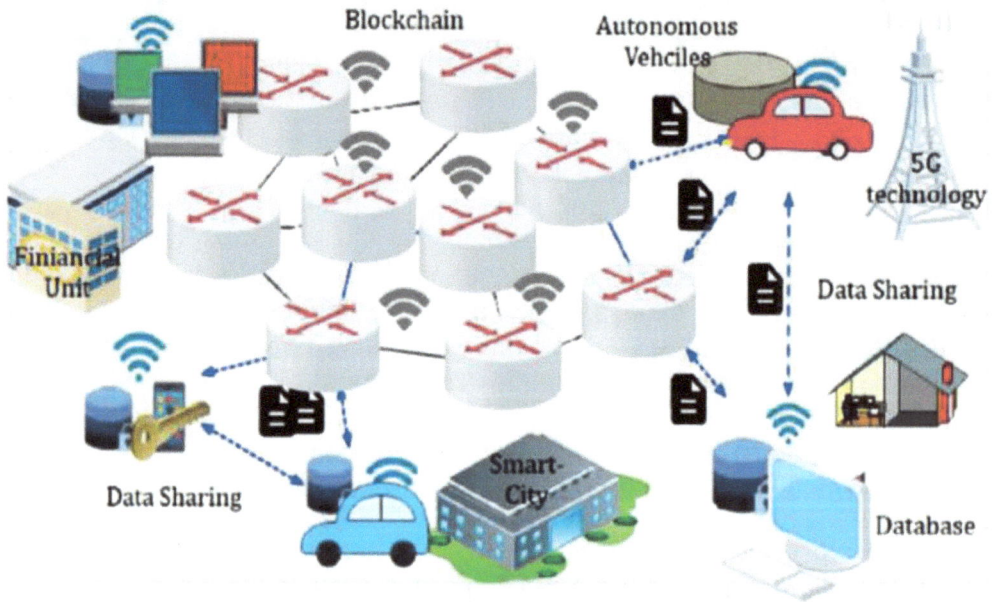

Fig. (6). Proposed Data-sharing Scheme [8].

The research [10] aims to discover a portfolio of risk factors for preventive healthcare and investigate the connection between behavioral patterns and chronic diseases. The data come from the Centers for Disease Control and Prevention's 2012 Behavioral Risk Factor Surveillance System database. The work employs neural networks and SPSS Modeler to identify strong positive and negative associations between certain chronic diseases and behavioral patterns. For 2012, the CDC's Behavioral Risk Factor Surveillance System database contained information for 475,687 records. Alcohol consumption, regular soda (sugar) consumption, smoking, weekly working hours, fruit and vegetable consumption, and exercise are all indicators of behavioral habits. Heart attack, stroke, asthma, and diabetes are all chronic diseases. Included are marital status, age, and income level as demographic variables. The data for the variables were extracted at the state level.

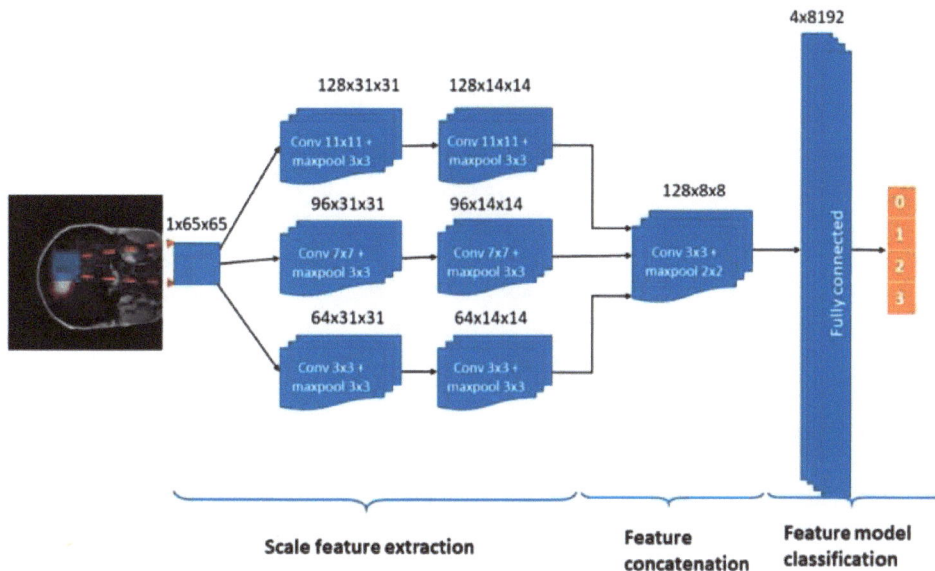

Fig. (7). Proposed Architecture [9].

A healthcare-domain ontology-based health-related Named Entity Recognition task [11] that can identify health-related entities from a large number of Twitter user messages is the recommendation. Three categories of entities are symptoms, pharmacologic substances, and diseases. The Micromed dataset also contains annotations for entities of this kind. For the term "pharmacologic substance," 409,268 tweets were found, with 848,871 medical and 8148 unique terms. The work uses the Pytorch library. When creating a word embedding, medical and non-medical pre-trained word embeddings are compared. Character embedding is done with CNN, and additional word features are done with POS tagging. BiLSTM generates word-level contextual representations that indicate the confidence score "CS" for each word by learning the contextual information from the concatenated word and character representations. The CRF layer uses contextual knowledge to determine the tagging scores for each input word. The Viterbi algorithm selects the tag sequence that yields the highest number of tagging scores. Fig. (**8**) represents the same.

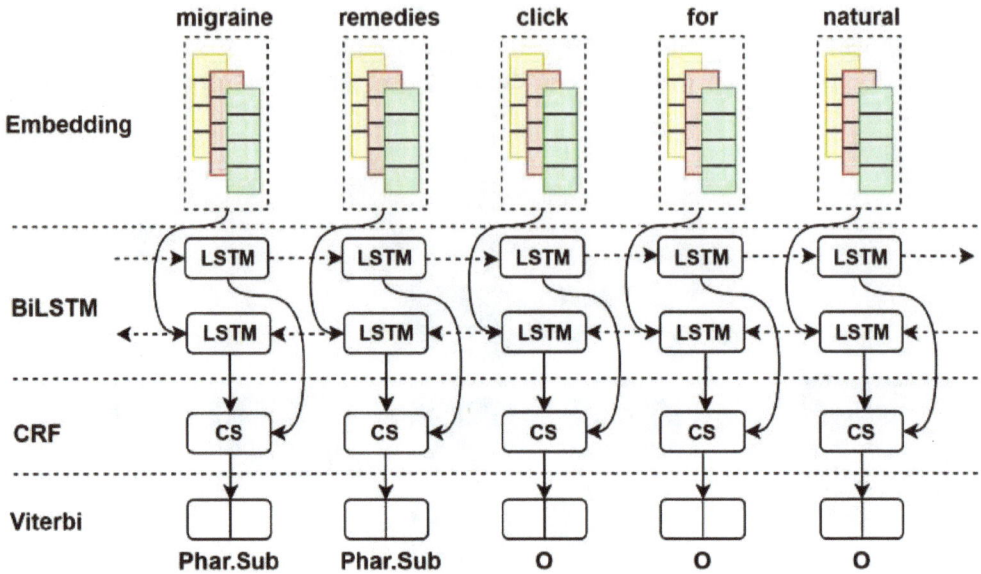

Fig. (8). BiLSTM-CRF model [11].

2.2.3. Naive Bayes Method

The Naive Bayes algorithm [12] is a supervised learning algorithm used to solve classification problems and is based on the Bayes theorem. It's mainly used to classify text using a high-dimensional training dataset. One of the most straightforward and efficient classification algorithms, the Naive Bayes Classifier, aids in developing rapid machine learning models capable of making fast predictions. It is a probabilistic classifier, which implies it predicts based on the likelihood of an item.

The clinical data used in this study [13] come from one of Chennai's leading diabetic research institutes and include the records of approximately 500 patients. Items related to diabetes are given clear, concise definitions in the clinical data set specification. The diabetes data set ensures that people with diabetes have up-to-date records of their risk factors, current management, treatment target accomplishments, and regular surveillance arrangements and outcomes for complications. It will assist them in monitoring their care and making informed decisions about managing their diabetes. Additionally, it will guarantee that patients with diabetes receive accurate, up-to-date, and comprehensive information when they meet with healthcare professionals for a consultation.

Weka is a collection of data mining-related machine learning algorithms. The algorithms can be called from your Java code or applied directly to a dataset. Data pre-processing, classification, regression, clustering, association rules, and visualization are all supported by Weka. It is well-suited for the creation of novel machine-learning schemes. The experiments are carried out with the help of the weak tool, and outcomes are obtained. Using 70% of the percentage split, we classified the data using the naive Bayes method.

A hybrid algorithm with two phases is used in the proposed method [14]. The Whale Optimization Algorithm is used as a feature selection method in the first phase to reduce the number of features for big data. The three main phases are the services layer, the data processing phase, and the data collection phase. In the first phase, data are gathered from a variety of sources. At this point, the diversity of data is an issue. The second phase receives the data to carry out the data management process. The data are stored in the second phase, optimized, and categorized in a way that makes it easier for the third phase to function appropriately and provide flawless services. It will describe the steps of the AHCA-WOANB approach in detail in the following sections. The Diabetes and Digestive and Kidney Diseases National Institute is the dataset's source. The purpose of the dataset is to determine whether a patient has diabetes based on specific measures in the dataset. Fig. (**9**) represents the same.

The study [15] focuses on this aspect of medical diagnosis by discovering patterns in the Swine Flu data. The Intelligent Swine Flu Prediction software prototype was created as a result of this study. It trained the program to calculate the probabilities of all classes under each condition using a set of 50 cases. It saved the results in the database. When the test data were presented, we inferred that the patient belonged to the class with the highest probability based on probabilities for the various courses for the given symptom values. From the databases of multiple hospitals, it validated 100 records with 17 medical attributes (factors). It created two datasets from equally divided records: datasets for training and testing records for each set were chosen randomly to prevent bias. All three models only used categorical attributes to maintain consistency. All medical qualities that were not categorical were changed into categorical data. It recognized the property "Clinical trial" as the anticipated property. It is expected that issues like missing information, conflicting information, and copied information have all been settled. The program uses the JAVA platform to access database data.

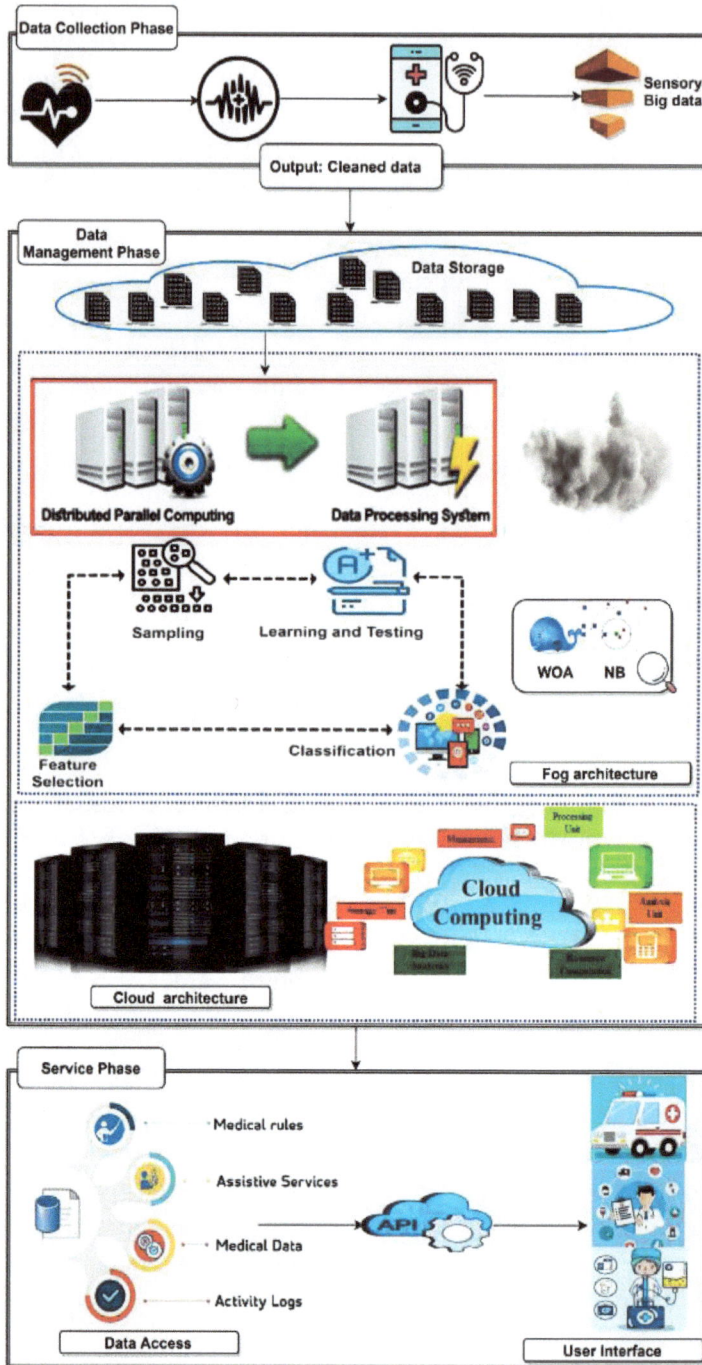

Fig. (9). Proposed architecture [14].

The multilayered feed-forward network architecture [16] of the neural network used in this study has 20 input nodes, ten hidden nodes, and ten output nodes. The finalized data determines the number of input nodes. The number of output nodes and the number of hidden nodes are determined by trial and error. Learning in a neural network requires adjusting the network's weights and biases to minimize The number of output nodes and the number of hidden nodes are determined by trial and error. Learning in a neural network requires adjusting the network's weights and biases to minimize the cost function. An error term, which indicates how closely the network's predictions match the class labels for the training set's examples, is always included in the cost function. A complexity term that responds to a prior distribution of the possible parameter values may also be included. JNCC2 loads data from ARFF files, which were created for WEKA and are in a plain text format.

The North Focal Malignant growth therapy for cellular [17] breakdown in the lungs and new persistent information are utilized to assess the role of SVM, NBs, and C4.5. It comprises three stages. Patient and NCCTG data are collected in the first phase, and features are extracted from the measured data to create derived features that are intended to be informative and non-redundant. When a patient is admitted for treatment, the following information is gathered for analysis: gender, age, smoking status, tumor location, t-stage, n-stage, stage, timing, and diabetes. These features are chosen based on responses from doctors and pathologists at various hospitals. In the second phase, the extracted feature set is added to three distinct MLT, and 14 of the 24 features are considered for data training and testing. In the third phase, the results of the SVM, C4.5, and NBs ML algorithms are compared, and the algorithm with the best-predicted result is considered. Implementation is done with the ORANGE tool.

The work [18] uses machine learning methods to predict diseases based on a patient's symptoms. The predictive analytics system is developed using the Naive Bayes Classification algorithm to predict patient conditions accurately. Cytoscape Web is used in the system's visual analytics technique to assist clinicians and doctors visually. The work produced DOCAID, a disease prediction system for typhoid, malaria, jaundice, tuberculosis, and gastroenteritis. This system uses the Naive Bayes Classification to make diagnosis based on the symptoms and complaints of the patient. There are 11 features in the input for the system. It uses a 300-record data set, with 80 percent as the training data set and 20 percent as the test data set.

The first step in developing the method [19] was to create a mining technique model employing a naive Bayes classifier and identify knowledge regarding the adult cardiovascular disease profile and the level of cardiovascular disease risk factors based on the medical record. Data testing was used to train and validate the proposed model. This model's accuracy, sensitivity, and specificity measurements revealed that, especially for adults, it could accurately detect cardiovascular disease at each of the three risk levels. Seventy percent of those who participated in the evaluation session strongly agreed that this model contributes to medical science by assisting in cardiovascular disease analysis and detection. Cardiologists, an internist, and the head nurse of the catheterization laboratory attended the evaluation sessions in the same private hospital.

2.2.4. K-nearest Neighbor

A supervised machine learning algorithm called K-nearest neighbors clustering is used for classification and predictive regression problems. A lazy learning algorithm uses all the training data during sort because there is no specific training phase. It does not make any assumptions regarding the underlying data. The distance is calculated to locate the designated centroid. Fig. (**10**) depicts the same.

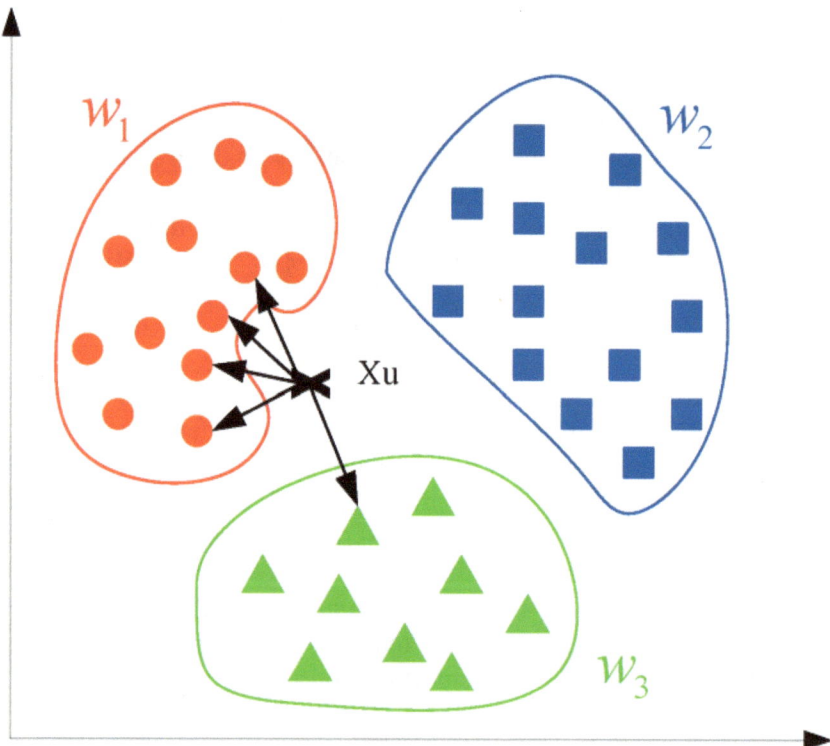

Fig. (10). k-nearest neighbour algorithm [20].

Using Paillier's homomorphic property [21], the K-NN model can be securely trained using polynomial addition and subtraction. The input terminal includes the encrypted version of the data. It also includes the name of the device from which the data is generated and the data provider's address. The output terminal stores an encrypted version of the data. It also contains the device from which the information is generated and the address of the data analyst. The addresses of the data provider and data analyst will serve as the hash value, and it will use homomorphic encryption to determine the encrypted data. The length of each encrypted data instance is set to 128 bytes and stored in the Blockchain, considering that the private key size is 128 bytes. The IoT device type has a segment length of 4 bytes. After assembling a new transaction, the node that serves as the data provider in the Blockchain network broadcasts it in a peer-to-peer system, where the miner nodes will verify the operation's accuracy. A particular excavator hub can bundle the exchange in another block and add the block to the current chain utilizing current agreement calculations. It can use a single block to register multiple transactions. As IoT data providers and data analysts simultaneously work, the experiments are carried out on a MacBook Pro with a 2.5 GHz Intel Core i5 processor and 4 GB of 1600 MHz DDR3 memory. The Platform incorporates the Secure K-NN, SPO, SBO, and SC. Fig. (**11**) represents the same.

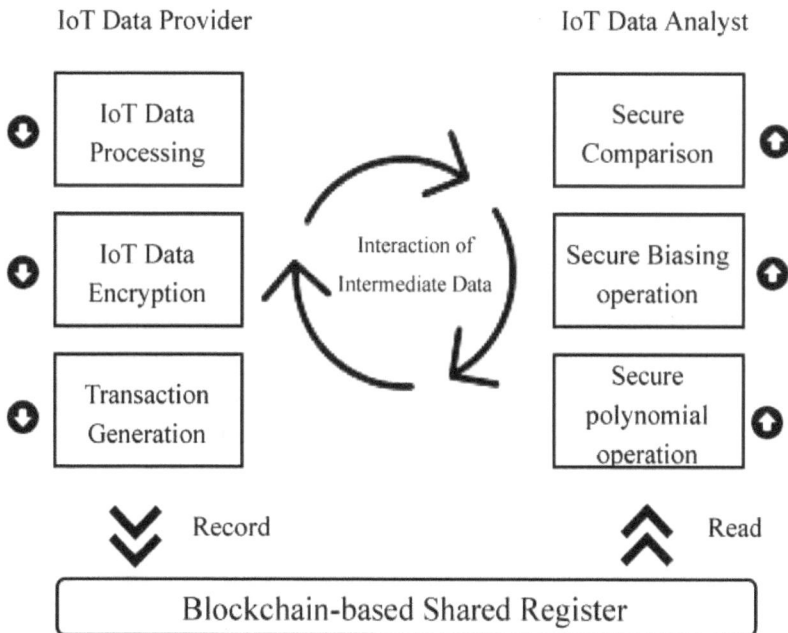

Fig. (11). System overview [21].

Different methods for predicting heart disease have been examined in this study [22]. It utilized the 303-record Heart Disease dataset from the UCI Machine Learning Repository. There are 14 attributes in this database. This study used the Naive Bayes, IBK (K-Nearest Neighbor), J48, Bagging classifiers, and ML techniques. In case 1, accuracy is calculated without feature reduction by applying all classifiers to the data. In case 2, feature/variable reduction reveals accuracy. In case 3, the most available features for predicting heart disease are removed to calculate accuracy. Seven attributes have been used to calculate the accuracy in case 4. In case 5, the Re-Sample filter was used with all 14 features and produced an accuracy of 79.20%. In case 6, it used the SMOTE option in Weka to calculate the accuracy.

Emotion recognition based on signals from multiple electroencephalogram channels is the recommendation [23]. It classified the emotional states in the valence and arousal dimensions using various EEG channel combinations. The first step was to normalize the DEAP default preprocessed data. Then, EEG signals were separated into four recurrence groups utilizing discrete wavelet change, and entropy and energy were determined as highlights of the K-closest Neighbor Classifier. EEG features are extracted through the use of discrete wavelet transform. It used the mother wavelet function to stretch and shift the EEG signals, resulting in wavelet coefficients. In this dataset, 32 people watched 40 videos that could make them feel different things. Each video lasts 60 seconds.

A technique for classifying objects based on their proximity to one another in the training set is the k-NN algorithm. The algorithm [24] compares the data of a patient to a training table of patients with various medical conditions and their respective medical attributes. The algorithm uses the k-NN method to classify patients as having or not having a particular situation and find the patient in the training set that best matches the subject. It uses that patient's diagnosis as our prediction for the issue is how the work determines whether a new topic is positive for a condition. The study uses the diagnosis for each k point to predict a patient's diagnosis by observing the k points closest to the patient's data. In particular, the diagnostic predictor will be the majority value among those k diagnoses. The Chronic Kidney Dataset, published as an open-source dataset by the UCI Machine Learning Repository, uses the data of 400 patients measuring 25 distinct attributes for two months to determine if a patient is suffering from chronic kidney disease. The k-NN algorithm takes into account all 25 features in the dataset. Using 76 attributes, the UCI Machine Learning Repository Heart Disease Dataset determines whether 303 subjects have heart disease.

E-health cloud servers, multiple medical data owners, and a patient inquirer make up the proposed PPkNN [25]. Numerous medical data owners outsource their medical datasets to e-health cloud servers to provide a medical diagnosis service. By doing so, they can use extensive computing resources and save money on management costs. The symptoms of a patient who wishes to have a medical examination are sent to the e-health cloud servers. As part of the medical diagnosis, the e-health cloud servers perform PPkNN classification and provide the patient with the result. PE-FTK performs the input-sharing phase by sending shares generated from their datasets to each cloud server on a global dataset owned by multiple data owners. It uses five cloud servers to select the top 100 of 1000 randomly generated 33-bit data, varying the number, length, and k of the data for each experiment 30 times. It ran each cloud server on its server and shared intermediate results over a 100 Mb/s network. An Intel Core i7, 2.4 GHz CPU, was utilized in a cloud server.

The method [26] uses a genetic algorithm and a KNN to improve the accuracy of the heart disease data set's classification. It ranks the attributes that contribute the most to the category and uses genetic search as a good measure to remove features that are redundant or irrelevant. The most minor ranked details are released, and the classification algorithm is built based on evaluated attributes. This classifier has been trained to categorize the heart disease data set as either healthy or sick. Six medical data sets and one non-medical data set are used to evaluate the work. It selected six of the seven data sets from the UCI Repository, and heart disease A.P. was gathered from various corporate hospitals in Andhra Pradesh. It chose attributes based on the advice of an expert doctor.

The voting method and KNN used to diagnose heart disease patients are discussed in study [27]. It is based on voting. It is based on majority or plurality voting, and each classifier gets one vote. The majority of voters determine the outcome. There is three to one subset of voting divisions used. There are 76 raw attributes in the dataset.

The methodology [28] is an optimal KNearest Neighbor learning-based prediction model based on patients' habitual attributes in various dimensions. With a low error rate, this method determines the optimal number of neighbors for a better prediction outcome in the resulting model. The work gathers real-world diabetes data from 500 patients at appropriate medical facilities. Diet, hypertension, vision issues, genetics, and other risk factors of diabetes are all included in the dataset. The diabetes dataset has undergone data pre-processing. It prepares and modifies the initial hospital-collected raw datasets. The algorithm stores the attribute or feature and class label of the training samples during the Training phase. This algorithm classifies the unlabeled test sample during the Classification phase using the value of "k." The test sample can be placed in the specified class by calculating feature similarity.

2.2.5. Decision Support System

A decision support system [29] is a computer program used to boost a company's decision-making capabilities. It presents an organization with the best options based on extensive data analysis. To provide users with information that goes beyond the usual reports and summaries, decision support systems combine data and knowledge from various fields and sources. It is meant to help people make better choices.

The proposed fusion-based machine learning architecture [30] is trained and tested using two datasets. The first dataset, which consists of 9858 records and eight features, is derived from the National Health and Nutrition Examination Survey, which is made available to the public. It obtained the second "Pima Indian diabetes" from the "Kaggle" online repository, which contains eight features and 769 records. Both datasets have the same features but differ in the number of records they hold. It has five layers. The process of associating and combining data from various sources is known as data fusion. It is characterized by constantly refining its estimates, determining whether or not additional data are required, and adapting its procedure to achieve higher-quality data. Pre-processing is initiated by the treatment of missing values, followed by standardization. Imputed values include missing or null values; Otherwise, the machine learning classifier's prediction accuracy is compromised. There are five folds in the dataset. In the inner loop where the grid search algorithm was used, K-1 folds are used for training and fine-tuning the hyper-parameters. The SVM model predicts the classes for a new sample. Fig. (**12**) represents the same.

The work [31] focuses on how data mining can use various classification methods to predict benign and malignant breast cancer. The attribute, clump thickness, was used as the evaluation class, and the Breast Cancer Wisconsin dataset from the UCI repository was used as the experimental dataset. It used twelve algorithms for classification. During the experiment, it tested ten dataset attributes. The model is trained with the Wisconsin Breast Cancer Diagnosis dataset from the UCI repository and other publicly accessible datasets.

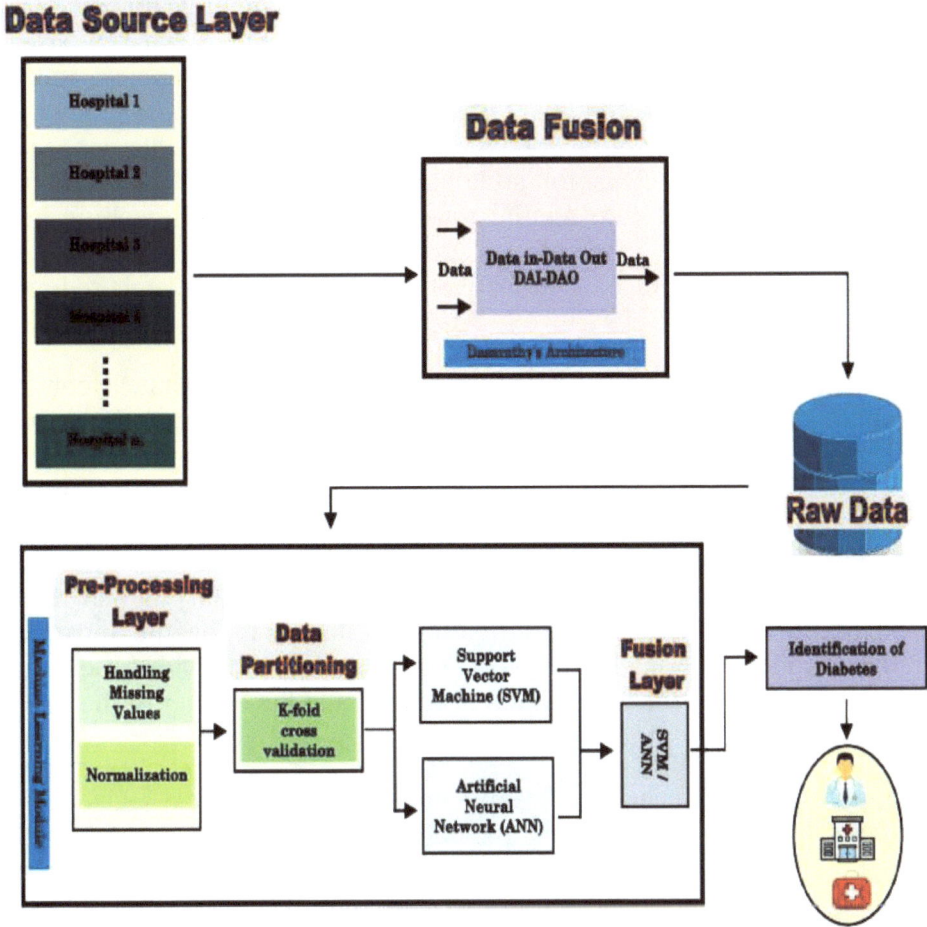

Fig. (12). Proposed model [30].

Any computer-based application that assists the user in making better decisions is considered decision support [32, 33]. To make clinical or administrative decisions, healthcare professionals can access literature. They can also ask questions about aggregates of patient data and receive warnings or suggestions when the data satisfies specific logical rules. They receive critiques when proposing therapies or ordering diagnostic tests, access programs that analyze tradeoffs and likelihoods of alternative outcomes, and access lists of differential diagnoses. Automated diagnoses will continue to be a research topic until we have sufficient clinical data, but practice guidelines, reminders, alerts, and suggestions will likely lead the way.

The ability to promptly provide appropriate, proactive, and value-added services to various client groups is crucial to the efficient provision of healthcare services. Healthcare services generally require systematic determination based on requirements; combining demographics, behavioral psychographics, and usage patterns; and distributed in an always present, proactive, and consistent way. It is difficult even to formulate or meet these constraints, which are interconnected by using conventional strategies for strategic planning. Hereafter, for improved effectiveness of medical care administration, there is an approaching need to demonstrate and quantify medical care processes utilizing authoritative medical services process models that are inductively obtained from the gathered medical care information.

A set of measures to recalibrate AI algorithms necessitates continuous surveillance of an AI system. IT System quality monitoring includes indicators like accessibility, reliability, flexibility, integration, response time, and ease of learning, in addition to surveillance aimed at AI development. These measures and pointers are designated for checking and advancing the whole socio-specialized framework where artificial intelligence is carried out. When AI components feed other interim processes, function quality is an essential component of system quality. Information quality may be the most crucial surveillance and monitoring domain for AI algorithms, along with system quality. It covers the quality of the information produced and the quality of the data used as an AI input.

Analyzing the significance of explainability for medical AI from the technological, legal, medical, and patient perspectives is a multidisciplinary approach. Supported clinical decision-making using established diagnostic tools and AI. Fig. (**13**) represents Decision Tree algorithm. Its goal is to identify factors necessary for determining the significance and necessity of explainability in each domain. Patient-centered care is listening to and respecting each patient's values and needs. It emphasizes patient's right to choice and control over medical decisions and views them as active partners in the care process. Shared decision-making aimed at determining the most suitable treatment for each patient is an essential part of patient-centered care.

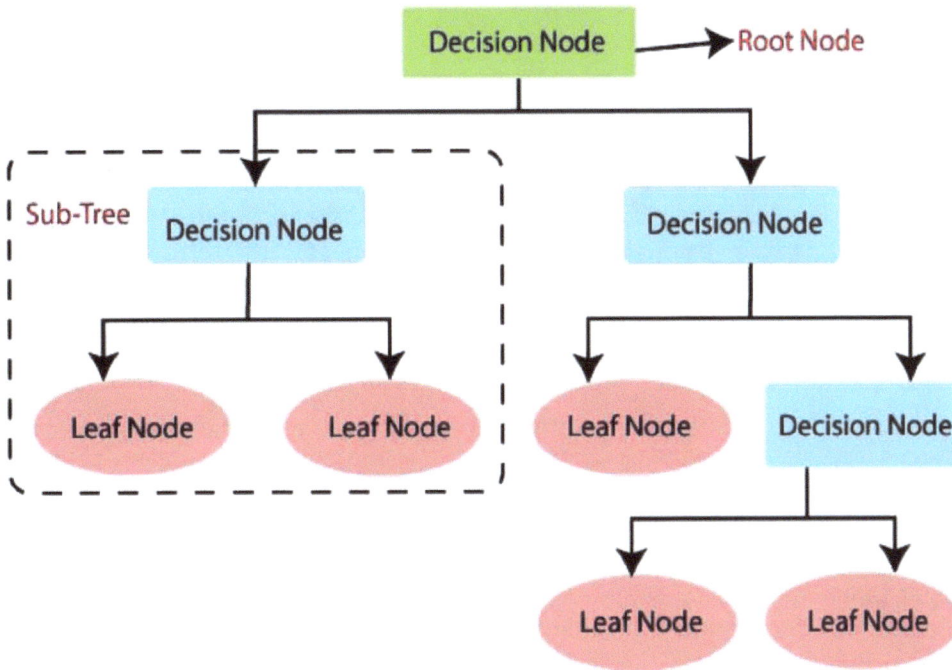

Fig. (13). Decision Tree algorithm [34].

A predictive machine-learning representation known as a decision tree uses various attribute values from the available data to decide a new sample's target value (dependent variable). In a decision tree, the multiple attributes are represented by the internal nodes, the probable importance of these attributes in the observed samples is shown by the branches between the nodes, and the terminal nodes produce the final value (or classification) of the dependent variable. The attribute's value will predict the importance of all the other qualities. It is recognized as the dependent variable. The dataset's independent variables are the other attributes that aid in predicting the value of the dependent variable.

The study [35] explains how medical data mining is used to choose how to perform medical operations. The C4.5 algorithm was used because it could be used to apply negotiation strategies, figure out how to deliver a baby, and be very accurate in medical applications. The work selects five attributes and then employs the decision tree C4.5 algorithm to locate value data among all patient records. The Weka3.6.6 software in our dataset gathers data on 80 pregnant women. Quinlan's highly effective decision tree algorithm is centered on the C4.5 algorithm, which employs a top-down, greedy search strategy to construct decision trees.

The review [36] proposes to research a crossover plot, given fluffy choice trees, as a productive choice for new classifiers that are applied freely. Breast cancer prognosis is based on SEER (Surveillance, Epidemiology, and End Results) data from 1973 to 2003. The SEER program asserts the quality and completeness of the data, and the data set is regarded as the most comprehensive source of information on cancer incidence in the United States. Each of the 433,272 records has 86 variables. Each record represents a single cancer incidence. After extensive preprocessing, it constructed a final data set with 162500 forms, 16 predictor variables, and one target variable. A binary target variable is created with values 0 (did not survive) and 1 (survived). For all of the experiments, the work uses binary C4.5. It works for partitioning the data, and an attribute with the lowest entropy is chosen through a test. When a feature contributes additional information about the class, the information gain is used to measure the entropy difference.

The review [37] presents another technique for investigating clinical information in light of the LogNNet brain organization, which utilizes complex mappings to change input data. The method effectively solves classification issues and calculates risk factors for a patient's disease presence by using a set of medical health indicators. During the balancing stage, it must sort the training set in sequential order, the number of objects in each class must be equal, and it must add copies of existing things to the categories. The model's constant parameters are set at the following stage. The LogNNet network's training begins with two nested iterations. By employing the backpropagation technique on the training set, the internal iteration trains the output LogNNet classifier. Particle swarm optimization of model parameters is used in the external iteration. The validation set determines the classification metrics following the linear classifier's training. A fetal cardiotocogram can be utilized as an observing device to distinguish high-risk ladies during labor. It uses approximately eight kB of RAM. Fig. (**14**) represents the same.

A practical hierarchical location-allocation model [38] based on supply and demand characterizes the trade-off between social, economic, and environmental factors. It is the framework for optimizing the location of healthcare facilities for developing Chinese cities. The township has sixteen patient areas and five central healthcare units. The number of sick beds in the existing hospitals is 527, which is not enough to meet the total needs of nearly 800. Governmental agencies and academic institutions provide numerical data about the population, medical demand, and healthcare information. It used a Windows 10 computer with 8 GB of RAM and an Intel Core i7 processor running at 2.8 GHz to perform the BLMOPSO algorithm.

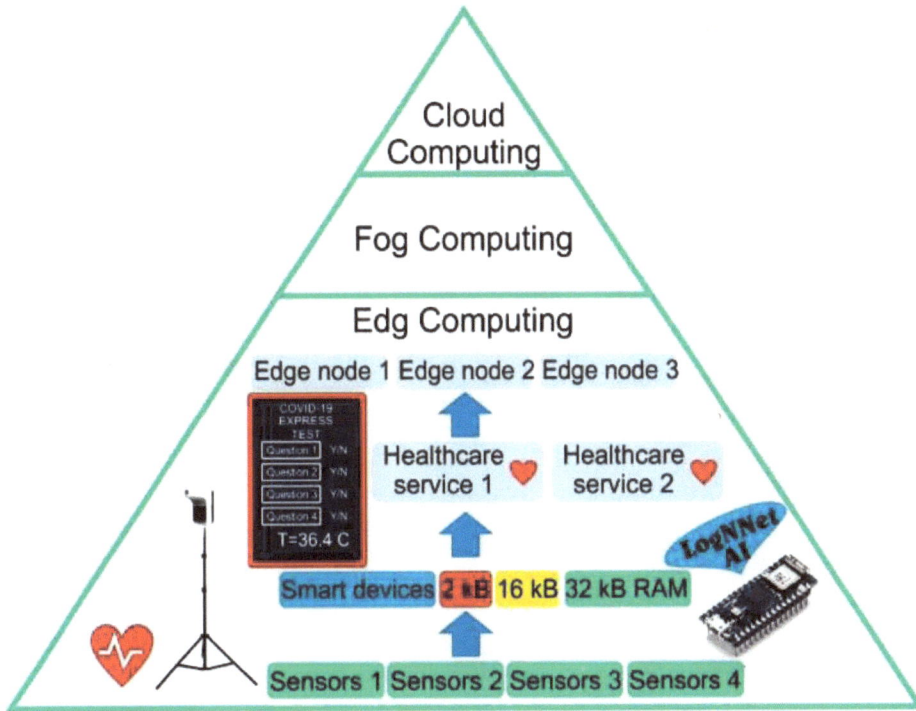

Fig. (14). Architecture of the system [37].

The project [39] is called "Integration of Pharmacogenetics into Primary Care". The prospective, observational, multicenter IP3 study aims to determine whether pharmacist-initiated pharmacogenetics testing in a clinical decision support system for primary care is feasible. In the delivery of healthcare, the general practitioner acts as a checkpoint. The general practitioner is consulted for all initial health issues and may recommend specialized care when necessary. Utilizing the Oragene DNA OG-250, pharmacists collected a 2-milliliter saliva sample from participating patients following the signing of an informed consent form. The examples were moved to the PGx lab in Leiden College Clinical Center by research staff or mail. Following the Oragene DNA OG-250 isolation procedure, DNA was extracted using a solution volume of 100 L rather than 200 L. The genotypes predicted phenotypes, including DPWG therapeutic recommendation for the drug of enrollment in a paper report sent to the patient's GP and pharmacist *via* mail or fax. For comparison, patients have been stratified into three groups. The first group is of those who did not experience an actionable drug-gene interaction for the drug of enrollment. The second one is of those who did experience an actionable drug-gene exchange for the prescription but whose healthcare providers followed the DPWG guideline. The last category is of those who did experience an actionable drug-gene interaction for the drug of enrollment but did not follow the DPWG guideline. Between November 2014 and July 2016, the IP3 study included 200 patients.

The project Framework [40] involves creating a digital health platform for a healthcare organization in Colombia that will combine advanced analytics with operational, clinical, and business data repositories to enhance population health management decision-making. The platform's implementation was an ambitious endeavor that required the definition of IT management procedures that were strong enough to support interoperability with other systems, the integration of health information from various sources, and the construction of numerous technological and functional components. Data related to patients, diagnostic reports, prescriptions, medical images, pharmacy records, research data, operational data, financial data, and human resources data were all part of the digital health information platform. The design and construction of a comprehensive health digital platform for a healthcare organization in Colombia, with the patient at its center and all of its information aggregated and summarized based on the standardized enterprise data repository, was pioneered by this innovative project. All technical complexity is hidden in this information, which can be accessed quickly and easily whenever and wherever needed. It also provides tools for longitudinal process management and professional decision support. The granular ingest of data from over fifty different source systems, including claims, clinical, financial, administrative, wearable, genomic, and socioeconomic data, is possible with the Digital Healthcare platform architecture. The platform can consume machine learning models whenever needed without requiring additional development. Open APIs enable access, reuse, and update of the data logic models on top of the raw data without modifying clinical or business logic. The platform successfully integrated both structured and unstructured data. It is common to see media of this kind that can integrate structured or unstructured data, but only some of them can do so successfully. APIs for open microservices were made for data pipeline management, authorization, identity management, and interoperability. The integration of third-party applications with the platform is made possible by these microservices. The initial strategy was building a significant data processing pipeline with a Microsoft Azure lambda architecture to support real-time and batch analytics. The architecture has a serving layer, a real-time layer, and a batch layer. The batch layer can scale horizontally and is in charge of persistent storage. The real-time layer handles dynamic computation and processes streaming data. The serving layer consumes the prediction models and query data from the repositories. The data lake allows for storing heterogeneous data in a single location by capturing data of any volume, type, or ingestion speed. A cloud-based data integration service orchestrates these data-driven workflows and the platform's automation, transformation, and data movement. The platform's security mechanisms support the OAuth 2.0 protocol for REST interface authentication and can provide protection and alert monitoring. Files, subfolders, and folders all support ACLs. A non-invasive neural network classification model for early neonatal sepsis detection was developed in this work. This study uses data from the Cartagena-Colombia Crecer's Hospital center. Fig. (**15**) represents the same.

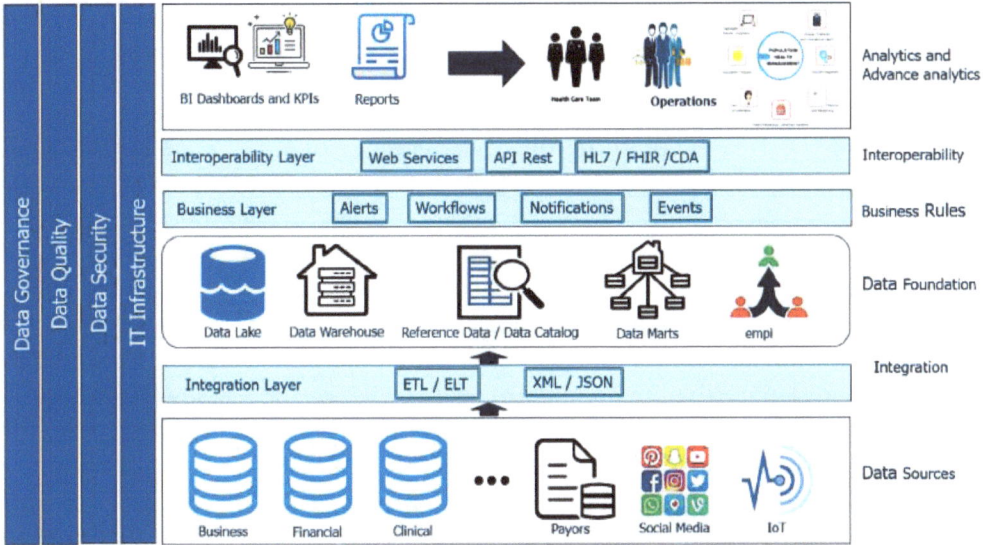

Fig. (15). Conceptual Framework [40].

Implementing a wide variety of pre-packaged, query-driven solutions or modules with pre-defined functionality that are user-customizable is known as SHDS info-structure [41]. The DM modules are made to interact with users to understand the problem better and provide decision-support services in return. A user-friendly and cognitively transparent top-level user interface for specifying a decision-support service and visualizing the DM outcome is the stratified design of the SHDS infrastructure. It is a collection of DM modules with varying functionalities spanning the entire range of healthcare-related decision-support services. The content sources, such as healthcare databases, data warehouses, and knowledge bases, make up the Content Layer. Data and knowledge resources are abstracted and specified in terms of metadata and ontologies, respectively, in the second layer, the Knowledge Description Layer. The Application Layer has two engines, one of which is geared toward DM tasks. The Services Layer user interface allows users to select and specify the SHDS required and receive the findings, recommendations, and results.

An innovative decision support system [42] is an intelligent module integrated into the system or attached. Intelligence strategies-based systems either use a single method to solve specific issues or a combination of two or more ways to solve more complex problems with some degree of ambiguity. It employs one or more artificial intelligence techniques to develop a diagnosis system for headache based on a set of signs and symptoms. Since there are multiple types of headaches, the system can assist doctors in determining which type to treat based on a set of symptoms. A clinical decision support system for the diagnosis of a headache is created by utilizing either Fuzzy-Rule-based or Fuzzy-Decision tree methods in combination. The questions need to be mentioned using a genetic algorithm as a feature selection for the initial data processing stage.

Centerstone [43] uses a combination of fee-for-service and case rate payment models, including Medicare, Medicaid, and commercial payers, to operate its fully functional electronic health record. Changes to a state-run payer in Tennessee compelled Centerstone to optimize the match between available services and the clinical needs of patients to minimize the provision of services that aren't needed and maximize outcomes. It necessitated the initial work described here. For data mining purposes, data were extracted from Centerstone's electronic health record into a specialized schema in the data warehouse. The subsequent CARLA outcome measure served as the target variable. Based on recovery levels utilized by Pike's Peak Mental Health Center and other level-of-care models such as ASAM, LOCUS, and the Ohio scale, clinical experts at Centerstone developed and validated the CARLA. A score of one indicates severe impairment in each dimension, and a score of four indicates little or no impairment. Clinicians use the CARLA to provide a systematic rating of the patient's symptoms, functioning, support, insight, and engagement in treatment. Preparation of the data is the first step. The change in CARLA scores over time was the primary focus of the initial analysis, which focused on clinical outcomes. Several models, including WEKA models and native KNIME models, were built on top of the dataset to determine the best performance. It uses a 10-fold cross-validation. The final step was to evaluate the model's performance to rule out the possibility that the statistical findings were an artifact of capitalizing on chance.

The work [44] assessed the significance of clinical features in predictions using deep Taylor decomposition for MLP, Shapley values for tree boosting, and model coefficients for logistic regression. Following the Helsinki Declaration, the study was approved by the Charité Universitätsmedizin Berlin's institutional ethics committee, and all patients gave written informed consent. Iv- tissue-plasminogen activators for thrombolysis therapy or conservative treatment were the outcomes of the patients' triage. Three months after the stroke, using the modified Rankin Scale, a telephone call was made to assess each patient's disability or dependence on daily activities. Five hundred fourteen patients in the database had undergone three imaging sessions.104 had no mRS values and were not eligible for follow-up. Due to matters outside the permissible parameter range, one patient had to be excluded. In addition, the outcome was predicted using machine learning techniques and clinical data due to the absence of visible diffusion-weighted imaging lesions and infratentorial stroke in 95 patients.

Implementing an AI-based decision support system in the emergency department of a large Canadian Academic Health Center is the focus of this study [45], particularly on the issue of end-user adoption. To better comprehend the particular difficulties presented by AI systems [46] in health care, it emphasizes the significance of considering the connections between technical, human, and organizational factors. To develop strategies for adequately testing, adapting, and ensuring that AI systems meet the needs of health professionals and patients, it further emphasizes the need to investigate actors' perceptions of AI. Using clinical data and scientific literature-based evidence, the DSS is a diagnostic technology based on a deep-learning algorithm. The DSS is presented as a questionnaire that patients visiting the emergency department can answer on a mobile tablet. The patient is first asked why they came to the emergency department. The patient's written text is then analyzed by a Natural Language Processing engine to determine the primary complaint. The DSS outputs a medical history printed by nurses or clerks and presented to the physician before encountering the patient. The patient is then asked a series of questions based on the chief complaint, with each question adapting to the previous response. Twenty semi-structured interviews were conducted using the snowball method to find participants. Thematic content analysis with NVivo 12 software was used to identify, classify, and refine the primary obstacles to physician adoption of the DSS.

The work [47] is a new hybrid methodology called Expert-based Cooperative Analysis, which aims to enhance healthcare decision support by eliciting implicit or tacit expert knowledge and incorporating explicit prior expert knowledge into data analysis techniques. The PSICOST research association has conducted two complex mental health care case studies. The first case study evaluated the technical efficacy of Spain's 12 distinct small health areas. The data for each catchment area were compiled in residential care, structured daycare, non-acute outpatient care, and emergency outpatient care. Case-mix schizophrenia based on functional dependency is the second case study. Expert-based cooperative analysis, or EbCA, is a method for iteratively eliciting implicit knowledge from experts that allow prior expert knowledge to be included in the data analysis. It is a method which gives functional definitions to fundamental profiles in an exceptionally complicated space. Inductive Learning from AI and clustering from statistics are combined in this hybrid method to extract knowledge from complex domains in the form of typical profiles. Selection of relevant variables to be considered, inclusion and exclusion criteria, data representation, missing data analysis, outlier detection and treatment, and other aspects of data collection and preparation are all included. The process of acquiring and designing the Prior Knowledge Base is Prior Expert Knowledge. Depending on the chosen underlying method, PKB-guided analysis can be used to guide the analysis in several ways—support-interpretation, which includes instruments for assessing results and identifying inconsistencies.

The work [48] consists of two parts-designing the components of an IoT healthcare platform and a decision support system. It achieves the objectives of an effective technology-led healthcare system, demonstrating the concept by applying it to cardiovascular diseases, and identifying risk groups from a sample set of individuals. Before beginning a new diagnosis, the IoT-based system keeps a pool of historical data about a patient's healthcare. It considered the physiological characteristics of 600 individuals. It used Framingham's Equation for Cardiovascular Diseases to calculate the Framingham Scores for each sample set. Two clusters have been established for the data.

A virtual human interviewer called SimSensei Kiosk [49] creates an engaging face-to-face interaction in which the user feels at ease talking and sharing information. It is based on a general modular virtual human architecture that abstractly defines a virtual human's capabilities and interactions. The acquisition and analysis of human-to-human interactions have comprised the primary focus of the first cycle. A corpus of 120 face-to-face interactions between a confederate interviewer and a paid participant was collected. It analyzed the interviewee's behaviors to identify potential indicators of distress and the interviewer's behaviors to identify appropriate questions and nonverbal behaviors to animate the virtual human. During the second cycle, a Wizard of Oz prototype allowed two human operators to dictate the virtual human's verbal and nonverbal responses. Ellie's behavior was jointly controlled by two wizards who had access to a predetermined set of 191 utterances and 23 nonverbal behaviors. It used this system to collect a corpus of 140 interactions between participants in the Wizard of Oz. The creation of our fully automatic system was the primary focus of the third cycle.

The most critical variables are identified through causal maps in the initial stage of the model [50]. The total time spent in the system is used to measure efficiency. Through the use of causal maps, the fundamental or critical variables of the system to be modeled are identified concerned with knowledge acquisition and problem structuring. A Bayesian Belief Network represents the key variables' conditional dependencies and uncertainties in the second stage. In the third stage, a sensitivity analysis employing a BBN is carried out to identify the variable with the most significant impact on the system. The developed BBN provides a framework for representing the uncertainty of variables in the map by representing conditional dependencies between and among those variables affecting the total time spent in the system. The tomography section of a private Turkish hospital's radiology department is now used with the proposed decision support model. The hospital has 279 skilled physicians, 1038 healthcare and support staff, and 42 branches, including clinical research, diagnostics, and outpatient and inpatient care. With a 210-bed capacity and an ISO 9001 quality certificate, the facility serves 162,423 polyclinic patients annually. Each year, 36,000 radiological tests are carried out.

A Video Capsule Endoscopy [51] is a noninvasive procedure. Observing a patient's gastroenterological tract produced the medical data set that is the subject of the current study. Coelho provided 3295 images in the Red Lesion Endoscopy data set, which are accessible to the general public. There are two sets of images in the data set. The main pack contains 1131 pictures with injuries and 2164 without sores, for 3295 photos. There are 600 appearances in the second set, including 439 with lesions and 151 without lesions. The work used Python to implement the LIME and SHAP explainable methods on the Triton high-performance computing cluster provided by Aalto University. In contrast, it used RStudio version 1.2.1335 to generate CIU explanations. Participants were divided into three groups: NoXAI and LIME explanations were given to the first group, noXAI and SHAP descriptions to the second group, and noXAI and CIU explanations to the third group. Fig. (**16**) depicts the same.

Face sketch synthesis is performed using a modified version of U-Net in this project. The initial segment is a compiler network [52], which depends on a lingering organization of two branches, and the skip associations are made in a twisting design. It creates a raw sketch for an input photo. The second part of the plan is a feature extractor based on a Vgg-19 network that has already been trained. Another intermediate entity, the feature sketch, is formed by these net and its components. This network is made up of two strains that are the same, and each strain has three stages. Convolutional layers make up the first part. The compiler network is an essential module throughout the framework's implementation and operation phases. This network receives the training photo images during the training phase, and at its conclusion, a pseudo sketch is created. The comparisons are made between this sketch and the remaining components of the overall plan. For each train photo, features of the top n candidates of viewed drawings are extracted from the reference dataset using a pre-trained Vgg-19 model. Maps or matrices of overlapping patches are created from identical photos and sketches. There were two phases of neural network training. The setup's first run used the CUFS reference style, and the second used the CUFSF reference style to train the system. Fig. (**17**) represents the same.

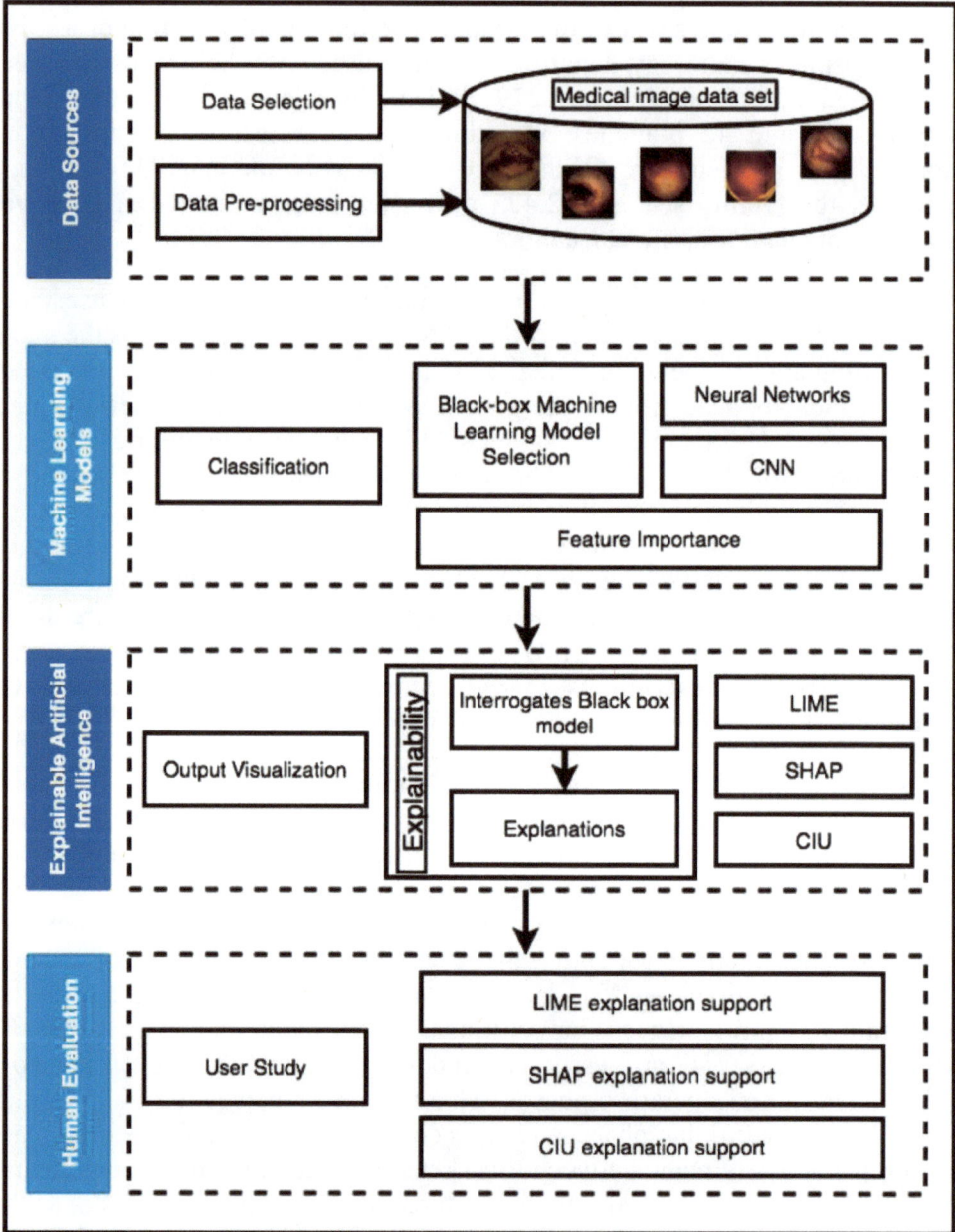

Fig. (16). Proposed System [51].

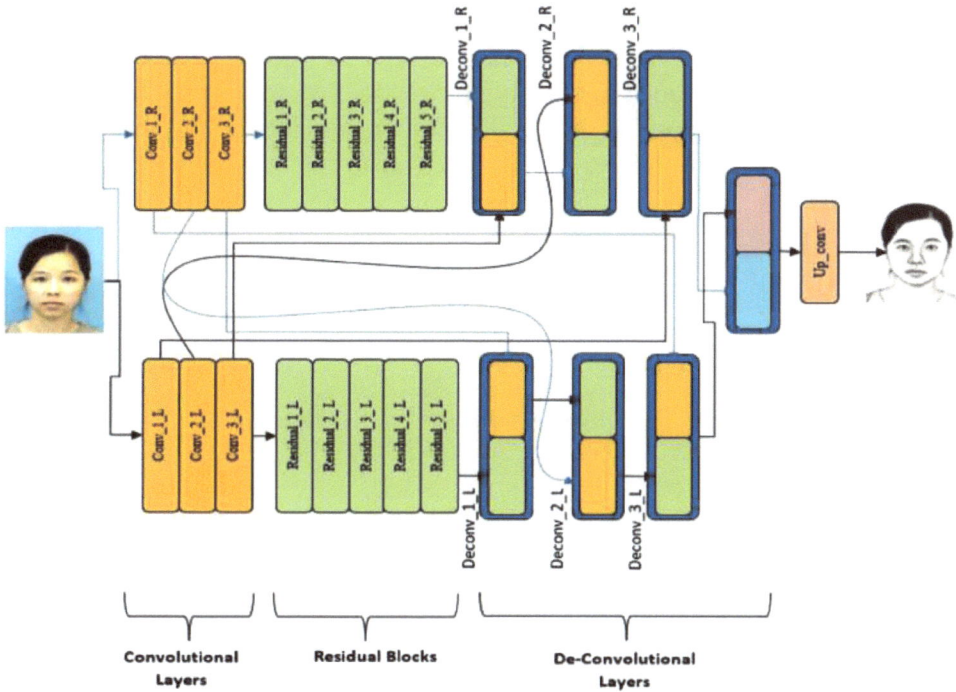

Fig. (17). Architecture of Spiral-Net [52].

2.2.6. One Rule (Oner)

OneR, which stands for "One Rule," is a straightforward yet precise classification algorithm that selects the rule with the slightest total error as its "one rule" after generating one rule for each predictor in the data. We construct a frequency table for each predictor and compare it to the target to create a rule for that predictor. It has been demonstrated that OneR produces human-readable rules that are marginally less accurate than the most recent classification algorithms.

An intelligent algorithm that was developed to intelligently determine whether a parameter has exceeded a threshold, which may or may not involve urgency, is included in the proposed architecture [53]. It has three main parts to it. The wearable device is controlled by Arduino Uno and connected to a smartphone. It is made up of several sensor modules, such as a glucose sensor, a motion sensor, and a temperature sensor. Bluetooth is used to connect smartphones to sensor devices in the system. The diabetic patient's glucose level, temperature, and movement are all recorded by the body sensors. A Bluetooth connection is used to send this data to the mobile device. The database server and mobile application make up the data acquisition module. The database server gathers the sensors' data. The handling unit comprises a specialist's portable and observing frameworks. Through a 4G network, the smartphone transmits data to the processing unit. The monitoring system analyzes the sensor data. Each diabetic patient can carry a developed or portable device that is attached to their hand and connected to their phone. The ESP8266 is an integrated circuit for a microcontroller that connects to Wi-Fi. Fig. (**18**) represents the same.

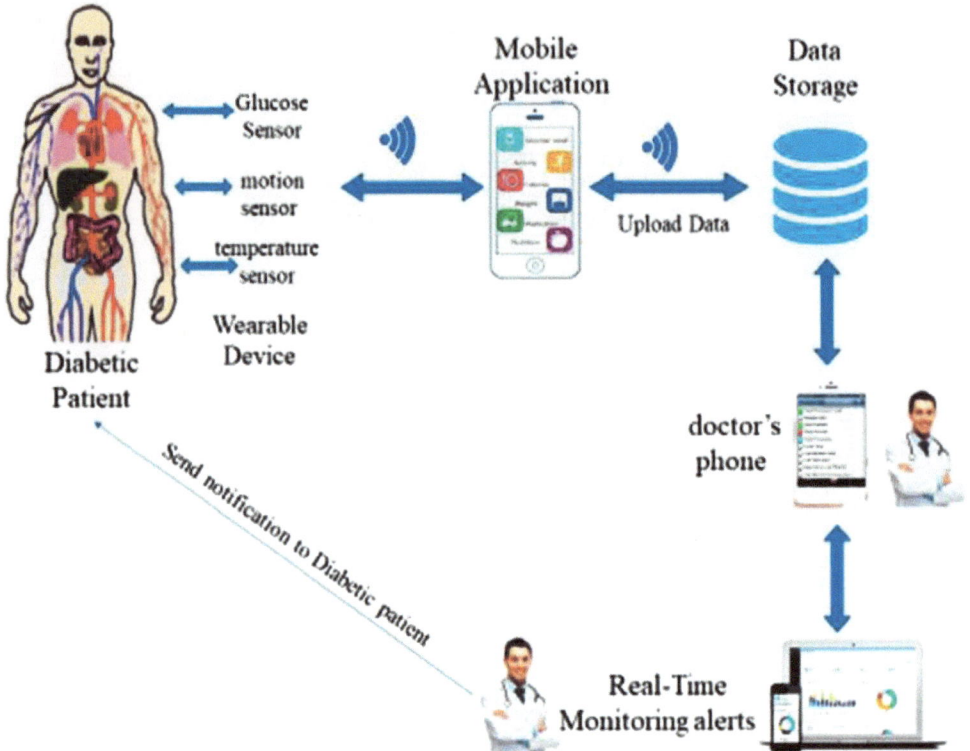

Fig. (18). Proposed Architecture [53].

Numerous intelligent algorithms are presented in this work [54] to support advanced analytics and provide diabetic patients with individualized medical assistance. This classification is based on the algorithms Naive Bayes J48, ZeroR, Sequential Minimal Optimization, Random tree, and OneR. Because of this disease prediction, patients can be treated before the disease gets worse or fails and their health is in danger. It used Weka's functions in every experiment. These methods are based on the JAVA environment. The system uses a database with the glucose levels of 40 diabetic patients, 30 men and ten women between the ages of 25 and 60, over 30 days.

2.2.7. Zero Rule (Zeror)

ZeroR is the most straightforward classification technique that disregards all predictors and relies on the target. The ZeroR classifier predicts the majority category (class). The target's frequency table is created, and the value with the highest frequency is chosen.

The system [55] provides information on blood glucose levels and readings in real-time. It regularly checks the status of glucose in the blood. The goal of the proposed method is to avoid significant fluctuations in glucose levels and high blood sugar. The system provides a precise outcome. The data collected and stored will be classified using several classification algorithms. Three distinct subsystems make up the designed blood glucose monitoring system. The first is devoted to using the glucose sensor to measure blood glucose levels. This sensor records the glucose level in the blood, its precise value is displayed, and the data is sent to an Android phone *via* the communication module. Because current mobile phones lack a means of directly interacting with analog signals from the outside world, this is necessary. The smartphone's data storage and processing service is part of the second subsystem. Decision-making and data analysis by domain experts comprise the third subsystem. For any electronic project that necessitates the utilization of dependable biometric measurements, the e-health sensor shield can be connected to an Arduino board. It makes available the data gathered by nine different biometric sensors. A Transistor-Transistor Logic to RS232 converter also links the GSM module to the Arduino board. The value is 115,200 bps for serial communication between the microcontroller, the sensor, and the GSM module. Fig. (**19**) represents the same.

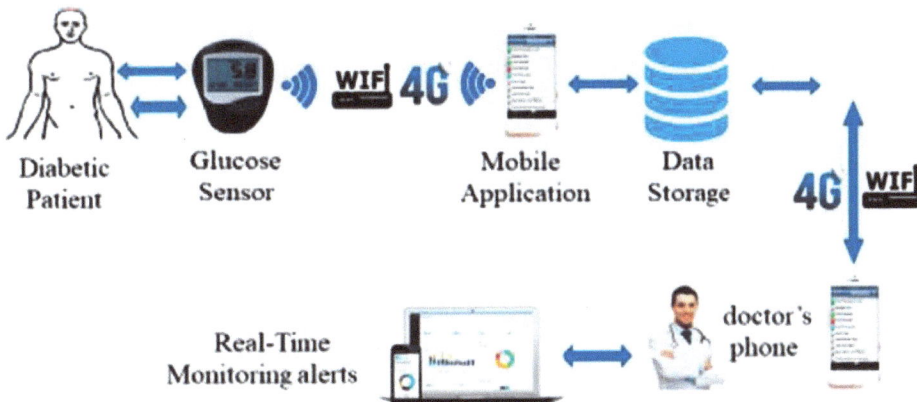

Fig. (19). proposed Architecture [55].

The system [56] suggests employing decision trees such as J48, Naive Bayes, ANN, ZeroR, 1BK, and the VFI algorithm to classify these diseases and contrast their efficiency and correction rate. WEKA, an open-source data mining tool, is utilized in work. Data pre-processing, feature reduction, classification, regression, clustering, and association rules are all implemented by WEKA. Tools for visualization are also included.

2.3. LINEAR REGRESSION

The value of one variable can be used to predict the value of another variable using linear regression analysis. The dependent variable is the one you want to predict. The independent variable is the one you use to indicate the value of the other variable. The coefficients of the linear equation with one or more independent variables that best predict the value of the dependent variable are estimated using this analysis method. Linear regression [57] produces a surface or straight line with the lowest possible difference between predicted and actual output values. Simple linear regression calculators use the "least squares" method to determine the best-fit line for a set of paired data. It gauges the worth of X (subordinate variable) from Y (free factor). Fig. (**20**) represents the Integrated Model.

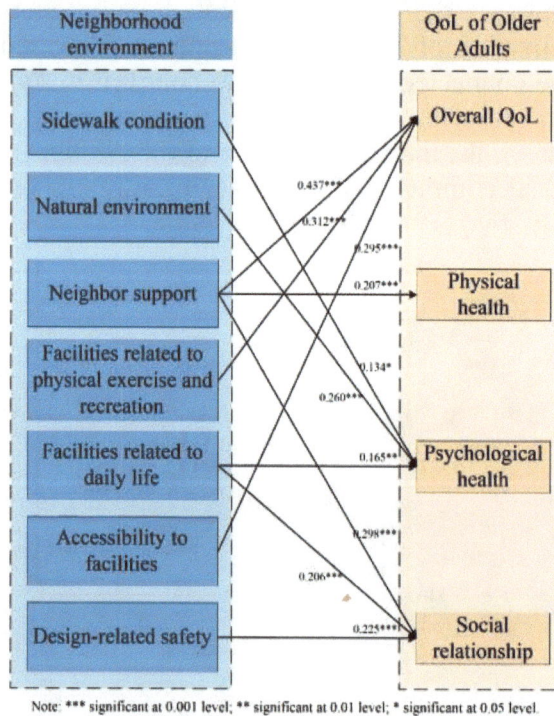

Note: *** significant at 0.001 level; ** significant at 0.01 level; * significant at 0.05 level.

Fig. (20). Integrated Model [58].

To overcome some limitations and develop a rigorous mathematical approach [59] to temporal variation analysis, the system study was conducted. The time series' temporal evolution could be accurately described using the proposed method, and the conclusions that could be drawn from merely comparing groups were strengthened. 2777 patients with proximal femoral fragility fractures were the subject of the study. 2117 of these patients had 2176 fractures before the HFU was started, and 660 of these patients had 671 fractures treated after the HFU was started. Demographic information on patients was also gathered. In the context of learning curve modeling, the study is an adaptation of a segmented linear regression method (EMV) previously published by one of the authors. The models ranged from a straightforward plateau to two straight lines that were adjacent to one another and had a single knot at the time that minimized the sum of the squares of the residuals. This range of models has a respectable level of complexity and is able to capture shifting trends throughout the study period. At the same time, the descriptions of movements remain clear and meaningful.

The model [60] is a piecewise linear function of the independent variable's time as a binary dependent variable. The values of the parameters of the proposed set of models are maximum likelihood estimates because they are derived to maximize the likelihood of the experimental data. A time series of data from a Level 1 Major Trauma Center in the United Kingdom was modeled using this method. It used the modeling technique on three-time series: Mortality rates among patients at 30, 120, and 365 days. It compared patient mortality before and after the intervention (pre-HFU) using statistical tests.

At the administrative county level, the study [61] aimed to investigate the spatial and temporal heterogeneous effects of various socioeconomic and environmental factors on healthcare resource disparities. One of China's seven geographical divisions, the study area of southwest China, is situated between $97°21'–110°11'$ east longitude and $21°08'–33°41'$ north latitude. The study gathered information on 32 potential socioeconomic and environmental covariates in southwest China between 2002 and 2011.

An artificial intelligence network-based regression-based model [62] for predicting health insurance premiums was trained and evaluated in this study. The authors prepared machine learning-based model and implemented it using Python programming to predict health insurance premiums. The initial steps were importing the Python libraries and packages as well as the dataset. It included over 1300 entries in the dataset, with seven columns for charges, smoking, location, children, BMI, sex, and age. The health insurance premium was predicted using this dataset. An exploratory data analysis was then carried out. The dataset was checked for null values in this step. It analyzed the dataset during the phase of performing the Data Analysis and Feature Engineering to verify the relationship between the various columns. It cleaned the dataset during the visualization step so the model could be trained and shown. The authors introduced the linear regression model during the "Training and Evaluating a Linear Regression Model" phase, but it cleaned the dataset first.

This strategy [63] focuses on investigating the required fundamental structural changes in healthcare systems. It emphasizes on the development of ML concepts for use in medicine, which may center on personalized diagnosis and treatment based on the patient's general information and collective experience. The authors asserted that an EHR's pattern detection training ML classifier would enable physicians to anticipate future events in high-risk patients. It obtains an accurate and complete diagnosis and provides a fast search engine for locating pertinent information within a patient's chart, resulting in less clicking, voice dictation, and improved predictive typing.

2.3.1. Random Forest

Random forests, also known as random decision forests [64], are ensemble learning for classification, regression, and other tasks. It works by building a lot of decision trees during training. The class most trees choose is what the random forest produces for classification tasks. The individual trees' mean or average prediction is returned for regression tasks. Irregular choice timberlands are suitable for choice trees' propensity for overfitting their preparation set. Though their accuracy is lower than that of gradient-boosted trees, random forests generally perform better than decision trees. However, their performance can be affected by data characteristics.

Density-based spatial clustering of applications with noise is one component of the proposal [65]. The other components are the Synthetic Minority Over-Sampling Technique to balance class distribution, Random Forest to classify diseases, and DBSCAN to remove outlier data. CKD, diabetes, and hypertension datasets are referred to as datasets I, II, and III, respectively. University of Virginia School of Medicine provided dataset I. There were 403 instances in the data. To learn more about the prevalence of obesity, diabetes, and other cardiovascular risk factors among African Americans in central Virginia, the subjects were questioned. On male subjects, the relationship between elevated blood pressure and BMI, WC, HC, and WHR is shown in dataset II. Apollo Hospital in Tamilnadu, India, has provided dataset III. The original dataset contained 400 instances of 24 features, each of which classified the subject as having or not having chronic kidney disease. 261 tested negative, 137 tested positives, and two unlabeled data make up the dataset. Fig. (**21**) represents the same.

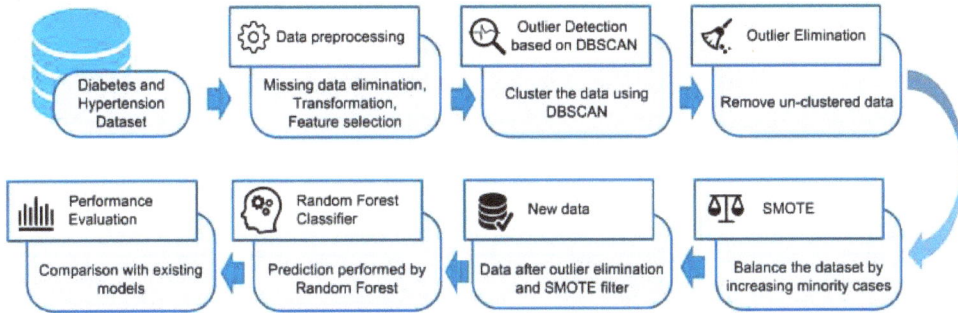

Fig. (21). Hybrid prediction model [65].

This study [66] aimed to determine the factors that could have prevented this complication. The "Unidad de Investigación Médica en Bioqumica, Centro Médico Nacional Siglo XXI, IMS" provided the dataset for this study. The dataset consists of 32 features, including clinical, para-clinical, and additional information about T2D patients. This study used 140 and 70 diabetic patients without microvascular complications (controls). The 32 features were normalized using the standard score. Boruta is a Random Forest-based method for selecting elements. The Boruta algorithm was used to determine characteristics and locate all relevant attributes. The selected variables are then used as the RF technique's input variables. The methodology was developed using a dataset with 32 features, 140 observations of 32 variables, and one output class. This study included 140 subjects and divided them into a non-DSPN group and a DSPN group.

This review [67] aims to improve the sensitivity and specificity of macrosomia prediction. It develops new predictive models using a random forest model to identify macrosomia.405 macrosomia and 3855 normal-weight newborns were the study subjects, which included 4260 newborns who met the criteria. When ntree was 500, it chose the number of decision trees used in this study to select the best model. The model's overall misjudgment rate was 6.34 percent using the OBB data. The importance ranking of the explanatory variables was determined to be in line with the average decline in the Gini coefficient for each risk factor used in the random forest model. The results of the random forest's screening of predictive macrosomia factors using the variable importance measure: interspinal diameter, transverse outlet diameter, intercristal diameter, sacral external diameter, age, number of pregnancies, and parity are all factors in this measurement.

eGAP [68] develops a Random Forest ensemble by employing the evolutionary game theoretic approach and replicator dynamics. It brings together two methods. Replicator dynamics was used on a diversified random forest with subforests produced by randomized subspaces to evolve subforests by allowing those with better performance to grow and those with lower performance to shrink. Clustering was the primary method used in to extreme prune random forests. In evolutionary game theory, the straightforward evolutionary model known as replicator dynamics is frequently used. The replicator equation calculates the proportion of each type in the subsequent period as a function of the type's payoff and its current share in the population. eGAP creates a pruned RF ensemble by incorporating replicator dynamics and clustering. An effective clustering technique is then used to group the trees in this forest into groups of similar trees. Each tree is represented as an ordered list of classification outputs for classification tasks for clustering. The Hamming distance between the two ordered lists calculates any tree's dissimilarity. Regression creates a real-number vector with the regressed values representing each tree. Fig. (**22**) represents the same.

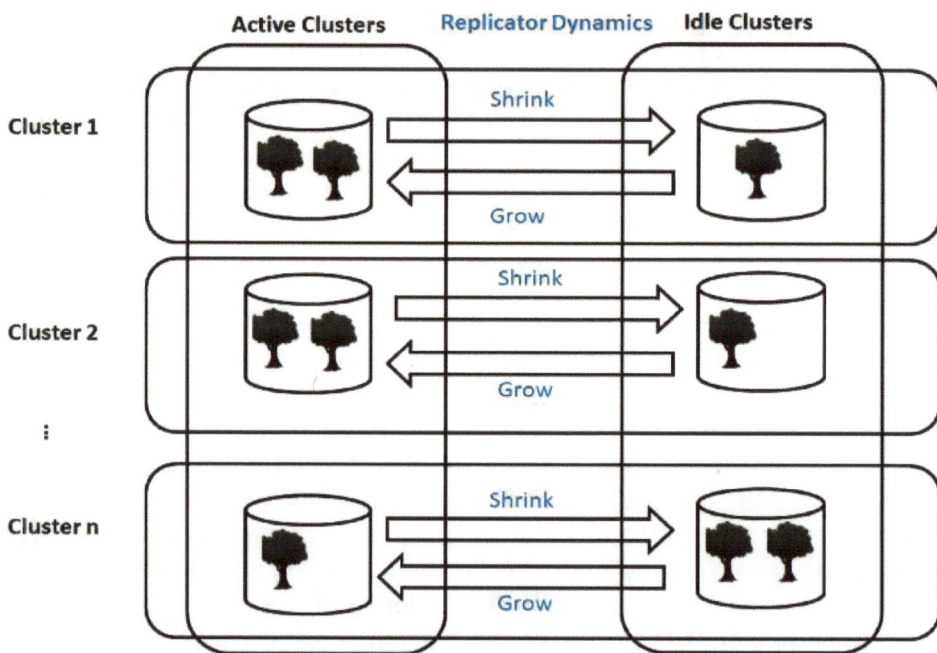

Fig. (22). eGAP system [68].

The cognitive authentication framework [69] uses adaptive machine and deep learning to process, extract, and classify cognitive/EEG signals. When managing and monitoring the brain wave authentication, the feedback from HCI *via* the initial EEG signal plays a significant role following the establishment of human-computer interaction. One of the most extensive and widely used databases, Physione, provided the EEG motor movement/imagery datasets used in the study. Individual 2-minute EEG recordings made by 109 subjects using the European Data Format web browser make up the selected datasets. Sixty-four scalp electrodes are used to perform a few tasks in the data. Out of 109 data recordings, 20 subjects are being considered. Fig. (**23**) represents the same.

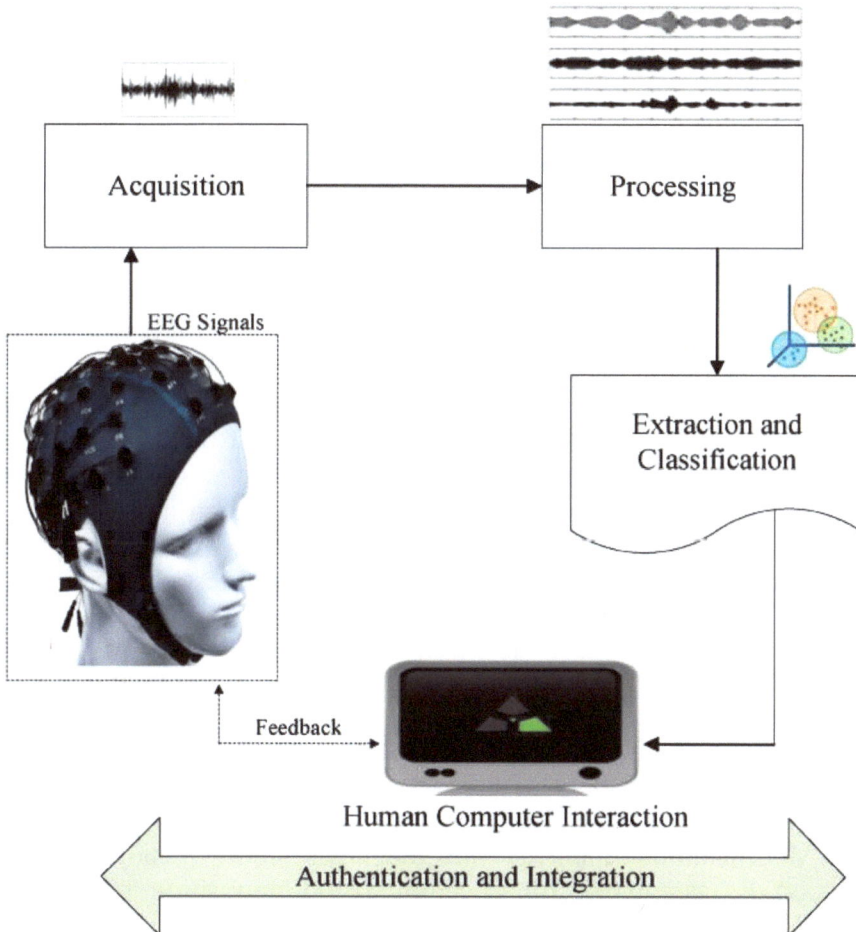

Fig. (23). Proposed framework [69].

After careful selection, the collected questionnaires were turned into binary code feature vectors in this study [70]. In Beijing's Xicheng district, a questionnaire survey with snowball sampling and convenient sampling was carried out with middle-aged and older adults as the primary target demographic. It can break down the information in the survey into four categories: personal information, eating habits, exercise situation, and family history, each of which has multiple issues. It provided a binary coding-based method for feature representation. It transformed the responses to each question in each sample into a feature vector, which served as the XGBoost model's input vector. The work was written in Python 3.8, modeled and trained on the Windows 10 Operating System (Microsoft, Redmond, WA, USA), and the CPU was an Intel Core I7-6700HQ with 3.5 GHz and 4 GB of memory. During this survey, 380 samples were collected for the study;368 models were left for analysis after 12 missing samples, and it removed inconsistent cases.

The authors [71] developed a system for real-time and remote health monitoring based on IoT infrastructure and cloud computing using a variety of machine learning methods and public health care datasets stored in the cloud. The system can make recommendations based on the cloud's historical and empirical data. The Internet of Things is a network of networks made possible by technology. The Internet of Things (IoT) makes it possible to connect things or machines that are stationary and mobile by utilizing wireless communications for inexpensive sensors supported by computing and storage devices. The physician will need help keeping up with the large amounts of data in the system. The health care information is initially transferred through a sensor network to mobile devices. Bluetooth, a Wi-Fi application, or a USB connection are all options for the sensor network. The IoT operator is a patient's cell phone, which is used to send their health data to the cloud. The precise information related to the query dataset of diseases is extracted from the database using a random forest classifier.

The Nationwide Inpatient Sample is a database [72] of hospital inpatient admissions from 1988 that is used to identify, track, and examine national trends in healthcare utilization, access, costs, quality, and outcomes. There are approximately 8 million records of hospital stays in the data set, each with 126 clinical and nonclinical data elements. There are 15 vectors of diagnosis codes in each history. The International Classification of Diseases, Ninth Revision, and Clinical Modification represent the diagnosis codes. The World Health Organization is responsible for developing and publishing the International Statistical Classification of Diseases. Hospitals, insurance companies, and other facilities use the ICD-9, an alphanumeric code with 3-5 characters, to describe the patient's health conditions. Each code represents a disease, condition, symptom, or cause of death. There are numerous codes, including 3,900 procedures and over

14,000 ICD-9 codes. It included the 7,995,048 records in the data set in a substantial ASCII file that was provided. The first steps were parsing the data set, selecting N records at random, and extracting a set of relevant features. However, HCUP provides a SAS program for parsing the data set. The work dragged the age, race, sex, and 15 diagnosis categories from each record. The training and testing data sets are created by dividing the data set into active and inactive instances using the Repeated Random Sub-Sampling method. Except for the final sub-sample, the training data is divided into sub-samples with equal representatives from each class.

The work [73] is an effective model incorporating multiple domain features, feature reduction, and a recognizer engine. The system has statistical and time-domain features integrated to guarantee performance measure robustness. Noise removal and preprocessing steps are included in the proposed model to ensure error-free data. It used the median filter for the IMU sensor, the band-pass filter for the EMG sensor, and the moving average filter for the MMG sensor to remove the noise from the various inertial sensor signals. After it removed the noise, it added windows with an interval of five seconds for each type of signal. There are three distinct phases to it. All three types of sensors' data have been filtered using median, band-pass, and moving average filters during the preprocessing and segmentation phases. After that, it broke up the de-noised data into overlapping windows based on how big each step of the physical activities was. In the element extraction stage, time-domain highlights and measurable elements are utilized. Lastly, during the phase of symbolization and classification, it used the bagged random forest method to classify feature vectors.

The proposition [74] utilizes a gathering relapse method given CLUB-DRF, a pruned Irregular Woods with these elements. CLUB-DRF is an enhancement of RF that produces a child RF. A K-means clustering algorithm takes as input the super-ordered list. The work consists of clusters, with each group containing ordered lists that are similar and likely to have the fewest discrepancies when clustering is finished. The algorithm's final step involves selecting a representative from each cluster. Diabetes, breast cancer, and Parkinson's disease are the goals of the work. The University of Waikato Repository housed the first data set, while the UCI Machine Learning Repository housed the second and third sets. The experiments were carried out on a laptop running Windows 7 Enterprise with 8 GB of RAM, a dual processor running at 2.60 GHz, and the Python programming language's Scikit-learn machine learning library.

2.3.2. Gradient Boosted Regression Tree

Regression and classification, among other tasks, are examples of machine-learning applications for gradient boosting [75]. An ensemble of weak prediction models, typically decision trees, is provided as a prediction model. The algorithm produced is referred to as a gradient-boosted tree when a decision tree serves as the weak learner. It typically performs better than random forest. Like other boosting techniques, a gradient-boosted trees model is constructed stage-by-stage, but it extends these techniques by allowing optimization of any differentiable loss function. Fig. (**24**) represents gradient boosting decision tree.

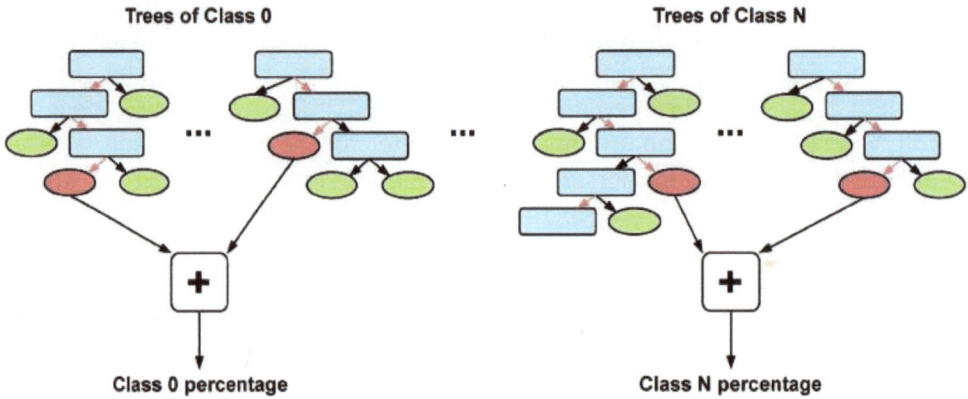

Fig. (24). Gradient boosting decision tree [76].

This study [77] proposes a CVD prediction model using machine learning (ML) algorithms and the National Health Insurance Service-Health Screening datasets. It used fourfold cross-validation of the datasets to measure the performance using the criteria of the area under the receiver operating characteristic curve (AUROC) scoring mechanism. The model repeated the same validation 30 times—the minimum number of iterations required to achieve the same result—to mitigate any effect of random sampling. The average AUROC values score represents each model's final performance comparison results. The CVD prediction model was constructed using 38 contributing factors, and it measured relative feature significance to determine how well the model performed. This study used data from the National Health Insurance Corporation (NHIC) dataset from 2009 to 2013. The study included 4699 patients over the age of 45 who were diagnosed with cardiovascular disease (CVD) using the international classification system (I20–I25). A non-CVD group included 4699 random subjects without a diagnosis of cardiovascular disease.

The study [78] aims to examine statistical modeling approaches for evaluating fictitious health benefits. It processes the four Medicare-derived datasets from Kaggle, which contain medical beneficiaries and their claims. Beneficiaries, outpatient claims, inpatient claims, and provider fraud are all described by four data sources. This dataset, which includes 700,000 shares, 200,000 beneficiaries, and 5,410 providers, is intended to compare healthcare providers while preserving specific information about beneficiaries and claims. The work uses a decision tree learning mechanism involving several steps.

An example of how it can use Artificial Intelligence in healthcare is the recommendation [79] to identify insurance fraud. Data on providers' Medicare claims submissions are the first source.CMS has provided this data. The second source is a list of healthcare providers that are not allowed to submit Medicare claims. Data on Medicare Part B insurance claims from 2012 to 2017 and data on Medicare Part D insurance claims from 2013 to 2017. These data are derived from several files that CMS makes available to the general public. The components of the Part B and Part D insurance claims data are described in CMS documents. These data are presented in character-separated value (CSV) format at a high level, with one file for each year. Each record in the data identifies a provider based on the provider's NPI and, in part, on a few other elements that provide information about the provider's name, demographics, and location. Additionally, a provider type in the records explains the nature of the provider's practice. There is one record in the Part-B PUF file for the year for each procedure for which the provider has submitted a claim to Medicare in the Part B data. A Healthcare Common Procedure Coding System (HCPCS) code represents this procedure. The LEIE data create a label for the Medicare Part B and Part D data for a specific year. Data can be handled by XGBoost, CatBoost, LightGBM, Random Forest, or Logistic Regression—the work uses one-hot encoding.

The work [80] develops a machine-learning screening approach to help healthcare professionals prioritize patient needs automatically. To sequence and predict elective patients, it utilized five machine learning methods: XGBoost, gradient-boosting decision tree (GBDT), extreme gradient boosting (XGBoost), and an ensemble model of the four models are all examples of logistic regression (LR). Information preprocessing is a center move toward working on the nature of crude information. It used machine learning algorithms to analyze the data following preprocessing to learn about the patient selection procedure and prioritized preadmission patients. The work deals with the missing values with high precision using multiple interpolations. The R software and the R package MICE were used to carry out the method. It uses transformation, such as normalizing the original values of those variables and discretizing them. Values were grouped and categorized with the help of an interval (min and max). The model is usually built with a training set; Performance is evaluated with the help of a verification set, allowing the user to make any necessary adjustments to the model parameters. A model's results are affected by various parameters, which we must adjust to select the best one. After an ideal model is obtained, a test set is utilized for expectation, permitting the client to assess the exhibition of the last model. It used samples from 2014 as a training set, from 2015 as a validation set, and from 2016 as a test set.

Predictive analysis can be used in the health care system, particularly for monitoring and prediction. The regulated and generated data serve as feedback to the system [81], providing the necessary decision support for professionals working in the healthcare industry. It constantly monitors health-related data and provides healthcare guidance based on the decision support made available from the DSS installed at the medical camp that operates as a not-for-profit organization. A medical center is considered to care for stressful work and other health issues. The applicability of various machine learning algorithms for healthcare prediction is investigated, and individual performance is compared. The platform for implementing experimental findings is R Studio. The setup, the Java runtime environment, and the Java Development Kit (JDK) were all installed on the Windows platform. All actual data have been gathered from Vidya Knockobter-2016 analytics.

2.3.3. Perception Back-Propogation

The method can break down the Backpropagation neural network's [82] operations into two steps: backpropagation and feedforward. An input pattern is applied to the input layer during the feedforward step, and its effect spreads through the network layer by layer until the output is produced. An error signal is then calculated for each output node after the actual output value of the network is compared to the expected outcome. The output error signals are sent backward from the output layer to each hidden layer node that immediately contributes to the output layer because all hidden nodes have contributed somehow to the errors visible in the output layer. After that, this process is repeated layer by layer until each node in the network receives an error signal that details its proportional share of the total error. When the mistake signal for every hub is partially set in stone, the blunders are then involved by the hubs to refresh the qualities for every association load. It happens until the organization joins an express that permits all the preparation examples to be encoded. It uses a method known as gradient descent or the delta rule. The Backpropagation algorithm seeks the error function's minimum value in weight space. The learning issue is likely solved by choosing weights that minimize the error function. The behavior of the network is comparable to a human being asked to categorize a set of data into predefined classes. It will develop "theories" about how the samples fit into the categories, like humans. The network's guesses are then verified by comparing these to the correct outputs. The weights change significantly in the most recent theory, indicating radical changes, while small changes could be considered minor adjustments to the approach. Fig. (**25**) represents the similar technology.

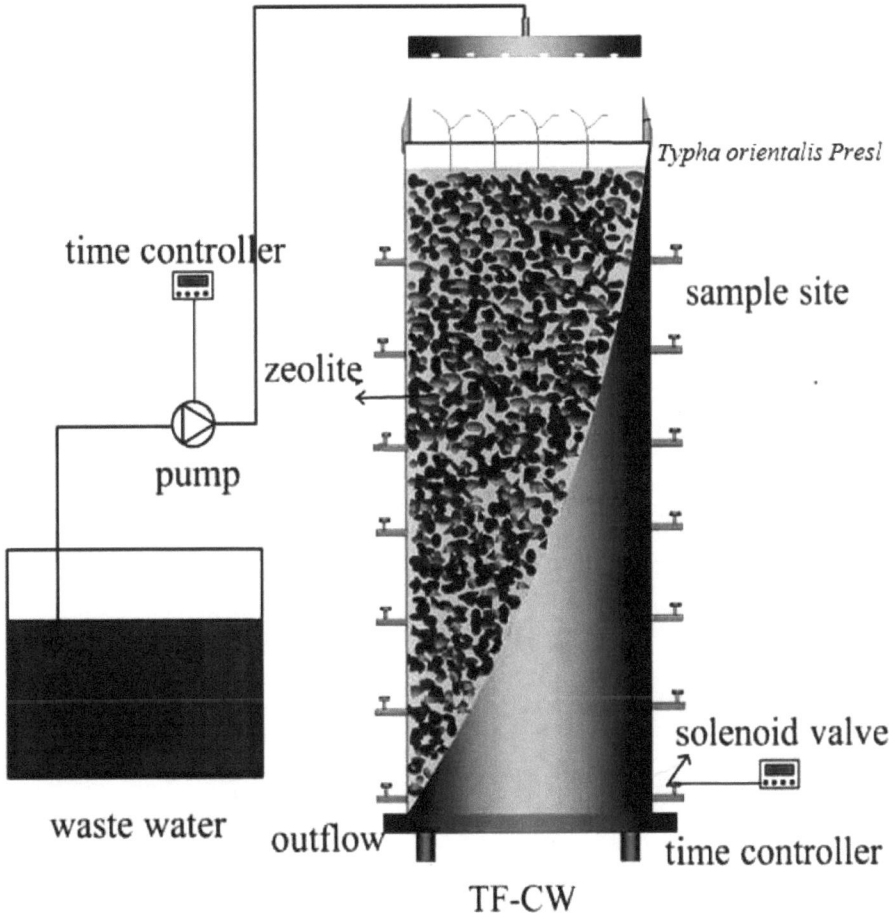

Fig. (25). Tidal flow well setup [83].

The work [84] is an analysis of Cleveland Clinic Foundation data that is stored in the UCI Machine Learning Repository. There are 303 instances with 14 attributes in the input dataset. The class label is the final attribute, and five possible heart disease diagnoses exist. Preprocessing techniques are used to remove all potential outliers and extreme values from the input data after it has been collected. A training dataset obtained from a repository serves as the foundation for the classification process. The training data are used to train a classifier model and are preprocessed to remove errors and inconsistencies. After the test data have been collected and preprocessed, the already-trained classifier is used in the classification process to get the needed results. The work used the Best-First Search method for feature selection, finding seven good attributes suitable for classification. The J48 decision tree classifier, which uses the C4.5 algorithm in Weka, is used in the study.

Utilizing back propagation and Multilayer Perceptron in selecting surgical procedures is the focus of this work [85]. The dataset of the caesarian area was gathered from the well-being focus of Tabriz. Age, number of pregnancies, length of labor, blood pressure, and heart condition are the five most important characteristics of delivery issues that make up the dataset's 80 instances. It chose the multilayer perceptron algorithm for its high accuracy in medical applications, ability to apply negotiation strategies, and ability to determine the delivery method for pregnant women. The study simulated the information of all pregnant women, and the indicator of the results that we obtained is that there was a direct correlation between the heart failure rate and deliveries that ended in a caesarian section.

Instead of the backpropagation learning algorithm, the recommendation [86] is adaptable LSTM trained with two optimizing algorithms. Genetic algorithm and biogeography-based optimization are the optimization algorithms. Two distinct neural networks separate the system. The MLP is initially applied to two Data sets. The algorithms update the weights and biases for BBO and GA optimization. Second, the consequences are updated with the same optimization algorithms, and LSTM is applied to the same data sets. The first data set is the Wisconsin Breast Cancer datasets from the UCI Machine Learning Repository. There are 32 attributes contained within the dataset. These qualities are ID, diagnosis, and a feature with 30 real-valued inputs. The dataset can be retrieved from the UCI Web Portal and downloaded from the UCI repository at the University of California, Irvine. Second, various methods, including testing and interviews, were used to collect the diabetes dataset for DM patients at the local clinic. For DM patients, 26 variables have been collected.

2.4. DRAWBACKS

Early demonstrative anticipation of SARS-CoV-2 can assist with decreasing the weight on the medical care framework and help with saving lives by foreseeing Coronavirus before the condition turns out to be very extreme. To predict the occurrence of COVID-19 infection, ML was utilized to analyze demographic and epidemiological parameters. Compared to radiographic and molecular tests, these results are readily available in shorter intervals and at a lower cost. Data imbalance persists in a lot of medical AI research. In every case, there are more healthy patients than infected ones. If an ML model cannot adapt to novel situations, it will struggle to perform well. Prepared models in directed learning could better distinguish significant changes in setting or information, which prompts wrong forecasts in light of out-of-scope information. At a point when the ML technique is mistakenly applied to a startling patient circumstance, it could cause a uniqueness between the learning and practical knowledge.

2.5. FUTURE DIRECTIONS

Although machine learning studies were conducted to combat COVID-19, there is potential for producing more effective outcomes. Due to the spread of COVID-19 and its impact on humanity, patients' data must be accessible to the general public. Researchers could analyze these data this way and produce valuable outcomes for the healthcare industry. Many investigations utilize basic characterization calculations with negligible endeavors to exploit later analyses. These results open the entryway for future exploration and urge researchers to chip away at further developed strategies, like growing new calculations or working on the existing ones. As a result, the application of machine learning algorithms is further hampered by the need for patient clinical features.

CONCLUSION

The Internet of Things (IoT) is a new information technology paradigm that aims to connect various physical and virtual "things" with the expanding mobile and sensor industries to create a dynamic global network infrastructure. The term "Internet of Things" (IoT) was first proposed to refer to radio-frequency identification (RFID)-enabled uniquely identifiable objects (things) and their virtual representations in an internet-like structure. Later on, it expanded the Internet of Things (IoT) concept to include a broader range of "things" with a variety of sensors, including mobile devices, global positioning system (GPS) devices, and actuators. System architecture, data processing, and applications are just a few of the areas in which these sensors' seamless integration and effective utilization in an Internet-connected platform have sparked numerous research questions. Although current artificial intelligence (AI) models are astonishingly accurate, accuracy is only one of the crucial aspects. A thorough comprehension of the model and its outputs is also essential for sensitive domains.

REFERENCES

[1]   A. Jaiswal, A.R. Babu, M.Z. Zadeh, D. Banerjee, and F. Makedon, "A Survey on Contrastive Self-Supervised Learning", *Technologies (Basel), vol.* 9, no. 1, p. 2, 2020.
        [http://dx.doi.org/10.3390/technologies9010002]

[2]   P. Cunningham, M. Cord, and S.J. Delany, Supervised learning. *Machine learning techniques for multimedia.* Springer: Berlin, Heidelberg, 2008, pp. 21-49.
        [http://dx.doi.org/10.1007/978-3-540-75171-7_2]

[3]   Z.A. Khan, M. Adil, N. Javaid, M.N. Saqib, M. Shafiq, and J.G. Choi, "Electricity theft detection using supervised learning techniques on smart meter data", *Sustainability.,* vol. 12, no. 19, p. 8023, 2020.
        [http://dx.doi.org/10.3390/su12198023]

[4]   A. Ismail, S. Abdlerazek, and I.M. El-Henawy, "Development of smart healthcare system based on speech recognition using support vector machine and dynamic time warping", *Sustainability,* vol. 12, no. 6, p. 2403, 2020.
        [http://dx.doi.org/10.3390/su12062403]

[5]   A. Amiri, M. Abtahi, N. Constant, and K. Mankodiya, "Mobile phonocardiogram diagnosis in newborns using support vector machine", *Healthcare,* vol. 5, no. 1, p. 16, 2017.
        [http://dx.doi.org/10.3390/healthcare5010016] [PMID: 28335471]

[6]   E. Barreiro, C.R. Munteanu, M. Gestal, J.R. Rabuñal, A. Pazos, H. González-Díaz, and J. Dorado, "Net-net automl selection of artificial neural network topology for brain connectome prediction", *Appl. Sci.,* vol. 10, no. 4, p. 1308, 2020.
        [http://dx.doi.org/10.3390/app10041308]

[7]   Z. Zhang, Artificial neural network. *Multivariate time series analysis in climate and environmental research.* Springer: Cham, 2018, pp. 1-35.
        [http://dx.doi.org/10.1007/978-3-319-67340-0_1]

[8]   A. Ali, M.A. Almaiah, F. Hajjej, M.F. Pasha, O.H. Fang, R. Khan, J. Teo, and M. Zakarya, "An industrial iot-based blockchain-enabled secure searchable encryption approach for healthcare systems using neural network", *Sensors,* vol. 22, no. 2, p. 572, 2022.
        [http://dx.doi.org/10.3390/s22020572] [PMID: 35062530]

[9]   F.J. Díaz-Pernas, M. Martínez-Zarzuela, M. Antón-Rodríguez, and D. González-Ortega, "A deep learning approach for brain tumor classification and segmentation using a multiscale convolutional neural network", *Healthcare,* vol. 9, no. 2, p. 153, 2021.
        [http://dx.doi.org/10.3390/healthcare9020153] [PMID: 33540873]

[10]   V. Raghupathi, and W. Raghupathi, "Preventive healthcare: A neural network analysis of behavioral habits and chronic diseases", *Healthcare,* vol. 5, no. 1, p. 8, 2017.
        [http://dx.doi.org/10.3390/healthcare5010008] [PMID: 28178194]

[11]   E. Batbaatar, and K.H. Ryu, "Ontology-based healthcare named entity recognition from twitter messages using a recurrent neural network approach", *Int. J. Environ. Res. Public Health,* vol. 16, no. 19, p. 3628, 2019.
        [http://dx.doi.org/10.3390/ijerph16193628] [PMID: 31569654]

[12]   S. Chen, G.I. Webb, L. Liu, and X. Ma, "A novel selective Naive bayes algorithm", *Knowl. Base. Syst.,* vol. 192, p. 105361, 2020.
        [http://dx.doi.org/10.1016/j.knosys.2019.105361]

[13]   K. Vembandasamy, R. Sasipriya, and E. Deepa, "Heart diseases detection using naive bayes algorithm", *Int. j. innov. sci. eng. technol,* vol. 2, no. 9, pp. 441-444, 2015.

[14]   M. Alwateer, A.M. Almars, K.N. Areed, M.A. Elhosseini, A.Y. Haikal, and M. Badawy, "Ambient healthcare approach with hybrid whale optimization algorithm and Naive bayes classifier", *Sensors,* vol. 21, no. 13, p. 4579, 2021.

[http://dx.doi.org/10.3390/s21134579] [PMID: 34283139]

[15]   B.A. Thakkar, M.I. Hasan, and M.A. Desai, "Health care decision support system for swine flu prediction using Naive bayes classifier", *International Conference on Advances in Recent Technologies in Communication and Computing.* Kottayam, India, 2010.
[http://dx.doi.org/10.1109/ARTCom.2010.98]

[16]   K. Srinivas, B.K. Rani, and A. Govrdhan, "Applications of data mining techniques in healthcare and prediction of heart attacks", *Int. J. Comput. Sci. Eng.,* vol. 2, no. 2, pp. 250-255, 2010.

[17]   K.R. Pradeep, and N.C. Naveen, "Lung cancer survivability prediction based on performance using classification techniques of support vector machines, C4. 5 and Naive Bayes algorithms for healthcare analytics", *International Conference on Computational Intelligence and Data Science.* Coimbatore, Tamil Nadu, 2018.

[18]   Z.T. Fernando, P. Trivedi, and A. Patni, "DOCAID: Predictive healthcare analytics using naive bayes classification", *in Second student research symposium (SRS), international conference on advances in computing, communications and informatics (ICACCI'13).* Mysore, India, 2013.

[19]   E. Miranda, E. Irwansyah, A.Y. Amelga, M.M. Maribondang, and M. Salim, "Detection of cardiovascular disease risk's level for adults using naive bayes classifier", *Healthc. Inform. Res.,* vol. 22, no. 3, pp. 196-205, 2016.
[http://dx.doi.org/10.4258/hir.2016.22.3.196] [PMID: 27525161]

[20]   G.F. Fan, Y.H. Guo, J.M. Zheng, and W.C. Hong, "Application of the weighted k-nearest neighbor algorithm for short-term load forecasting", *Energies,* vol. 12, no. 5, p. 916, 2019.
[http://dx.doi.org/10.3390/en12050916]

[21]   R.U. Haque, A.S.M.T. Hasan, Q. Jiang, and Q. Qu, "Privacy-preserving k-nearest neighbors training over blockchain-based encrypted health data", *Electronics,* vol. 9, no. 12, p. 2096, 2020.
[http://dx.doi.org/10.3390/electronics9122096]

[22]   N. Khateeb, and M. Usman, "Efficient heart disease prediction system using K-nearest neighbor classification technique", *in BDIOT2017: International Conference on Big Data and Internet of Thing.* London United Kingdom, 2017.
[http://dx.doi.org/10.1145/3175684.3175703]

[23]   M. Li, H. Xu, X. Liu, and S. Lu, "Emotion recognition from multichannel EEG signals using K-nearest neighbor classification", *Technol. Health Care,* vol. 26, no. S1, pp. 509-519, 2018.
[http://dx.doi.org/10.3233/THC-174836] [PMID: 29758974]

[24]   S. Tayeb, M. Pirouz, J. Sun, K. Hall, A. Chang, J. Li, C. Song, A. Chauhan, M. Ferra, T. Sager, and J. Zhan, "Toward predicting medical conditions using k-nearest neighbors", *in IEEE International Conference on Big Data.* Boston, MA, USA, 2017.
[http://dx.doi.org/10.1109/BigData.2017.8258395]

[25]   J. Park, and D.H. Lee, "Privacy preserving k-nearest neighbor for medical diagnosis in e-health cloud", *J. Healthc. Eng.,* vol. 2018, pp. 1-11, 2018.
[http://dx.doi.org/10.1155/2018/4073103] [PMID: 30410714]

[26]   B.L. Deekshatulu, and P. Chandra, "Classification of heart disease using k-nearest neighbor and genetic algorithm", *Procedia Technol.,* vol. 10, pp. 85-94, 2013.
[http://dx.doi.org/10.1016/j.protcy.2013.12.340]

[27]   M. Shouman, T. Turner, and R. Stocker, "Applying k-nearest neighbour in diagnosing heart disease patients", *Int. J. Inf. Educ. Technol.,* vol. 2, no. 3, pp. 220-223, 2012.
[http://dx.doi.org/10.7763/IJIET.2012.V2.114]

[28]   I.H. Sarker, M.F. Faruque, H. Alqahtani, and A. Kalim, "K-nearest neighbor learning based diabetes mellitus prediction and analysis for eHealth services", *EAI Endorsed Transactions on Scalable Information Systems,* vol. 7, no. 26, pp. e4-e4, 2020.
[http://dx.doi.org/10.4108/eai.13-7-2018.162737]

[29]   G.M. Marakas, United States. *Decision support systems in the 21st century* vol. 134. Prentice Hall: Upper Saddle River, 2003.

[30]   M.W. Nadeem, H.G. Goh, V. Ponnusamy, I. Andonovic, M.A. Khan, and M. Hussain, "A fusion-based machine learning approach for the prediction of the onset of diabetes", *Healthcare.*, vol. 9, no. 10, p. 1393, 2021.
[http://dx.doi.org/10.3390/healthcare9101393] [PMID: 34683073]

[31]   V. Kumar, B.K. Mishra, M. Mazzara, D.N. Thanh, and A. Verma, Prediction of malignant and benign breast cancer: A data mining approach in healthcare applications. *Advances in data science and management.* vol. 37. Springer: Singapore, 2020, pp. 435-442.
[http://dx.doi.org/10.1007/978-981-15-0978-0_43]

[32]   E.S. Berner, Clinical decision support systems. *Science+ Business Media* vol. 233. Springer: New York, 2007.

[33]   Robert Greenes, *Clinical decision support: the road ahead* Elsevier: Amsterdam, Netherlands, 2011.

[34]   M.A. Hafeez, M. Rashid, H. Tariq, Z.U. Abideen, S.S. Alotaibi, and M.H. Sinky, "Performance improvement of decision tree: A robust classifier using tabu search algorithm", *Appl. Sci.*, vol. 11, no. 15, p. 6728, 2021.
[http://dx.doi.org/10.3390/app11156728]

[35]   F. SoleimanianGharehchopogh, P. Mohammadi, and P. Hakimi, "Application of decision tree algorithm for data mining in healthcare operations: A case study", *Int. J. Comput. Appl.*, vol. 52, no. 6, pp. 21-26, 2012.
[http://dx.doi.org/10.5120/8206-1613]

[36]   M.U. Khan, J.P. Choi, H. Shin, and M. Kim, "Predicting breast cancer survivability using fuzzy decision trees for personalized healthcare", *Annu. Int. Conf. IEEE Eng. Med. Biol. Soc.*, pp. 5148-5151, 2008.
[http://dx.doi.org/10.1109/IEMBS.2008.4650373] [PMID: 19163876]

[37]   A. Velichko, "A method for medical data analysis using the lognnet for clinical decision support systems and edge computing in healthcare", *Sensors.*, vol. 21, no. 18, p. 6209, 2021.
[http://dx.doi.org/10.3390/s21186209] [PMID: 34577414]

[38]   L. Wang, H. Shi, and L. Gan, "Healthcare facility location-allocation optimization for china's developing cities utilizing a multi-objective decision support approach", *Sustainability.*, vol. 10, no. 12, p. 4580, 2018.
[http://dx.doi.org/10.3390/su10124580]

[39]   C.H. van der Wouden, P.C.D. Bank, K. Özokcu, J.J. Swen, and H.J. Guchelaar, "Pharmacist-initiated pre-emptive pharmacogenetic panel testing with clinical decision support in primary care: record of pgx results and real-world impact", *Genes.*, vol. 10, no. 6, p. 416, 2019.
[http://dx.doi.org/10.3390/genes10060416] [PMID: 31146504]

[40]   F. López-Martínez, E.R. Núñez-Valdez, V. García-Díaz, and Z. Bursac, "A case study for a big data and machine learning platform to improve medical decision support in population health management", *Algorithms,* vol. 13, no. 4, p. 102, 2020.
[http://dx.doi.org/10.3390/a13040102]

[41]   S.S.R. Abidi, "Knowledge management in healthcare: Towards 'knowledge-driven' decision-support services", *Int. J. Med. Inform.*, vol. 63, no. 1-2, pp. 5-18, 2001.
[http://dx.doi.org/10.1016/S1386-5056(01)00167-8] [PMID: 11518661]

[42]   A.J. Aljaaf, D. Al-Jumeily, A.J. Hussain, P. Fergus, M. Al-Jumaily, and K. Abdel-Aziz, "Toward an optimal use of artificial intelligence techniques within a clinical decision support system", *in Science and Information Conference (SAI).* London, UK, 2015.
[http://dx.doi.org/10.1109/SAI.2015.7237196]

[43]   C.C. Bennett, T.W. Doub, and R. Selove, "EHRs connect research and practice: Where predictive

modeling, artificial intelligence, and clinical decision support intersect", *Health Policy Technol.,* vol. 1, no. 2, pp. 105-114, 2012.
[http://dx.doi.org/10.1016/j.hlpt.2012.03.001]

[44]   E. Zihni, V.I. Madai, M. Livne, I. Galinovic, A.A. Khalil, J.B. Fiebach, and D. Frey, "Opening the black box of artificial intelligence for clinical decision support: A study predicting stroke outcome", *PLoS One,* vol. 15, no. 4, p. e0231166, 2020.
[http://dx.doi.org/10.1371/journal.pone.0231166] [PMID: 32251471]

[45]   C. Petitgand, A. Motulsky, J.L. Denis, and C. Régis, "Investigating the barriers to physician adoption of an artificial intelligence-based decision support system in emergency care: An interpretative qualitative study", *Stud. Health Technol. Inform.,* vol. 270, pp. 1001-1005, 2020.
[http://dx.doi.org/10.3233/SHTI200312] [PMID: 32570532]

[46]   B. Saravi, F. Hassel, S. Ülkümen, A. Zink, V. Shavlokhova, S. Couillard-Despres, M. Boeker, P. Obid, and G. Lang, "Artificial intelligence-driven prediction modeling and decision making in spine surgery using hybrid machine learning models", *J. Pers. Med.,* vol. 12, no. 4, p. 509, 2022.
[http://dx.doi.org/10.3390/jpm12040509] [PMID: 35455625]

[47]   K. Gibert, C. García-Alonso, and L. Salvador-Carulla, "Integrating clinicians, knowledge and data: Expert-based cooperative analysis in healthcare decision support", *Health Res. Policy Syst.,* vol. 8, no. 1, p. 28, 2010.
[http://dx.doi.org/10.1186/1478-4505-8-28] [PMID: 20920289]

[48]   P. Chatterjee, L.J. Cymberknop, and R.L. Armentano, "IoT-based decision support system for intelligent healthcare—applied to cardiovascular diseases", *in 7th International Conference on Communication Systems and Network Technologies (CSNT).* Nagpur, India, 2017.
[http://dx.doi.org/10.1109/CSNT.2017.8418567]

[49]   D. DeVault, R. Artstein, G. Benn, T. Dey, E. Fast, A. Gainer, K. Georgila, J. Gratch, A. Hartholt, M. Lhommet, and G. Lucas, "SimSensei kiosk: A virtual human interviewer for healthcare decision support", *in international conference on Autonomous agents and multi-agent systems.* 2014.

[50]   E. Aktaş, F. Ülengin, and Ş. Önsel Şahin, "A decision support system to improve the efficiency of resource allocation in healthcare management", *Socioecon. Plann. Sci.,* vol. 41, no. 2, pp. 130-146, 2007.
[http://dx.doi.org/10.1016/j.seps.2005.10.008]

[51]   S. Knapič, A. Malhi, R. Saluja, and K. Främling, "Explainable artificial intelligence for human decision support system in the medical domain", *Machine Learning and Knowledge Extraction,* vol. 3, no. 3, pp. 740-770, 2021.
[http://dx.doi.org/10.3390/make3030037]

[52]   I. Azhar, M. Sharif, M. Raza, M.A. Khan, and H.S. Yong, "A decision support system for face sketch synthesis using deep learning and artificial intelligence", *Sensors.,* vol. 21, no. 24, p. 8178, 2021.
[http://dx.doi.org/10.3390/s21248178] [PMID: 34960274]

[53]   A. Rghioui, J. Lloret, M. Harane, and A. Oumnad, "A smart glucose monitoring system for diabetic patient", *Electronics.,* vol. 9, no. 4, p. 678, 2020.
[http://dx.doi.org/10.3390/electronics9040678]

[54]   A. Rghioui, J. Lloret, and A. Oumnad, The Role of Artificial Intelligence in Diabetes Management. *Advanced Bioscience and Biosystems for Detection and Management of Diabetes.* Springer: Cham, 2022, pp. 243-257.
[http://dx.doi.org/10.1007/978-3-030-99728-1_12]

[55]   A. Rghioui, J. Lloret, L. Parra, S. Sendra, and A. Oumnad, "Glucose data classification for diabetic patient monitoring", *Appl. Sci.,* vol. 9, no. 20, p. 4459, 2019.
[http://dx.doi.org/10.3390/app9204459]

[56]   T.R. Baitharu, and S.K. Pani, "Analysis of data mining techniques for healthcare decision support system using liver disorder dataset", *Procedia Comput. Sci.,* vol. 85, pp. 862-870, 2016.

[http://dx.doi.org/10.1016/j.procs.2016.05.276]

[57] S. Weisberg, *Applied linear regression.* vol. Vol. 528. John Wiley & Sons, 2005.
      [http://dx.doi.org/10.1002/0471704091]

[58] F. Zhang, and D. Li, "Multiple linear regression-structural equation modeling based development of
      the integrated model of perceived neighborhood environment and quality of life of community-
      dwelling older adults: A cross-sectional study in nanjing China", *Int. J. Environ. Res. Public Health,*
      vol. 16, no. 24, p. 4933, 2019.
      [http://dx.doi.org/10.3390/ijerph16244933] [PMID: 31817493]

[59] E.M. Valsamis, D. Ricketts, H. Husband, and B.A. Rogers, "Segmented linear regression models for
      assessing change in retrospective studies in healthcare", *Comput. Math. Methods Med.,* vol. 2019, pp.
      1-9, 2019.
      [http://dx.doi.org/10.1155/2019/9810675] [PMID: 30805023]

[60] E.M. Valsamis, H. Husband, and G.K.W. Chan, "Segmented linear regression modelling of time-series
      of binary variables in healthcare", *Comput. Math. Methods Med.,* vol. 2019, pp. 1-7, 2019.
      [http://dx.doi.org/10.1155/2019/3478598] [PMID: 31885678]

[61] C. Song, Y. Wang, X. Yang, Y. Yang, Z. Tang, X. Wang, and J. Pan, "Spatial and temporal impacts of
      socioeconomic and environmental factors on healthcare resources: A county-level bayesian local
      spatiotemporal regression modeling study of hospital beds in southwest China", *Int. J. Environ. Res.
      Public Health,* vol. 17, no. 16, p. 5890, 2020.
      [http://dx.doi.org/10.3390/ijerph17165890] [PMID: 32823743]

[62] K. Kaushik, A. Bhardwaj, A.D. Dwivedi, and R. Singh, "Machine learning-based regression
      framework to predict health insurance premiums", *Int. J. Environ. Res. Public Health,* vol. 19, no. 13,
      p. 7898, 2022.
      [http://dx.doi.org/10.3390/ijerph19137898] [PMID: 35805557]

[63] Z. Ahmed, K. Mohamed, S. Zeeshan, and X. Dong, "Artificial intelligence with multi-functional
      machine learning platform development for better healthcare and precision medicine", *Database,* vol.
      2020, p. baaa010, 2020.
      [http://dx.doi.org/10.1093/database/baaa010] [PMID: 32185396]

[64] L. Breiman, "Random forests", *Mach. Learn.,* vol. 45, no. 1, pp. 5-32, 2001.
      [http://dx.doi.org/10.1023/A:1010933404324]

[65] M. Ijaz, G. Alfian, M. Syafrudin, and J. Rhee, "Hybrid prediction model for type 2 diabetes and
      hypertension using DBSCAN-Based outlier detection, synthetic minority over sampling technique
      (SMOTE), and random forest", *Appl. Sci.,* vol. 8, no. 8, p. 1325, 2018.
      [http://dx.doi.org/10.3390/app8081325]

[66] V. Maeda-Gutiérrez, C.E. Galván-Tejada, M. Cruz, A. Valladares-Salgado, J.I. Galván-Tejada, H.
      Gamboa-Rosales, A. García-Hernández, H. Luna-García, I. Gonzalez-Curiel, and M. Martínez-Acuña,
      "Distal symmetric polyneuropathy identification in type 2 diabetes subjects: A random forest
      approach", *Healthcare,* vol. 9, no. 2, p. 138, 2021.
      [http://dx.doi.org/10.3390/healthcare9020138] [PMID: 33535510]

[67] F. Wang, Y. Wang, X. Ji, and Z. Wang, "Effective macrosomia prediction using random forest
      algorithm", *Int. J. Environ. Res. Public Health,* vol. 19, no. 6, p. 3245, 2022.
      [http://dx.doi.org/10.3390/ijerph19063245] [PMID: 35328934]

[68] K. Fawagreh, and M.M. Gaber, "eGAP: An evolutionary game theoretic approach to random forest
      pruning", *Big Data Cogn. Comput.,* vol. 4, no. 4, p. 37, 2020.
      [http://dx.doi.org/10.3390/bdcc4040037]

[69] A.H. Sodhro, C. Sennersten, and A. Ahmad, "Towards cognitive authentication for smart healthcare
      applications", *Sensors,* vol. 22, no. 6, p. 2101, 2022.
      [http://dx.doi.org/10.3390/s22062101] [PMID: 35336276]

[70]   L. Wang, X. Wang, A. Chen, X. Jin, and H. Che, "Prediction of type 2 diabetes risk and its effect evaluation based on the XGBoost model", *Healthcare,* vol. 8, no. 3, p. 247, 2020.
[http://dx.doi.org/10.3390/healthcare8030247] [PMID: 32751894]

[71]   P. Kaur, R. Kumar, and M. Kumar, "A healthcare monitoring system using random forest and internet of things (IoT)", *Multimedia Tools Appl.,* vol. 78, no. 14, pp. 19905-19916, 2019.
[http://dx.doi.org/10.1007/s11042-019-7327-8]

[72]   M. Khalilia, S. Chakraborty, and M. Popescu, "Predicting disease risks from highly imbalanced data using random forest", *BMC Med. Inform. Decis. Mak.,* vol. 11, no. 1, p. 51, 2011.
[http://dx.doi.org/10.1186/1472-6947-11-51] [PMID: 21801360]

[73]   M. Javeed, A. Jalal, and K. Kim, "Wearable sensors based exertion recognition using statistical features and random forest for physical healthcare monitoring", *in International Bhurban Conference on Applied Sciences and Technologies (IBCAST).* Islamabad, Pakistan, 2021.
[http://dx.doi.org/10.1109/IBCAST51254.2021.9393014]

[74]   K. Fawagreh, and M.M. Gaber, "Resource-efficient fast prediction in healthcare data analytics: A pruned Random Forest regression approach", *Comput.,* vol. 102, no. 5, pp. 1187-1198, 2020.
[http://dx.doi.org/10.1007/s00607-019-00785-6]

[75]   J.H. Friedman, "Stochastic gradient boosting", *Comput. Stat. Data Anal.,* vol. 38, no. 4, pp. 367-378, 2002.
[http://dx.doi.org/10.1016/S0167-9473(01)00065-2]

[76]   A. Alcolea, and J. Resano, "FPGA accelerator for gradient boosting decision trees", *Electronics,* vol. 10, no. 3, p. 314, 2021.
[http://dx.doi.org/10.3390/electronics10030314]

[77]   J.O.R. Kim, Y.S. Jeong, J.H. Kim, J.W. Lee, D. Park, and H.S. Kim, "Machine learning-based cardiovascular disease prediction model: A cohort study on the korean national health insurance service health screening database", *Diagnostics,* vol. 11, no. 6, p. 943, 2021.
[http://dx.doi.org/10.3390/diagnostics11060943] [PMID: 34070504]

[78]   N.A. Akbar, A. Sunyoto, M.R. Arief, and W. Caesarendra, "Improvement of decision tree classifier accuracy for healthcare insurance fraud prediction by using extreme gradient boosting algorithm", *in International Conference on Informatics, Multimedia, Cyber and Information System (ICIMCIS).* Jakarta, Indonesia, 2020.
[http://dx.doi.org/10.1109/ICIMCIS51567.2020.9354286]

[79]   J.T. Hancock, and T.M. Khoshgoftaar, "Gradient boosted decision tree algorithms for medicare fraud detection", *SN comput. sci.,* vol. 2, no. 4, pp. 1-12, 2021.
[http://dx.doi.org/10.1007/s42979-021-00655-z]

[80]   L. Luo, J. Li, C. Liu, and W. Shen, "Using machine-learning methods to support health-care professionals in making admission decisions", *Int. J. Health Plann. Manage.,* vol. 34, no. 2, pp. e1236-e1246, 2019.
[http://dx.doi.org/10.1002/hpm.2769] [PMID: 30957270]

[81]   A.K. Mishra, P.K. Keserwani, S.G. Samaddar, H.B. Lamichaney, and A.K. Mishra, A decision support system in healthcare prediction. *Advanced Computational and Communication Paradigms.* vol. 475. Springer: Singapore, 2018, pp. 156-167.
[http://dx.doi.org/10.1007/978-981-10-8240-5_18]

[82]   L.B. Almeida, Backpropagation in perceptrons with feedback. *Neural computers.* vol. 41. Springer: Berlin, Heidelberg, 1989, pp. 199-208.
[http://dx.doi.org/10.1007/978-3-642-83740-1_22]

[83]   W. Li, L. Cui, Y. Zhang, Z. Cai, M. Zhang, W. Xu, X. Zhao, Y. Lei, X. Pan, J. Li, and Z. Dou, "Using a backpropagation artificial neural network to predict nutrient removal in tidal flow constructed wetlands", *Water,* vol. 10, no. 1, p. 83, 2018.

[http://dx.doi.org/10.3390/w10010083]

[84]   C.L. Krishna, and P.V.S. Reddy, "An efficient deep neural network multilayer perceptron based classifier in healthcare system", *in 3rd International Conference on Computing and Communications Technologies (ICCCT).* Chennai, India, 2019.
[http://dx.doi.org/10.1109/ICCCT2.2019.8824913]

[85]   M.Z. Amin, and A. Ali, "Application of multilayer perceptron (MLP) for data mining in healthcare operations", *3rd Conference on Biotechnology,* 2017.

[86]   T.A. Rashid, M.K. Hassan, M. Mohammadi, and K. Fraser, Improvement of variant adaptable LSTM trained with metaheuristic algorithms for healthcare analysis. *Advanced classification techniques for healthcare analysis* IGI Global: US, 2019, pp. 111-131.
[http://dx.doi.org/10.4018/978-1-5225-7796-6.ch006]

CHAPTER 3

Semi-Supervised Algorithms

Abstract: Semi-supervised learning, or SSL, falls somewhere between supervised and unsupervised learning. The algorithm is provided with some supervision data in addition to unlabeled data. There are two primary learning paradigms in it. Transductive education aims to use the trained classifier on unlabeled instances observed during training. This kind of algorithm is mainly used for node embedding on graphs, like random walks, where the goal is to label the graph's unlabeled nodes at the training time. Inductive learning aims to develop a classifier that can generalize unobserved situations during a test. This chapter details different semi-supervised algorithms in healthcare.

Keywords: Semi-supervised algorithms, Logistic regression, Unlabeled data, Linear regression.

3.1. INTRODUCTION

The subfield of machine learning, known as semi-supervised learning, uses both labeled and unlabeled data for specific learning tasks. In semi-administered learning research, an extra presumption frequently included is group suspicion. The information addresses similar classes. The primary objective of semi-supervised learning is to use unlabeled data to improve learning methods. The relative performance of various machine learning algorithms is influenced by numerous decisions when evaluating and comparing them. Additional factors play a role in semi-supervised learning. First, it must decide which to label data points and which should remain unlabeled in many benchmarking scenarios. Second, one can evaluate the learner's performance on a test set that is entirely disjointed or on the unlabeled data used for training, which is, by definition, the case in transductive learning. In addition, it is essential to establish high-quality supervised baselines to evaluate the unlabeled data's added value accurately. Fig. (**1**) portrays the same.

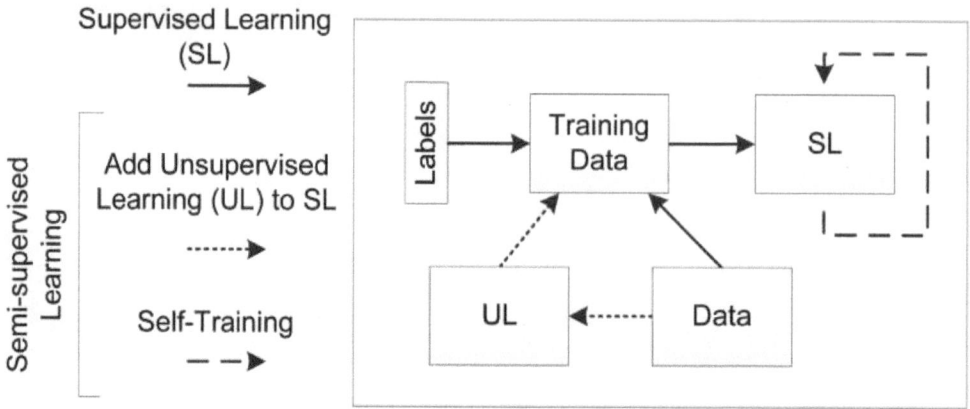

Fig. (1). Relation of semi-supervised learning (SSL) approaches to standard supervised learning [1].

3.2. SEMI-SUPERVISED ALGORITHMS IN HEALTHCARE

A type of Machine Learning (ML) technique is called semi-supervised learning (SSL). It is somewhere between administered and solo learning, *i.e.*, the dataset is somewhat named. It eliminates the disadvantages of supervised and unsupervised learning. Compared to unlabeled data, the labeled data should be shorter. The idea behind semi-supervised learning is that performance significantly shifts when labeled and unlabeled data are used together. The training set that is being used is more temporary. Usually, it is used to find outliers. Various information has materialized in medical care, including clinical information, sensor information, Omics information, *etc*. This kind of data requires multiple algorithms to be trained to make better predictions, and various mining techniques are used to find the most relevant features. Fig. (**2**) represents the Conceptual schematic for artificial intelligence in cardiovascular genetics.

The study [3] is a brand-new semi-supervised model for medical image classification. It uses an improved version of focal loss at the supervision loss to reduce sample misclassification. It incorporates a self-attention mechanism into the backbone network to learn more meaningful features for image classification tasks. It contains samples of intrinsic relationship characteristics. The mechanisms have student and teacher models. The model can spontaneously extract richer inherent information from representatives of unlabeled data and capture more crucial features of the current classification task. Finally, the improved focus loss is incorporated into the supervision loss, resulting in misjudged samples dominating the model's minimization goal and consequently improving the model's performance. For single-label classification, the ISIC 2018 dataset is utilized. It contains 10,015 examination images of seven common skin lesions labeled as instances. Fig. (**3**) represents the same.

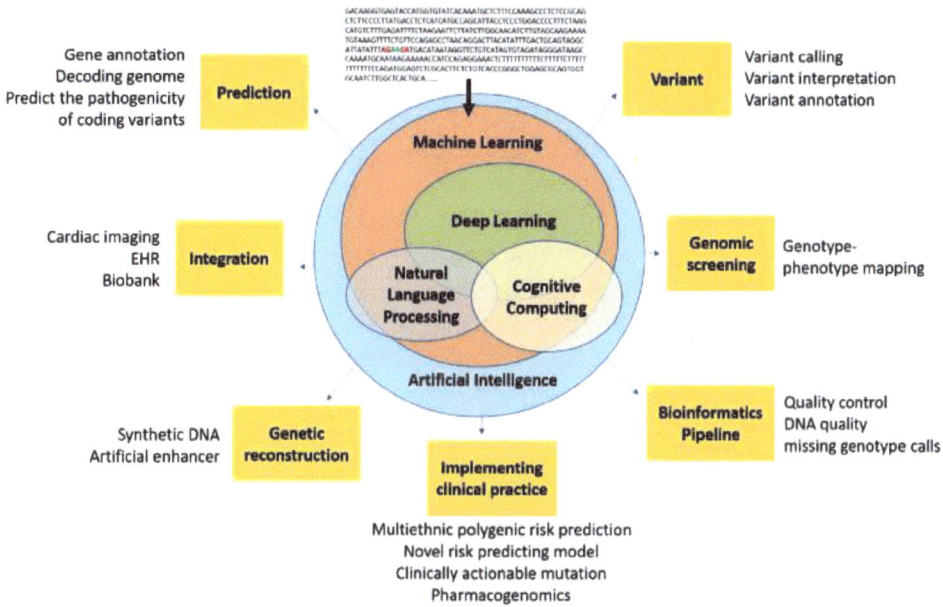

Fig. (2). Conceptual schematic for artificial intelligence in cardiovascular genetics [2].

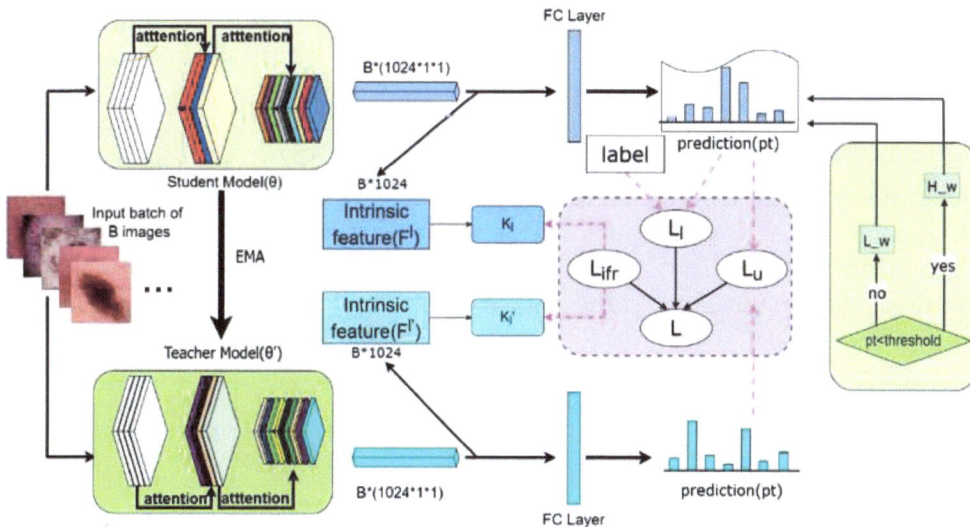

Fig. (3). Semi-supervised framework for medical image classification [3].

The work [4] first learns a kernel before integrating it with other kernel learners. The learned kernel enables semi-supervised learning. There are two primary phases. To learn a linear combination of a set of fundamental kernel functions, we propose a supervised multiple kernel learning algorithm as the initial step. A point cloud regularization term changes the learned kernel for the second step. In the second step, a point cloud norm is used to change the intellectual kernel function to force the contour to follow the distribution of all seen data samples. The KDD data mining cup provided two healthcare datasets for the study. The first is a clinical dataset for pulmonary embolism, and the second is a clinical dataset for breast cancer. A skilled chest radiologist reviewed each case and marked the PEs for Dataset 1 out of 69 collected. The subjects were arbitrarily partitioned into preparing and test sets. The remaining 23 issues are in the test set, while the training set has 38 positive and eight negative cases. The test group is isolated and will only be used to assess the final system's performance. For Dataset 2, a breast cancer screening typically includes four X-rays: two pictures of each breast taken from different angles. There are multiple candidates for each image. There is an image ID and a location for the patient ID for each candidate, many features, and a class label indicating whether or not it is malignant.

The MFSS-SVM calculation [5] uses the accelerometer signal's pinnacle energy and relationship coefficient. Laboratory tests on falling, walking, free jumping, rhythmic jumping, bag dropping, and ball dropping make the proposed algorithm effective. The SVM plays out the errand of twofold grouping by planning input vectors into a hyperplane. It is a high-layered space developed to isolate input vectors. The well-known generalization measure known as the Vapnik Chervonenkis dimension is maximized by this hyperplane if it exists. Experiments were carried out in the intelligent structural hazard mitigation laboratory at San Francisco State University to collect vibration signals from human falling and other everyday activities to test the proposed MFSS-SVM algorithm. The data acquisition system was a National Instrument cDAQ-9171 with 32-bit and 24-bit resolution NI 9234 input module. This study looked at six activities: falling, walking, free jumping, rhythmic jumping, bag dropping, and ball dropping. Two dummy human models weighing 70 kg and 48 kg were used for the falling experiments. Based on the direction of the falls, the falls were divided into forward and backward falls. There were a total of 260 basketball fall tests performed. Fig. (**4**) represents the same.

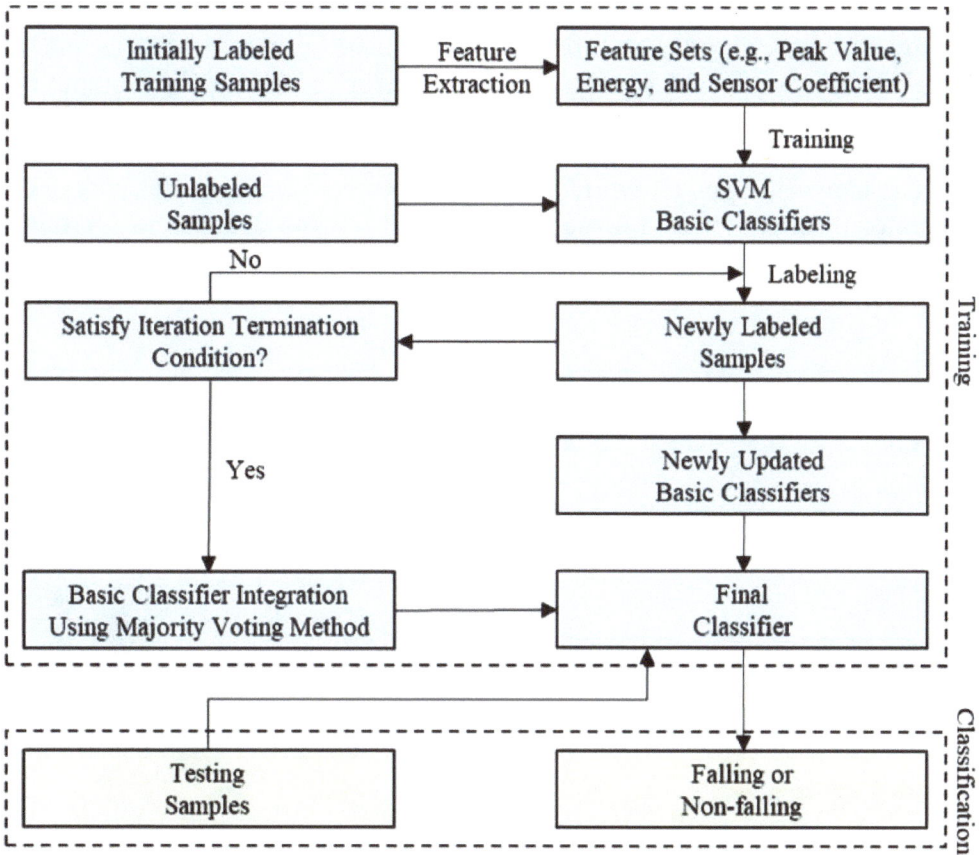

Fig. (4). Proposed Framework [5].

It is a semi-supervised generative adversarial network [6]. It serves as the foundation for the work's defecation pre-warning system and bowel sound acquisition system. The physiological signal acquisition system can gather bowel sounds, gastric electrical signals, and ECG signals. The 3M company's Littmann 3200 electronic stethoscope is the sensor for recording bowel sounds. It is a piezoelectric stethoscope with a 4 kHz sampling rate that can record electrical signals and convert sound energy. The generator and discriminator apply the zero-sum game theory. Random noise is fed into generator G while training the network to produce output that resembles accurate data or a picture. The discriminator's job returns the discriminant result to the generator. It differentiates the generated sample from the absolute example. The discriminant results are used to guide the training of the generator during the GAN training process. The generator's goal is to learn the distribution of accurate data and generate actual data or images so that the discriminator cannot determine whether the input is generated data or fundamental data. The discriminator's goal is constantly to improve the discriminant's ability. It distinguishes actual data from generated data. Random noise serves as the generator network's input, and the output is fake data with the same shape as the actual data after preprocessing. In contrast to the two-dimensional neural networks typically utilized in image processing, the internal network layer is a one-dimensional convolutional neural network. The generator receives random noise with a shape of 10,000 1, passing through the entire connection layer of 160,000 1. It gathered the data at the South China University of Technology and Beijing Bo'ai Hospital. Fig. (**5**) represents the same.

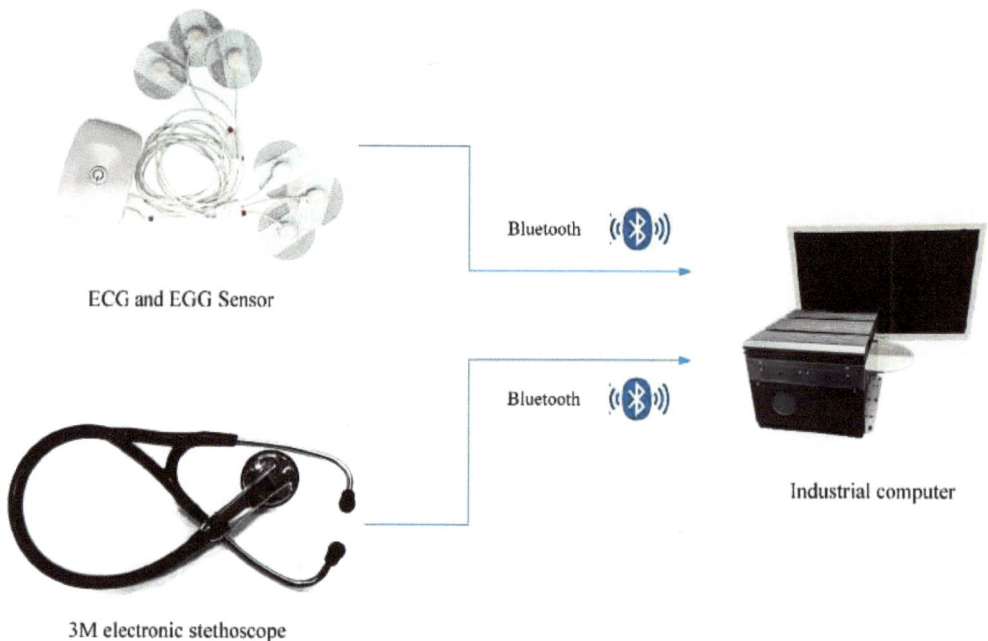

Fig. (5). Physiological signal Acquisition system [6].

Convolutional neural networks illustrate a novel semi-supervised classification model for EEG recognition [7]. It classifies motor imagery data after creating in-depth features using CNN models on motor imagery samples. A laplacian matrix is constructed using label data and added to the optimal reverse prediction model to obtain a cartesian k-means model that is more discriminative. It uses the in-depth CNN feature, which employs fully connected layers to combine all extracted convolutional features. It will receive an output 2D feature map from the across-time samples fed into EEG channels. The multilayer feature extraction and fusion phase follow the conclusion of the feature learning phase. The saw-cropped input EEG signal is taken in the first phase of this model, and Laplacian matrix construction is used to process these features. After max pooling, the elements used in the quantization process are taken from the convolution layers to keep the relevant information extracted by the convolutional layers complete while reducing the feature size. Consequently, the element maps are entirely removed from the Pool-1, Pool-2, Pool-3, and Pool-4 layers. Pooling layers represent convolutional layers at various levels of CNN architecture abstraction. The semi-supervised cartesian k-means model enhances the previous K-means performance and incorporates the sample's label information into the quantization step using the optimal reverse prediction model as the quantization distortion function. The work quantifies the data into 8 bits, resulting in 256 clusters; however, the actual label count typically does not equal 256. It has 12 cores and 64 GB of RAM and runs on Intel Xeon E5-2680 2.40 GHz CPUs.

A convolutional neural network and variational auto-encoder were combined to create the proposed framework [8]. CNN aims to extract discriminative features and generate low-dimension latent codes, variational auto-encoder. It seeks to remove the relevant characteristics of human activity data and provide valuable criteria for compressed sensing reconstruction. The architecture uses compressed samples from the latent vector in a deconvolutional decoder to reconstruct the input time series. For intelligent health systems, it trains the classifier to recognize human actions. It uses the Actitracker dataset, which includes six daily activities—walking, jogging, standing, sitting, and going up and down stairs. This dataset was gathered from 36 users in a controlled laboratory setting. These user's cell phones are used to collect the dataset, which consists of 29,000 frames at a 20Hz sampling rate.

The ART system [9] examines a few explicit launches and approves them on benchmark and genuine medical services information. Framework learns a projection direction by solving an optimization problem to partition the data at each node of the indexing tree. The tradeoff between these two terms is also adaptive because the unsupervised term will receive more weight in a more balanced partitioning if there is more unlabeled data in a single node. For approximate nearest neighbor search, it employs clever indexing methods rather than the tree's uniform distance measure for all patients in the indexing tree. The work creates a more precise indexing tree for retrieving similar patients. It meets two UCI standards: *e.g.*, diabetes and breast cancer datasets. 569 data vectors with a dimensionality of 30 are included in the Breast Cancer data set. A digital image of a breast mass taken by fine needle aspiration is used to calculate each data vector. These features describe the characteristics of the image's cell nuclei. All of the samples will be classified as benign or malignant. The Pima Indians Diabetes dataset contains 768 patients who are females no less than 21 years of age of Pima

Indian heritage.3 Every patient is addressed by an eight-layered vector. In the end, each patient will be categorized as diabetic or not.

A semisupervised privacy-preserving clustering algorithm [10] is proposed in this work. With only a small amount of labeled data, the training data provider would first use the supervised information to train the LMNC metric. Then it would use the learned metric to add multiplicative perturbation to the raw data to protect privacy and improve clustering accuracy. The perturbed data would then be uploaded to the cloud miner by the training data provider for clustering analysis and knowledge discovery. However, other horizontally distributed data providers could benefit from the LMNC metric regarding privacy protection and clustering accuracy if the training data provider shared the LMNC metric with the cloud miner. The work used the HDFT dataset gathered by the PBC in 2009 as the standard dataset. The HDFT dataset contains approximately 300,000 fiber streamlines for each brain scan performed twice on three individuals using a cutting-edge MRI-based diffusion imaging method. It used a desktop PC with an Intel® CoreTM i7-4770 CPU, and the benchmark dataset was downloaded from the 2009 PBC site using the Matlab programming language.

The proposed structure [11] broadens Reptile, a model freethinker meta-learning calculation, to a unified setting. There are two parts of it. The server's initialization of the shared global model and client selection for training are the server's responsibilities. After each activity round, the server sends the most recent parameters of the shared global model to the chosen clients. Each client computes the international model's parameter updates and local training. These parameter updates are sent to a server, where they are compiled and used in the shared global model. There is a labeled and an unlabelled dataset in client processing. The client receives the global model from the server during a training round. Separately, the proposed framework is trained for phenotype classification, mortality prediction, and decompensation prediction. In the second scenario, NGL-FedRep is taught to predict mortality and decompensation and simultaneously classify phenotypes. The performance of the task-specific centralized neural networks is contrasted with that of each task. The datasets examined in this study are all labeled in the third scenario.

The ability of a semi-supervised learning-based adaptive neuro-fuzzy inference system (ANFIS) [12] to classify lousy debt in the healthcare industry is the subject of this investigation. The dataset contains 6117 cases with an extraordinary total of $2,381,453. It used different membership functions in computer simulation for ANFIS. Unique and preliminary insights into the interactions between the input variables and the probability of default or recovery were provided by interpreting the ANFIS-generated control surfaces.

A semi-supervised adaptive HAR system [13] combines offline and online recognition methods to provide intelligent real-time support for frequently performed user activities to resolve these issues. Instead of video data or wearables, the system uses passive and ambient sensors embedded throughout the house. The system's short-term memory stores and analyzes sensor data. Offline HAR and online HAR are the two parts of the HAR system. There are three steps in each of these parts. The offline HAR system's goal is to find activity clusters in unlabeled user data at the end of each day and compare them to activity clusters from the previous days to find repeated activities. It creates a model of each identified repetitive activity. This model can perform online or real-time HAR for automated assistance or prompts and updates the activity model based on user actions. These steps are repeated daily to create and update the activity models database. Old routines and activities are removed from the database because of the deletion of any data more older than the specified amount of system memory. For seven months, the Aruba CASAS study installed multiple motion sensors in each room of an older female participant's home, providing labeled activity data. From this dataset, four week's worth of kitchen data—two from each of two distinct months—were selected randomly and divided into two weeks for offline HAR training, development, and testing. The kitchen data was chosen so that it could be complemented by additional complementary data from the Bristol Robotics Laboratory's Assisted Living Studio (ALSt) kitchen. The ALSt was equipped with Fibaro FGMS-001 motion sensors, Everspring SM810 magnetic contact sensors for cabinets, and TKB TZ69E wall plugs as part of an open HAB-based Z-wave sensor network. On various days, a total of six activity sessions were recorded by four participants. All processing of the data was done in Matlab.

The study's hybrid model [14] uses the mechanistic model's underlying biological knowledge and imaging data from unbiopsied brain regions to predict brain tumor density spatially. Following institutional review board protocol, patients with clinically suspected GBM were recruited and subjected to preoperative stereotactic MRI before any treatment. The Declaration of Helsinki obtained approval from the Mayo Clinic in Arizona and Barrow Neurological Institute institutional review boards. Before being enrolled, each patient gave written and informed consent. Each of the 18 GBM patients had between two and fourteen biopsy samples, totaling 82.

The obtained pseudo-labeled samples are used as the training samples for the best accuracy, which is the convergence condition in the study [15]. A base model is trained to label unlabeled samples using labeled samples. In gene selection, combined marked and pseudo-labeled representatives may perform better. Three public cancer datasets from the U.S. National Library of Medicine's National Center for Biotechnology Information are used in this study. The Boston

University Medical Center is the source of the lung cancer dataset, GSE4115. There are 97 lung cancer samples and 90 healthy samples, and each instance contains 22,215 genes. The French Institut Bergonie's breast cancer dataset (GSE21050) includes 310 samples, 54,677 genes as the model input, from 183 lung cancer and 127 standard lung samples. The MIT Whitehead Institute is the source of the prostate cancer dataset. The prostate dataset contains 12,600 genes in two classes—tumor and expected—that account for 52 and 50 samples, respectively, after preprocessing. A portion of the three disease datasets is used in the experiments as unlabeled samples to test the proposed method's classification accuracy. The labeled and unlabeled samples are randomly chosen in each program run. The methodology of the tests includes 10-fold cross-validation to evaluate the learning of the techniques. It tracks the variation in their performance.

Event detection models are trained using noisy guesses of the event's ending times in the study [16]. It uses a mathematical model to explain and estimate the evolution of classification performance for increasingly noisy end-time estimates. The training set may contain samples that have been mislabeled, depending on how conservative these guesses are. It uses the Berkeley MHAD and HMBD51 video datasets and adapts sequential CIFAR-10 and MNIST versions. It makes use of CIFAR-10 images in a toy dataset. The training set's images are evenly divided into training, and validation sets, with the testing images, kept separate. A compact ResNet serves as the model for the architecture. The initial two convolutional layers have 32 channels each, and the last two have 64 channels each. ReLU activations follow the zero-padded convolutions.

The approach [17] looks into ways to automatically improve activity classifiers once implemented in an application. To determine which of three semi-supervised learning strategies—self-learning, En-Co-Training, and democratic co-learning—show promise for this purpose, it compares active learning. Walking, running, and staying in one place were all options. These exercises were available to all members since they required no particular hardware. The elements utilized for arrangement were GPS speed, and speed increase determined one time. The subjects used an HTC Android Dev Phone 1 to collect data for the classifier. The application on the phone allowed to keep track of how much time they had spent doing each activity. For the base classifiers, 17 participants first collected labeled training data. The initial classifier can be more robust thanks to the diverse training data provided by this relatively large group size. After that, 15 additional subjects collected data for the tests to use as unlabeled data, though it labeled the data to check the accuracy of the results. Each participant received 90 minutes of data or 30 minutes of each activity. The algorithms used Weka's implementation of machine learning algorithms.

3.2.1. Linear Regression

Predicting a variable's value from the value of another variable is done with linear regression analysis. The dependent variable is the one you want to predict. The independent variable is the one you use to indicate the value of the other variable. One or more independent variables that best predict the value of the dependent variable are used in this type of analysis to estimate the coefficients of the linear equation. Linear regression produces a surface or straight line with the lowest possible difference between predicted and actual output values. For a set of paired data, straightforward linear regression calculators employ the "least squares" method to determine the best-fit line. Fig. (**6**) is the Flow chart of the Regression process.

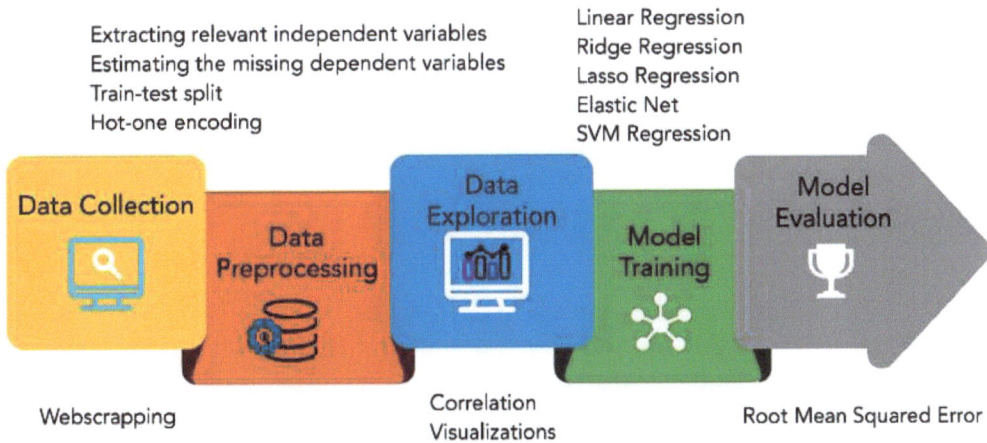

Fig. (6). Flow chart of Regression process [18].

The work [19] presents a novel modeling approach that employs least squares regression to fit time series with progressively more complex linear sections. The method compares the goodness of fit between the periods before and after implementation Using F-tests. It overcomes limitations and analyzes temporal variation, and a rigorous mathematical approach is being developed. The subjects were two thousand seven hundred seventy-seven patients with proximal femoral fragility fractures. It could accurately describe the time serie's temporal evolution using the proposed approach and strengthened the conclusions it could draw from merely comparing groups.

A novel stability selection method [20] is recommended. The technique applies GA iteratively to a subset of records and features Using GA-based feature selection. Each GA individual is a binary vector containing selected features in the subsample. Cross-validation of the subsamples is used to train and evaluate GA-selected features. It is in an unregularized logistic linear regression model. During a GA run, fitness is evaluated using the area under the curve and optimized. AUC is assessed with an unregularized strategic relapse model on different subsampled medical services records, gathered under the Medical care Cost and Usage Task, using the Public (Cross country) Long term Test data set. The reported results enhance these AUC results by averaging feature importance from the top four SS and the SS using GA.

This study [21] investigated the factors influencing consulting costs in online healthcare services. The prices of online health care consulting, economic factors and online and offline reputation are all considered in an integrated multilevel model. According to the empirical findings, doctors will charge more for consulting services if they hold higher clinic titles, work in higher-level hospitals, have better online reputations, or have made more sales. The wage level determines the doctor's opportunity cost in the city where they work, which also influences consulting fees. The study first used descriptive statistics to examine the factors that influence consulting prices using a large sample of 16,008 Chinese doctors. It used web crawler technology to look at the profiles of over 423,000 doctors on the Haodf website.

In a community-based sample, this study [22] found a correlation between subjective complaints of daytime sleepiness, insufficient sleep, and insomnia, objective measures of the severity of SDB, and an indirect measure of healthcare utilization. A multicenter investigation of the cardiovascular effects of SDB recruited participants from various ethnic group cohort studies of cardiovascular or respiratory disease. Participants in the parent cohorts who met the inclusion criteria were invited to participate in the SHS's initial examination. The study's logistics and the participant's characteristics influenced each location's selection and recruitment processes. To maximize statistical power by increasing the prevalence of SDB among younger participants, people who had a history of snoring were oversampled from people younger than 65. Between December 1995 and February 1998, 6,440 of the 11,053 participants in the parent cohorts that were found to be potentially eligible underwent a successful unattended baseline PSG. SPSS was used for the analyses. It finds out how CDS is related to each variable using linear regressions.

A non-constant variance linear regression model [23] is suggested. The controlled preliminary of the PC-created DUR was directed in the essential consideration arrangement of Indiana College Clinical Group–Primary Care, which contains a few ghettoes rehearses that serve an overwhelmingly destitute populace in Indianapolis, Indiana, USA. Wishard Memorial Hospital, a public teaching hospital with 300 beds, is affiliated with IU Medical Group Primary Care. The computer-based DUR randomized control trial displayed guideline-based treatment recommendations to enrolled patient's primary care physicians and pharmacists working in Wishard's outpatient pharmacy, where more than 90% of study patients obtained their prescriptions. The clinical trial used a two-power, two-factorial design in which patients were randomly assigned to one of four groups. The usual care was one group, and primary care physicians and pharmacists did not see the computer-generated treatment recommendations when they saw their patients. The physician-targeted DUR was the second type of DUR. This type only showed the treatment recommendations for the enrolled patients to the primary care physicians as they wrote prescriptions on microcomputer workstations. A third group was the pharmacist-targeted DUR, in which only pharmacists could see the treatment recommendations for enrolled patients while filling outpatient prescriptions. It gave the treatment recommendations to the enrolled patient's primary care physicians and pharmacists in the fourth group. The work examined whether there was a statistically significant difference in patient's total healthcare costs between the DUR study's control and intervention groups.

The work [24] applies regression techniques suitable for healthcare cost analysis of an experimental cardiovascular treatment and an observational diabetes hospital care setting. The degree to which the underlying assumptions of each method and the particular characteristics of the healthcare issue are compatible determines whether or not the methods yield distinct outcomes. It must take care when comparing healthcare cost models to a study's analytical goals and data characteristics.

Anomaly detection in medical wireless body area networks for the ubiquitous patient and healthcare monitoring is described in detail, as is the preliminary testing of the proposed framework [25]. Modern sensor fusion techniques are combined with advanced data mining and machine learning algorithms in the architecture. It recognizes unusual qualities to diminish phony problems that came about because of broken estimations while separating deficiencies from patient well-being corruption. Linear regression and the decision tree are the foundations of the proposed method. It creates a decision tree and searches typical vital signs for linear coefficients within a limited interval range of the monitored attributes. There are two phases to the proposed strategy: detecting and training classification models for SVM and linear regression methods are built during the training phase, and abnormal inputs are labeled deviant during the testing phase if they depart from the established model. The SVM then uses the attribute data of each instance in the test set to classify them using this model. Maximizing the distance between two parallel boundaries, or hyperplanes, defined by support vectors is the central idea behind linear SVMs. SVM searches for the greatest edge hyperplane, which isolates the preparation information into two classes. The margin errors are used to prevent problems with overfitting. They are favorable for points on the wrong side of the classifier inside or outside the margin and 0 for issues on the right side of the classifier. Data is collected using wireless motes with limited resources; a portable collection device with more resources and better transmission capabilities than motes is used to analyze the data and alert the emergency team of abnormal patterns.

The economic burden of RTIs and their impact on population health are highlighted in this study [26]. Policymakers, researchers, and the general public could benefit from learning more about the Kingdom's rising traffic accidents. Public health interventions are needed to make roads safer and save money on healthcare. Patients aged 18 or older who were admitted to the emergency department following RTIs between January 1, 2017, and December 31, 2017, were eligible. Also included were patients who were dead upon arrival or admission. It used the trauma registry at the KAMC to identify the patients. Each patient was followed retrospectively by the research team. Each patient's demographics, injury details, length of stay in the ward and intensive care unit, medical procedures and treatments, and health outcomes were all recorded. It included 381 of the total number of injured people in the analysis because they met the inclusion criteria. STATA version 12 was used to analyze the data.

It is a postal survey [27] of patients treated in an inpatient setting. They were asked to complete the Picker Inpatient Survey questionnaire regarding specific aspects of their care. Patients were also asked to evaluate their overall experience with this episode of care. The Picker Institute in Boston, USA, was responsible for the initial instrument development. It used a literature review, in-depth interviews, and focus groups with patients to develop the instrument's questions, which were then reviewed and formatted into a questionnaire by an expert advisory group. It resulted in creating a pilot version of the device, which was then revised and put through its paces using cognitive interviews with patients. Over a year, 3592 questionnaires were mailed to patient's homes within one month of their hospital discharge. Patients over 18 who had been discharged received questionnaires *via* mail within one month. In Scotland, one NHS trust surveyed nine provider units covering five hospital specialties. It sent two reminders to non-responders; the patients were selected at random from the Hospital Information System and stratified by provider unit, age, and sex. 65 percent of the questionnaires were returned.

The analyses [28] were restricted to patients who presented within 12 hours of symptom onset. It had documented ST-segment elevation on their admission electrocardiogram. It received thrombolysis within 12 hours of hospital arrival. The focus was on patients with unequivocal evidence-based indications for thrombolysis. 8838 of the 22 896 AMI patients in the registry met the eligibility criteria for ST-segment elevation myocardial infarctions presenting within 12 hours of symptom onset.7630 of these patients did not have any missing data on important variables. Because the province of Ontario has the data-linkage capabilities to follow patients longitudinally using administrative databases, this study was limited to the 57 participating Ontario hospitals. The gender, admission date, and date of birth patient records were deterministically linked to a Canadian Institute for Health Information discharge abstract database. It included the information in the CIHI discharge abstracts and the Fastrak registry.

From the perspectives of physicians and nurses, this study [29] aimed to identify critical demographic variables that significantly impact the culture of patient safety in a Taiwanese regional teaching hospital. The investigated hospital can accommodate approximately 700 patients and offers all primary medical specialties and services. All doctors and medical caretakers in this emergency clinic were welcome to partake in the ongoing review. The valid number of participants in this study, which includes 42 physicians and 334 nurses, was 376 after it removed the invalid parentheses. The 2014 SAQ-C from JCT was used to collect data internally, in this case, the hospital. It had 46 questions about the attitudes of medical staff members toward eight dimensions, including teamwork climate, safety climate, job satisfaction, stress recognition, management perceptions, working conditions, emotional exhaustion, and work-life balance. The core staff of each organization is made up of doctors and nurses. They might have different perceptions of patient safety culture because of various demographic factors. This study used linear regression with forward selection, which began with an empty set and continuously added one attribute at a time to predict the dependent variables from the predictor variables. It included only the attribute with the highest performance in the selection at each step. SPSS version 18 was used for all of the statistical analyses.

The work [30] calculated historical annual age-adjusted PAMV incidence rates using estimated population statistics from the U.S. Census Bureau using data from the Agency for Healthcare Research and Quality's National Inpatient Sample/Health Care Utilization Project from 2000 to 2005. It adjusts linear regression models to the changes in the incidence rate over time to make predictions about future growth by age group. It used the U.S. Census Bureau's population projections to calculate age-adjusted estimates. It chose the year 2000 as our starting point for the observation period because the Census Bureau conducts a detailed U.S. population census every ten years, and that year was the year of the most recent actual census. Age-adjusted projections are available by decade through 2050 and are calculated using previous patterns of events like births, deaths, and migration.

One of 38 doctors from 28 general practices in Aarhus County, Denmark, treats one thousand seven hundred eighty-five patients with a new health issue [31]. The area under study is a mix of rural and urban areas with 600,000 people and 431 doctors in 271 practices. An educational program and a subsequent randomized controlled intervention study on assessing and treating patients with functional somatic symptoms and somatization were open to all physicians. Before the consultation, patients completed a questionnaire regarding their perceptions of their illness and emotional distress. The doctors for each patient conducted a diagnostic and prognostic questionnaire. Register information on essential medical care usage three years prior and two years after it acquired the pattern. Odds ratios were used to estimate the relationships between illness perceptions and previous healthcare utilization. It determines whether illness perceptions predict the subsequent use of health care. Linear regression analysis was used. For the study, 38 doctors from 28 practices offered their services. Compared to nonparticipating physicians in the county, the participating physicians did not differ in age, gender, type of clinic, or postgraduate psychiatric training.

Based on various definitions of residuals, the authors propose [32] several R-squared measures for the fundamental Poisson regression model and more general models with overdispersed data, such as negative binomial. The linear regression model considers calculations based on an unweighted residual sum of squares, also known as R-squared. In the intercept-only model with a fitted mean, the residual sum of squares serves as the standard. The deviance residual is the foundation for the preferred R-squared. The performance and utility of the various R-squareds are demonstrated by applying them to counts of data on healthcare service utilization.

The study [33] looked at secondary data from a survey of 7,076 registered nurses who worked in 161 Pennsylvania hospitals in 2006. it merged three data sources: the results of the nurse survey, the hospital infection data from the 2006 Pennsylvania Health Care Cost Containment Council (PHC4) report, and the hospital characteristics data from the AHA Annual Survey. Instead of using administrative patient discharge data codes to identify infections in the PHC4 data, conditions are specified using the Centers for Disease Control and Prevention definitions. All of the hospitals in the sample provided information on disorders related to health care to the PHC4 in 2006. IT decided to look at two kinds of conditions: diseases caused by surgical sites and infections caused by catheters in the urinary tract. The PHC4 reported these two infections as the most common, and patients are at risk of contracting them in any hospital unit. Bed size, teaching status, and technology were among the hospital characteristics used as controls obtained from the AHA's Annual Survey. It used the total number of licensed beds in a hospital to define bed size. The number of medical residents and fellows distinguished nonteaching hospitals, minor teaching hospitals, and major teaching hospitals as teaching institutions. If a hospital offered facilities for open-heart surgery, major organ transplants, or both, it was considered high-tech. The nurses surveyed and employed in 161 acute care included Pennsylvania hospitals in the sample. These hospitals provided PHC4 with infection data. Nearly half of the hospitals were designated as teaching hospitals, with an average of 227 beds per facility.

The work [34] used an administrative definition to identify cases of CD and UC using an administrative database containing 87 health plans. It found that IBD patients and matched controls received inpatient, office-based, emergency, and endoscopy services between 2003 and 2004. It found 10,364 UC patients and 9,056 CD patients. it calculated the excess utilization for each case by dividing the mean number of control visits by the number of case visits. It discovered the sociodemographic factors associated with excessive utilization through multivariable logistic and linear regressions. It analyzed the PharMetrics Patient-Centric Database's inpatient and outpatient insurance claims in a cross-sectional study from January 1, 2003, to December 31, 2004. Previous epidemiological studies of inflammatory bowel disease utilized this patient-level, longitudinal database, which aggregates claims from 87 different health plans in 33 states.

3.2.2. Multiple Regression

It can utilize the statistical method known as multiple regression to examine the connection between a single dependent variable and several independent variables. Using known independent variables to predict the value of a single dependent variable is the goal of multiple regression analysis. The weights of each predictor value indicate their proportional contribution to the overall prediction. Fig. (7) illustrates the general architecture for the multivariate-multiple regression model.

The motivation behind this study [36] was to decide on patient fulfillment with medical care benefits and the doctor's way of behaving as a balance between understanding fulfillment and medical care administrations. The study aims to measure how satisfied patients are with various healthcare services in Pakistan's public health sectors, including prenatal care, laboratory and diagnostic services, and preventive care. According to the model presented in this study, improved healthcare services like preventive healthcare, prenatal care, and care for diagnostic and laboratory tests raise patient satisfaction. OPD patients from

Pakistan's three public hospitals made up most of the study's participants. These facilities were Ayyub Teaching Hospital Abbottabad, Khyber Teaching Hospital Peshawar, and King Abdullah Hospital Mansehra. The patient's participation in this study was voluntary. Participants completed self-administered questionnaires for this study's primary data collection. The demographic data and general information about the survey participants were analyzed using a frequency analysis.

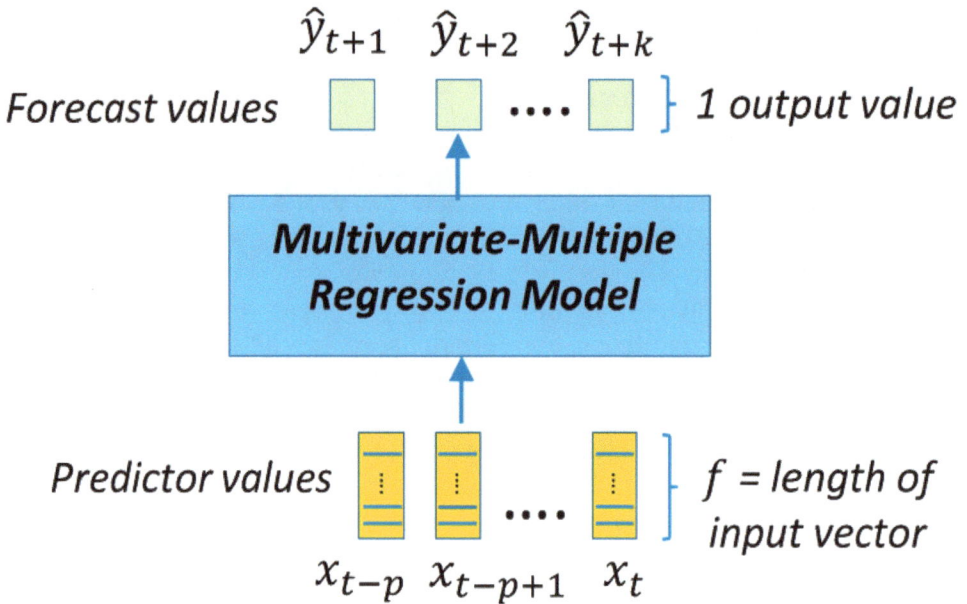

$$\hat{y}_{t+1} \quad \hat{y}_{t+2} \quad \hat{y}_{t+k}$$

Forecast values   ☐   ☐ ····   ☐ } *1 output value*

Multivariate-Multiple Regression Model

Predictor values   ▦ ▦ ···· ▦] *f = length of input vector*

$$x_{t-p} \quad x_{t-p+1} \quad x_t$$

Fig. (7). General architecture for the multivariate-multiple regression model [35].

Healthcare workers at a public hospital in South Korea provided the study's data [37]. Before collecting the data, the researchers went to the hospital to explain the purpose and method to the staff. Following Brislin's recommendation for a translation, the survey was carried out in Korean. It included a consent form for voluntary participation in the study in the survey packet distributed at work sites proportional to the number of employees in each ward and department. The completed surveys had to be sent in a sealed envelope to a designated collection box, where the researchers later collected them.711 of the 1001 questionnaires that were distributed were returned. Six hundred and ninety-four responses were used in the analysis, with cases with missing data being excluded through data cleaning. It used STATA 14.1 to conduct every one of the data analyses. It tested the study's hypotheses through a series of regression analyses.

This study [38] aimed to determine whether volunteer clown doctor's psychological health was positively correlated with self-efficacy and optimism, as well as whether empathy contributed to some incremental variance in this outcome. It completed the online survey by 160 volunteer healthcare clown doctors. The participants ranged in age from 20 to 60. The majority of them were women. Almost half of them had a high school diploma, had been volunteering as clown doctors for anywhere from one month to eleven years, and about a third had never done any other volunteering before starting their clown activity. The participants filled out an online sociodemographic form, and their gender, age, education, duration of volunteer service, and prior volunteer experience were all included. The study's objective was evaluated Using multiple linear regression analysis.

It gathered cross-sectional data from 457 nurses and 127 doctors employed in 37DHQ Pakistani hospitals for this empirical research [39]. The data were analyzed using descriptive statistics, correlation, and multiple regression methods. It ensures the clarity, suitability, and relevance of the research instrument. A pilot study was conducted on 15 doctors and 35 nurses. It selected 37 Pakistani government hospitals for final data collection. With the assistance of the human resources departments of these hospitals. It compiled a list of 170 doctors and 1700 nurses. The final workable responses from nurses were 457, and those from doctors were 127 after many sessions.

A secondary cross-sectional analysis was used in the study, which included 132 general practitioner's practices in four primary care trusts in the North West of England. These data are compiled by the prescription pricing authority and made available to GP practices and primary care trusts through prescribing analysis and cost (PACT) data. PACT data are available for all GP practices in England and permit in-depth examination of prescribed medications, including their dosages, pack sizes, and formulations. Statins, ACE inhibitors, beta-blockers, aspirin, and bendrofluazide were the drugs for which it gathered these data. For each GP practice in this study, 24 HCNIs were created, all of which were entered into multiple regression models. In addition to the combined dataset, multiple linear regression modeling was carried out for each drug group in each PCT. The prescribing rate was the dependent variable in each model, and the study's 24 HCNIs were the independent variables.

This study [40] aimed to clarify the structural differences between workers without pain and those with chronic pain in the factors that affect psychological job stress. The design of this study was cross-sectional. A core hospital's medical staff comprised the sample, and questionnaires were used to collect data in February 2018. The questionnaire survey was distributed to medical staff in all departments who had worked there for at least six months. It used a randomly selected identifier to identify the participants. 72% of the 284 members of the medical staff who were initially contacted responded with valid responses.

In the healthcare industry, a work [41] aims to identify components of patient-perceived total quality service. The infrastructure dimension looks at how satisfied patients are with the hospital's physical facilities. It includes the cleanliness, upkeep, and accessibility of services like waiting rooms, diagnostic test rooms, operation rooms, wards, food, beds, resident rooms, ambulance services, technological capability, pharmacies, and blood banks, among other places. Customers in retail rated the atmosphere, layout, and design of buildings as necessary. Customers gave the convenient location, building appearance, and staff appearance the highest ratings. The patient's experience with the hospital's doctors, nurses, paramedical and support staff, and administrative staff is the focus of the personnel quality dimension. Several facets of the quality of care provided by healthcare workers have been the focus of research. The doctor care dimension measures the patient's experience with the quality of care provided by doctors. It has been demonstrated that the medical encounter between a patient and a doctor requires extensive levels of interaction and significantly impacts patient satisfaction. The nursing care aspect of nursing-care quality surveys the view of the patient regarding the nature of nursing care given during their visit to the emergency clinic. One of the most crucial aspects of hospital services is the nursing service. Under the Paramedical and support staff quality dimension, the patient's perceptions of the quality of care, attention, empathy, and skill received at the hospital are examined. The study recommended that doctors be aware of the principles that influence the overall outcome of doctor-patient communication and the complexity of the communication process. The patient's experience with the various procedures that are a part of their stay in the hospital is an essential aspect of the quality of health care. In a hospital setting, administrative processes include the admission procedures, the hospital stay procedures, and the exit and discharge procedures of a patient's hospital stay. Patient's perceptions of a hospital's quality are influenced by the safety measures taken to protect patients physically.

3.2.3. Logistic Regression

Classification and predictive analytics frequently use this kind of statistical model, also known as the logit model. Based on a given dataset of independent variables, logistic regression calculates the probability that an event, such as voting or not voting, will occur. The dependent variable is limited to 0 and 1, as the outcome is a probability. A logit transformation is applied to the odds in logistic regression, which is the probability of success divided by the probability of failure. The natural logarithm of odds and the log odds are other names for this. It optimizes for the best fit to log odds. This method performs multiple iterations of testing various beta values. The log-likelihood function results from all of these iterations, and the goal of logistic regression is to find the best parameter estimate by maximizing this function. Fig. (**8**) represents Logistic Regression model.

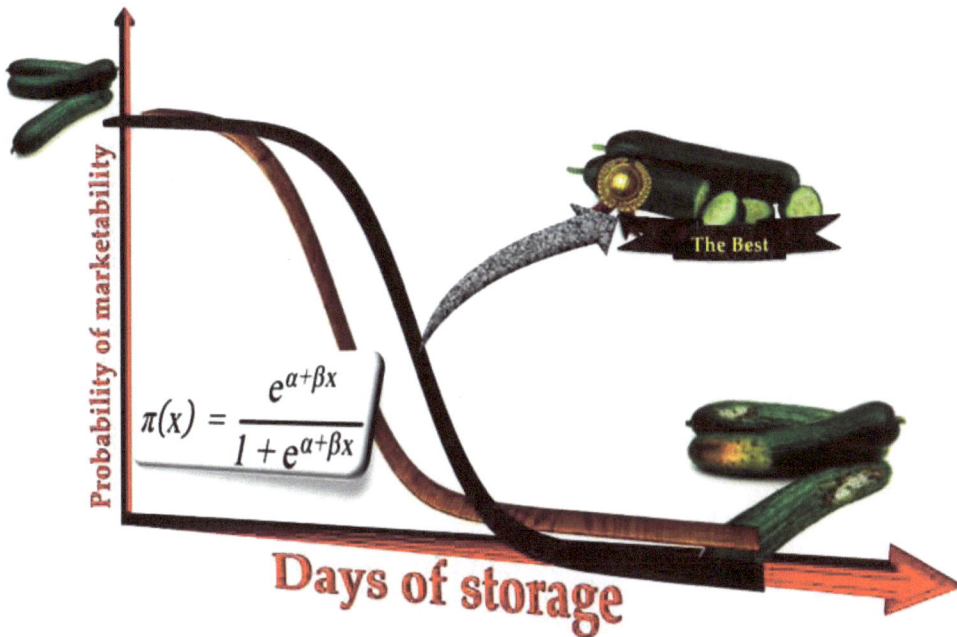

$$\pi(x) = \frac{e^{\alpha+\beta x}}{1 + e^{\alpha+\beta x}}$$

Fig. (8). Logistic Regression model [42].

The work [43] is an innovative use of logic regression in the delivery of kidney cancer treatment. Patients diagnosed with incident kidney cancer between 1995 and 2005 were identified using data from the SEER Program of the National Cancer Institute and the Centers for Medicare and Medicaid Services (Medicare). From 1995 to 2005, it identified 15,744 patients with nonurothelial, nonmetastatic kidney cancer. It determined demographic and cancer-specific information by utilizing SEER data. To distinguish the essential specialist for each case, we used scrambled Exceptional Doctor Identifier Numbers submitted with Federal health insurance doctor claims. It connected the extensive list of UPINs for surgeons to the American Medical Association Physician Masterfile, which contains information about the demographics, education, and certifications of over one million residents and doctors in the United States. Using claims from 1995 to 2005, it determined the average annual volume of partial or radical nephrectomies performed by each surgeon. The authors empirically defined high-volume surgeons among the SEER-Medicare population as achieving at least three cancer-related yearly nephrectomies.

This observational cross-sectional study [44] followed the Strengthening the Reporting of Observational Studies in Epidemiology guidelines. It included 485 recruited patients who were at least 20 years old, had been prescribed medication for at least a year and had been diagnosed with one or more chronic diseases. It used Jordanian secondary and tertiary care clinics to recruit chronically ill participants. There are two main components to Jordan's healthcare system: both the public and private sectors. Both sectors comprise hospitals, primary care clinics, pharmacies, and other auxiliary services. In Jordan, primary healthcare clinics provide quick access to various medical services, including vaccination, maternity and child care, and services for managing chronic diseases. Cardiovascular, respiratory, internal medicine and endocrinology are among the specialties represented by the clinics that are the subject of the current research. From patient records, it confirmed chronic disease diagnoses. It gathered the participant's sociodemographic information through questions in the first section of the questionnaire. It evaluated the participant's levels of adherence to their prescribed medications with the help of a self-reported questionnaire (MARS-5) that was included in the second section of the questionnaire. It had a self-report questionnaire in the third section -the Medicines Beliefs Questionnaire. It used version 21 of IBM SPSS Statistics to conduct the analysis. The adherence level was chosen as the independent variable in a stepwise binary logistical regression model to determine the associated variables of adherence to chronic medications.

Based on their work characteristics, age, and sex, this study [45] aimed to investigate the effects of prolonged VDT working time on the physical and mental health disadvantages of healthcare workers in tertiary hospitals. The non-doctor/nurse and doctor/nurse groups had 945 and 1868 participants who participated in the study. This cross-sectional study was carried out in both the Taipei and New Taipei branches of MacKay Memorial Hospital, a tertiary teaching center with 2000 beds in Taiwan. Technicians, administrative staff, pharmacists, radiologists, nutritionists, and others made up the non-doctor/nurse group. The questionnaires were completed by 1868 and 945 members of the doctor/nurse and non-doctor/nurse groups, respectively, out of a total of 3038 participants. Structured questionnaires designed by the Institute of Labor, Occupational Safety and Health, and Ministry of Labor were used to collect data. The participants had three shifts, regular class and night shift. The definition of the regular class was that it did not have a rotation and started work in the morning. Work moves that began in the first part of the day, evening, or night and turned were arranged into three movements. However, they have considered night shifts if they continue past midnight. It adjusted inquiries on MSDs from the

Nordic Outer muscle Poll. The Mackay Memorial Hospital Human Research Ethics Committee evaluated and approved the study protocol. Each participant provided written informed consent.

The recommendation [46] offered a perspective for the Centers for Disease Control and Prevention to improve the Medicaid program and make political justice for the Medicaid gap, exposed healthcare geographical inequity and provided quantitative evidence for the Medicaid gap in Texas to extend Medicaid. From 2013 to 2020, 63,083 cases, including eight years of questionnaires, were the subject of data collection. This study focuses on the three insurance types of above-poverty, Medicaid, and the Medicaid gap in 13 Texas areas. Medical research, in which the dependent variable has a binary outcome of either 0 or 1, true or false, yes or no, high or low, is a popular application for logical regression.

In this case-control study [47], there were 5120 people in the POAG group and 1489 people in the NTG group. For 2008–2013, patient data were obtained from Taiwan's Longitudinal Health Insurance Database 2010. The information utilized in this study comes from one of the NHIRD information subsets, the Longitudinal Health care coverage Data set 2000, which contains all case information for 1 million delegate recipients haphazardly chosen from the NHIRD from 2002 to 2013. It can link these data to other research data sets or government surveys. Patients under the age of 20 were excluded from the case group. Patients with NTG or POAG had multiple outpatient and discharge diagnoses in the ophthalmology department. There were 5120 people in the comparison group, while 1489 were in the case group.

Two case studies in this work [48] use high-performance generalized additive models with pairwise interactions. The first one has data on pneumonia. 14,199 patients with pneumonia are in this dataset. Forty-six characteristics describe each patient. These include age and gender in the past, simple physical measurements like heart rate, blood pressure, and respiration rate, lab tests like white blood cell count and blood urea nitrogen, and chest x-ray features like lung collapse or pleural effusion. In the second case study, GA2M is applied to a current dataset for 30-day hospital readmission that is significantly larger. The information comes from cooperation with an enormous medical clinic. The train set contains 195,901 patients, the test set contains 100,823, and each has 3,956 features. Highlights incorporate lab test results, synopses of specialist notes, and subtleties of past hospitalizations. The purpose of this dataset is to predict whether or not any patients will need to return to the hospital in a brief period. Hospitals that have abnormally high rates of 30-day readmission are subject to financial penalties.

Over 6,000 people worked in a city-based hospital for the study [49]. Two hundred fifty employees from the four main occupational groups—nurses, doctors, administrative and ancillary staff—were selected through stratified random sampling. It found 746 people after excluding employees who had left, been on maternity or long-term sick leave, or had moved without a trace. In terms of age and gender, these were typical of the staff. It sent the 12-item general health questionnaire to them. It used a cut-off score of four or higher to identify potential cases of minor psychiatric disorders. Each respondent with a GHQ score of 4 or higher was invited to a research interview within four weeks of completing the questionnaire. The discussion covered the revised clinical interview schedule 28, the life events and difficulties schedule 21, and an objective measure of work problems. A semi-structured clinical interview schedule is used to diagnose minor psychiatric disorders in the general population. Each response was assigned a score, with a maximum of four points awarded for each section. Seven variables were included in the initial analysis: age, gender, family history of mental illness, lack of a confidant, significant difficulty outside of work, and several objective work problems. In the second logistic regression, nine distinct variables represented the objective work problems and three indicated vulnerability to psychiatric disorder, three defined domains of substantial difficulties outside of work, and a difference between cases and non-cases in univariate analysis.

The study's [50] focus was the prospective cohort data that were gathered as part of the Ambulatory Care Quality Improvement Project (ACQUIP). This randomized, multicenter trial aimed to investigate the efficacy of quality-of-care interventions based on primary care in a VA patient population. Participants received a Health Checklist when they signed up, which asked about their sociodemographic characteristics and any illnesses they had with each other. 54% of the enrolled patients returned the Health Checklist, produced by 35,383 of them. The 36-item Medical Outcomes Study Short Form, an instrument that measured general health status, was sent to patients who returned the Health Checklist. At least one SF-36 was produced by 61% of these participants during the study. The primary outcome was all-cause mortality in the year following the baseline health status assessment. The VA Beneficiary Identification in Record Locator Subsystem database, which keeps track of patients whose families apply for veteran's death benefits, was used to determine death.

It is a cross-sectional study [51] using a questionnaire. It used the convenience sampling method to recruit mental health nurses and mental health assistant nurses who worked in the mental health ward of a university hospital or one of seven mental health hospitals on the island of Kyushu in Japan. Age between 20 and 79 was the eligibility threshold. Candidates who were unable to comprehend the Japanese questionnaires were disqualified. Participants were encouraged to complete the questionnaires alone outside of work hours. It gathered sociodemographic information like sex, age, marital status, occupation, number of years as a registered nurse or assistant nurse, and the kind of workplace used at the time. Five hundred ninety-nine nurses and assistant nurses out of 650 eligible nurses participated in the study. JMP Pro, for the Windows version, was used for all statistical analyses. It examined 14—the continuous variable's normal distributions with the help of the Shapiro–Wilk test.

These disorders and other non-atopic comorbidities in AD are studied [52] to see how the severity of eczema affects their development. It used information from the NSCH survey of 91,642 households from 2007 to 2008 to estimate the prevalence of various physical, emotional, and behavioral factors related to child health issues. After picking the phone numbers randomly, It identified the households with at least one child under the age of 18. It then selected one child at random for an interview. Each state's non-institutionalized child population was considered when weighing the survey results. It adjusted weights for age, sex, race, ethnicity, household size, and educational attainment. Bureau of the Census to produce a dataset more representative of the population of non-institutionalized children under 18 in each state. It used SAS 9.2 for all data processing and statistical analyses.

The databases Medline, Embase, Psycinfo, and Biomed Central, as well as a random sample of postal or electronic surveys of healthcare workers from 1996 to 2005, were used to select the respondents [53]. Three hundred fifty studies were included in the analysis. It chose these databases because they covered the entire world and covered both medical and psychosocial fields. Based on data from studies of health professionals and the general population, the number of survey participants, the type of healthcare professional, the length of the questionnaire, the use of reminders, and financial incentives were chosen as predictors of response rate. It selected the publication type to investigate the possibility of publication bias. Because country-specific factors like the healthcare system and net compensation may moderate the effects of financial incentives, it included the population of the study country. The non-reaction examination was considered present because specialists looked at segment factors among respondents and non-respondents, showed test representativeness, or reached an example of the individuals who didn't answer. The relationship between response rate, publication type, healthcare profession, country, number of survey participants, questionnaire length, and use of reminders was examined using multilevel, multivariable logistic regression.

The work [54] identifies risk factors for headache development. It administered a survey to healthcare workers. The study was conducted at a tertiary hospital. The healthcare workers in high-risk areas like intensive care units, isolation wards, emergency rooms, operating rooms, and general medical wards were required to wear the N95 face mask during the SARS outbreak from March 2003 to March 2004. The study did not include healthcare professionals who did not wear the N95 face mask and was not exposed to these high-risk areas. A year following the primary revealed instance of SARS in our country, it haphazardly conveyed 250 arrangements of polls to respondents working in these high-risk regions in Spring 2004. The medical services laborers finished a self-administered survey. Age, gender, ethnicity, and occupation were among the demographic data gathered. Pre-existing headaches and their nature, if any, were questioned by respondents. It used the SPSS software for every statistical analysis.

Compared to doctors and nurses in other specialties, the work [55] evaluates the burnout and job satisfaction of dermatologists and nurses who work with dermatological patients. In February and March of 2003, an anonymous self-completed questionnaire was given to the staff of two hospitals in Rome, Italy: a dermatological hospital and a general hospital that are both operated by the same general management and are part of the same non-profit organization. With nine dermatological units, approximately 12,500 discharges, and 170,000 outpatient visits annually, the IDI hospital is a skin disease research and treatment facility. Every year, there are about 11,500 discharges and 46000 visits to the outpatient clinic. The IDI employs 221 nurses and 162 doctors as clinical staff. There are 287 nurses and 134 doctors working at the GH. It included two standard instruments: the Maslach Burnout Inventory and a 21-item questionnaire to measure burnout and job satisfaction. Principal components factor analysis was used to investigate the 21 variables related to job satisfaction. Tertiles were created by adding the variables' scores in each factor. The people in the upper tertile were satisfied with each element. Both clinical and non-clinical IDI staff received 929 questionnaires, and the GH staff received 494 questionnaires.

The REverse Time Attention (RETAIN) model [56] was developed using data from electronic health records. The patient had skin issues, a skin disorder, a benign neoplasm, and an excision of a skin lesion before being diagnosed with heart failure. The EHR data for each patient can be represented as a time-labeled sequence of multivariate observations. The patient also had cardiac dysrhythmia, heart valve disease, and coronary atherosclerosis. It is a strategy to decipher the start-to-finish conduct of Hold. Sutter Health's electronic health records make up the dataset. The prediction model studies participants are ranging in age from 50 to 80. It extracted visit records containing diagnosis, medication, and procedure codes from encounter records, medication orders, procedure orders, and problem lists. RETAIN was made possible by Theano 0.8. The mini-batch of 100 patients was used to train the model with Adadelta. It used a computer with an Intel Xeon

E5-2630 processor, 256GB of RAM, two Nvidia Tesla K80 graphics cards, and CUDA 7.5 for the training.

This study [57] aimed to ascertain patterns and predictors of adult lesbian, gay, and bisexual disclosure of sexual orientation to healthcare providers. A sample of participants, equal numbers of men and women, LGBT and straight, White, Black, and Latino individuals aged 18 to 59, were recruited at various locations. Participants from 128 different New York City zip codes, representing a variety of neighborhoods, were included in the successful recruitment. There are 396 LGB people in this sample. At baseline and one-year follow-up, trained interviewers conducted interviews with participants. It looked at recurring or ongoing instances of unfair treatment, such as being threatened or harassed, or treated with less respect. The participant's lifetime frequency of discriminatory experiences was assessed using eight statements. Respondents were asked to indicate whether it related their experiences of unfair treatment to their sexual orientation, gender, ethnicity, race, age, religion, physical appearance, income, social class, or some other form of discrimination. Items were adapted so that each statement applied to all of the minority groups in the study.

This study [58] aimed to find out what caused frontline healthcare workers to experience psychological morbidity and stress due to this catastrophe. In three hospitals, frontline healthcare workers received self-administered questionnaires. It identified psychological distress with the help of the General Health Questionnaire. It determined the variables associated with psychological morbidity, sociodemographic and stress variables were entered into a logistic regression analysis. The study found that nurses experienced more psychological morbidity and higher stress levels during the outbreak than other professionals. The Statistical Package for the Social Sciences (SPSS) was used to analyze the data. In June 2003, 1621 questionnaires were distributed to frontline healthcare workers. A total of 650 questionnaires were returned.

Based on 16 common self-reported chronic conditions, the study [59] examined the connections between multimorbidity, health-related quality of life (HRQL), and healthcare use. The Health Quality Council of Alberta (HQCA) 2010 Patient Experience Survey provided the basis for the study. A sample of adult Albertans over 18 who are representative of the general adult population was evaluated in this cross-sectional survey regarding their experiences and level of satisfaction with the quality of health services they have received over the past year. It used Random-Digit Dialing to administer the telephone-based survey. Households from smaller health regions were oversampled by the sampling design. At the analysis, it used sampling weights to account for oversampling.

The work [60] looks into whether a management change has improved outcomes. Children who were admitted to St. Mary's Hospital's pediatric intensive care unit (PICU) between June 1992 and December 1997 were included in the study. They were given the MD diagnosis based on the detection of meningococcal DNA by polymerase chain reaction. If there was no other bacterial or viral cause for the illness, patients with MD characteristics who had diagnostic tests that returned negative were included. Between 1992 and 1997, 331 children with meningococcal disease who were admitted to the PICU in a row were studied. It used the pediatric risk of mortality (PRISM) score to determine the disease's severity at admission. Corrections for age, gender, and clinical severity were made using logistic regression analysis; death was the outcome, and the primary exposure was the year of admission, a temporal trend variable.

During the COVID-19 outbreak, this study [61] aims to determine which key populations may require psychological intervention and investigate the prevalence of depression and anxiety among physicians, healthcare professionals, and USs. Between March 22 and March 28, 2020, a cross-sectional study using an online survey was conducted in Jordan to investigate the GP, HCP, and US mental health (depression and anxiety) during the COVID-19 outbreak. Because a more extended period may impact the study population's mental health, the data collection period was limited to one week. Through social media (Facebook and WhatsApp), the GP, HCPs, and USs were invited to participate in this study. Because each population has specific demographic questions, a separate survey link was used to ask each population about the study. As a result of their voluntary participation in the study, they were not required to give written informed consent. There was a total of 4,126 participants in the study.

3.3. DRAWBACKS

It could be made better with semi-supervised learning. Because a semi-supervised model can learn from unlabeled and labeled images simultaneously, the number of labeled images required for satisfactory performance is significantly reduced. The main drawback of this method is that it can take a lot of work to get an adversarial model to converge on a solution.

CONCLUSION

Every day, the healthcare industry produces a significant amount of medical data. The healthcare industry is experiencing this expansion because it generates a substantial amount of data daily: medical imaging data, electronic medical records (EMRs), routine medical examinations, lab tests, and medical expert's notes. In the healthcare world, joining labeled and unlabelled data to improve the performance of learned hypotheses has received much attention.

REFERENCES

[1]   S. Uhlmann, S. Kiranyaz, and M. Gabbouj, "Semi-supervised learning for Ill-posed polarimetric SAR classification", *Remote. Sens.,* vol. 6, no. 6, pp. 4801-4830, 2014.
[http://dx.doi.org/10.3390/rs6064801]

[2]   C. Krittanawong, K.W. Johnson, E. Choi, S. Kaplin, E. Venner, M. Murugan, Z. Wang, B.S. Glicksberg, C.I. Amos, M.C. Schatz, and W.H.W. Tang, "Artificial intelligence and cardiovascular genetics", *Life.,* vol. 12, no. 2, p. 279, 2022.
[http://dx.doi.org/10.3390/life12020279] [PMID: 35207566]

[3]   Z. Zhou, C. Lu, W. Wang, W. Dang, and K. Gong, "Semi-supervised medical image classification based on attention and intrinsic features of samples", *Appl. Sci.,* vol. 12, no. 13, p. 6726, 2022.
[http://dx.doi.org/10.3390/app12136726]

[4]   G. Zhang, S.X. Ou, Y.H. Huang, and C.R. Wang, "Semi-supervised learning methods for large scale healthcare data analysis", *Int. J. Comput. Healthc.,* vol. 2, no. 2, pp. 98-110, 2015.
[http://dx.doi.org/10.1504/IJCIH.2015.069788]

[5]   C. Liu, Z. Jiang, X. Su, S. Benzoni, and A. Maxwell, "Detection of human fall using floor vibration and multi-features semi-supervised SVM", *Sensors,* vol. 19, no. 17, p. 3720, 2019.
[http://dx.doi.org/10.3390/s19173720] [PMID: 31466268]

[6]   Y. Zou, S. Wu, T. Zhang, and Y. Yang, "Research on a defecation pre-warning algorithm for the disabled elderly based on a semi-supervised generative adversarial network", *Sensors,* vol. 22, no. 17, p. 6704, 2022.
[http://dx.doi.org/10.3390/s22176704] [PMID: 36081167]

[7]   M. Liu, M. Zhou, T. Zhang, and N. Xiong, "Semi-supervised learning quantization algorithm with deep features for motor imagery EEG Recognition in smart healthcare application", *Appl. Soft Comput.,* vol. 89, p. 106071, 2020.
[http://dx.doi.org/10.1016/j.asoc.2020.106071]

[8]   A. Zahin, L.T. Tan, and R.Q. Hu, "Sensor-based human activity recognition for smart healthcare: A semi-supervised machine learning", In: *International conference on artificial intelligence for communications and networks* Okinawa: Japan, 2019.
[http://dx.doi.org/10.1007/978-3-030-22971-9_39]

[9]   F. Wang, "Adaptive semi-supervised recursive tree partitioning: The ART towards large scale patient indexing in personalized healthcare", *J. Biomed. Inform.,* vol. 55, pp. 41-54, 2015.
[http://dx.doi.org/10.1016/j.jbi.2015.01.009] [PMID: 25656756]

[10]   M. Huang, Y. Chen, B.W. Chen, J. Liu, S. Rho, and W. Ji, "A semi-supervised privacy-preserving clustering algorithm for healthcare", *Peer-to-Peer Netw. Appl.,* vol. 9, no. 5, pp. 864-875, 2016.
[http://dx.doi.org/10.1007/s12083-015-0356-9]

[11]   A. Thakur, P. Sharma, and D.A. Clifton, "Dynamic neural graphs based federated reptile for semi-supervised multi-tasking in healthcare Applications", *IEEE J. Biomed. Health Inform.,* vol. 26, no. 4, pp. 1761-1772, 2022.
[http://dx.doi.org/10.1109/JBHI.2021.3134835] [PMID: 34898443]

[12]   D. Shi, J. Zurada, and J. Guan, "A Neuro-fuzzy system with semi-supervised learning for bad debt recovery in the healthcare industry", In: *Hawaii International Conference on System Sciences* Kauai, HI: USA, 2015.
[http://dx.doi.org/10.1109/HICSS.2015.376]

[13]   P. Gupta, and P. Caleb-Solly, "A framework for semi-supervised adaptive learning for activity recognition in healthcare applications", In: *International Conference on Engineering Applications of Neural Networks*, 2018.UWE Bristol, UK.
[http://dx.doi.org/10.1007/978-3-319-98204-5_1]

[14]   N. Gaw, "Novel semi-supervised learning models to balance data inclusivity and usability in

healthcare applications", Arizona State University, 2019.

[15]   C. Yin, and Z. Chen, "Developing sustainable classification of diseases via deep learning and semi-supervised Learning", *Healthcare.*, vol. 8, no. 3, p. 291, 2020.
[http://dx.doi.org/10.3390/healthcare8030291] [PMID: 32846941]

[16]   F. Dubost, E. Hong, N. Bhaskhar, S. Tang, D. Rubin, and C. Lee-Messer, "Semi-supervised learning for sparsely-labeled sequential data: Application to healthcare video processing", In: *IEEE/CVF Winter Conference on Applications of Computer Vision*, 2020.

[17]   B. Longstaff, S. Reddy, and D. Estrin, "Improving activity classification for health applications on mobile devices using active and semi-supervised learning", In: *4th International Conference on Pervasive Computing Technologies for Healthcare* Munich: Germany, 2010.
[http://dx.doi.org/10.4108/ICST.PERVASIVEHEALTH2010.8851]

[18]   M. Ahmed, Z. Mao, Y. Zheng, T. Chen, and Z. Chen, "Electric vehicle range estimation using regression techniques", *World Electr. Veh. J.*, vol. 13, no. 6, p. 105, 2022.
[http://dx.doi.org/10.3390/wevj13060105]

[19]   E.M. Valsamis, D. Ricketts, H. Husband, and B.A. Rogers, "Segmented linear regression models for assessing change in retrospective studies in healthcare", *Comput. Math. Methods Med.*, vol. 2019, pp. 1-9, 2019.
[http://dx.doi.org/10.1155/2019/9810675]

[20]   A. Zamuda, C. Zarges, G. Stiglic, and G. Hrovat, "Stability selection using a genetic algorithm and logistic linear regression on healthcare records", In: *Genetic and Evolutionary Computation Conference Companion* Berlin: Germany, 2017.
[http://dx.doi.org/10.1145/3067695.3076077]

[21]   Y.L. Chiu, J.N. Wang, H. Yu, and Y.T. Hsu, "Consultation pricing of the online health care service in China: Hierarchical linear regression approach", *J. Med. Internet Res.*, vol. 23, no. 7, p. e29170, 2021.
[http://dx.doi.org/10.2196/29170] [PMID: 34259643]

[22]   V.K. Kapur, S. Redline, F.J. Nieto, T.B. Young, A.B. Newman, and J.A. Henderson, "The relationship between chronically disrupted sleep and healthcare use", *Sleep,* vol. 25, no. 3, pp. 289-296, 2002.
[PMID: 12003159]

[23]   X.H. Zhou, K.T. Stroupe, and W.M. Tierney, "Regression analysis of health care charges with heteroscedasticity", *Appl. Stat.*, vol. 50, no. 3, pp. 303-312, 2001.
[http://dx.doi.org/10.1111/1467-9876.00235]

[24]   D. Gregori, M. Petrinco, S. Bo, A. Desideri, F. Merletti, and E. Pagano, "Regression models for analyzing costs and their determinants in health care: An introductory review", *Int. J. Qual. Health Care.*, vol. 23, no. 3, pp. 331-341, 2011.
[http://dx.doi.org/10.1093/intqhc/mzr010] [PMID: 21504959]

[25]   O. Salem, A. Guerassimov, A. Mehaoua, A. Marcus, and B. Furht, "Anomaly detection in medical wireless sensor networks using SVM and linear regression models", *Int. J. E-Health Med. Commun.*, vol. 5, no. 1, pp. 20-45, 2014.
[http://dx.doi.org/10.4018/ijehmc.2014010102]

[26]   S. Alghnam, M. Alkelya, M. Aldahnim, N. Aljerian, I. Albabtain, A. Alsayari, O.B. Da'ar, K. Alsheikh, and A. Alghamdi, "Healthcare costs of road injuries in Saudi Arabia: A quantile regression analysis", *Accid. Anal. Prev.*, vol. 159, p. 106266, 2021.
[http://dx.doi.org/10.1016/j.aap.2021.106266] [PMID: 34225170]

[27]   C. Jenkinson, A. Coulter, S. Bruster, N. Richards, and T. Chandola, "Patients' experiences and satisfaction with health care: Results of a questionnaire study of specific aspects of care", *Qual. Saf. Health Care.*, vol. 11, no. 4, pp. 335-339, 2002.
[http://dx.doi.org/10.1136/qhc.11.4.335] [PMID: 12468693]

[28]   P.C. Austin, J.V. Tu, P.A. Daly, and D.A. Alter, "The use of quantile regression in health care

research: A case study examining gender differences in the timeliness of thrombolytic therapy", *Stat. Med.,* vol. 24, no. 5, pp. 791-816, 2005.
[http://dx.doi.org/10.1002/sim.1851] [PMID: 15532082]

[29]   C.Y. Chi, H.H. Wu, C.H. Huang, and Y.C. Lee, "Using linear regression to identify critical demographic variables affecting patient safety culture from viewpoints of physicians and nurses", *Hosp. Pract. Res.,* vol. 2, no. 2, pp. 47-53, 2017.
[http://dx.doi.org/10.15171/hpr.2017.12]

[30]   M.D. Zilberberg, M. de Wit, J.R. Pirone, and A.F. Shorr, "Growth in adult prolonged acute mechanical ventilation: Implications for healthcare delivery", *Crit. Care Med.,* vol. 36, no. 5, pp. 1451-1455, 2008.
[http://dx.doi.org/10.1097/CCM.0b013e3181691a49] [PMID: 18434911]

[31]   L. Frostholm, P. Fink, K.S. Christensen, T. Toft, E. Oernboel, F. Olesen, and J. Weinman, "The patients' illness perceptions and the use of primary health care", *Psychosom. Med.,* vol. 67, no. 6, pp. 997-1005, 2005.
[http://dx.doi.org/10.1097/01.psy.0000189164.85653.bc] [PMID: 16314606]

[32]   A.C. Cameron, and F.A. Windmeijer, "R-squared measures for count data regression models with applications to health-care utilization", *J. Bus. Econ. Stat.,* vol. 14, no. 2, pp. 209-220, 1996.

[33]   J.P. Cimiotti, L.H. Aiken, D.M. Sloane, and E.S. Wu, "Nurse staffing, burnout, and health care–associated infection", *Am. J. Infect. Control,* vol. 40, no. 6, pp. 486-490, 2012.
[http://dx.doi.org/10.1016/j.ajic.2012.02.029] [PMID: 22854376]

[34]   M.D. Kappelman, C.Q. Porter, J.A. Galanko, S.L. Rifas-Shiman, D.A. Ollendorf, R.S. Sandler, and J.A. Finkelstein, "Utilization of healthcare resources by U.S. children and adults with inflammatory bowel disease", *Inflamm. Bowel. Dis.,* vol. 17, no. 1, pp. 62-68, 2011.
[http://dx.doi.org/10.1002/ibd.21371] [PMID: 20564532]

[35]   M. Lopez-Martin, A. Sanchez-Esguevillas, L. Hernandez-Callejo, J.I. Arribas, and B. Carro, "Additive ensemble neural network with constrained weighted quantile loss for probabilistic electric-load forecasting", *Sensors.,* vol. 21, no. 9, p. 2979, 2021.
[http://dx.doi.org/10.3390/s21092979] [PMID: 33922814]

[36]   F. Manzoor, L. Wei, A. Hussain, M. Asif, and S.I.A. Shah, "Patient satisfaction with health care services: An application of physician's behavior as a moderator", *Int. J. Environ. Res. Public Health,* vol. 16, no. 18, p. 3318, 2019.
[http://dx.doi.org/10.3390/ijerph16183318] [PMID: 31505840]

[37]   M.Λ. Opoku, H. Yoon, S.W. Kang, and M. You, "How to mitigate the negative effect of emotional exhaustion among healthcare workers: The role of safety climate and compensation", *Int. J. Environ. Res. Public Health,* vol. 18, no. 12, p. 6641, 2021.
[http://dx.doi.org/10.3390/ijerph18126641] [PMID: 34205508]

[38]   A. Dionigi, G. Casu, and P. Gremigni, "Associations of self-efficacy, optimism, and empathy with psychological health in healthcare volunteers", *Int. J. Environ. Res. Public Health,* vol. 17, no. 16, p. 6001, 2020.
[http://dx.doi.org/10.3390/ijerph17166001] [PMID: 32824812]

[39]   J. Waheed, W. Jun, Z. Yousaf, M. Radulescu, and H. Hussain, "Towards employee creativity in the healthcare sector: Investigating the role of polychronicity, job engagement, and functional flexibility", *Healthcare.,* vol. 9, no. 7, p. 837, 2021.
[http://dx.doi.org/10.3390/healthcare9070837] [PMID: 34356214]

[40]   Y. Sakamoto, T. Oka, T. Amari, and S. Shimo, "Factors affecting psychological stress in healthcare workers with and without chronic pain: A cross-sectional study using multiple regression analysis", *Medicina.,* vol. 55, no. 10, p. 652, 2019.
[http://dx.doi.org/10.3390/medicina55100652] [PMID: 31569824]

[41]   M. Duggirala, C. Rajendran, and R.N. Anantharaman, "Patient-perceived dimensions of total quality service in healthcare", *Benchmarking.,* vol. 15, no. 5, pp. 560-583, 2008.

[http://dx.doi.org/10.1108/14635770810903150]

[42]   M. Díaz-Pérez, Á. Carreño-Ortega, J.A. Salinas-Andújar, and Á.J. Callejón-Ferre, "Application of logistic regression models for the marketability of cucumber cultivars", *Agronomy,* vol. 9, no. 1, p. 17, 2019.
[http://dx.doi.org/10.3390/agronomy9010017]

[43]   M. Banerjee, C. Filson, R. Xia, and D.C. Miller, "Logic regression for provider effects on kidney cancer treatment delivery", *Comput. Math. Methods Med.,* vol. 2014, pp. 1-9, 2014.
[http://dx.doi.org/10.1155/2014/316935] [PMID: 24795774]

[44]   A.Q. Al Bawab, W. Al-Qerem, O. Abusara, N. Alkhatib, M. Mansour, and R. Horne, "What are the factors associated with nonadherence to medications in patients with chronic diseases?", *Healthcare,* vol. 9, no. 9, p. 1237, 2021.
[http://dx.doi.org/10.3390/healthcare9091237] [PMID: 34575011]

[45]   M.T. Tsou, "Influence of prolonged visual display terminal use on physical and mental conditions among health care workers at tertiary hospitals, Taiwan", *Int. J. Environ. Res. Public Health,* vol. 19, no. 7, p. 3770, 2022.
[http://dx.doi.org/10.3390/ijerph19073770] [PMID: 35409467]

[46]   J. Zhang, and X. Wu, "Predict health care accessibility for texas medicaid gap", *Healthcare.,* vol. 9, no. 9, p. 1214, 2021.
[http://dx.doi.org/10.3390/healthcare9091214] [PMID: 34574988]

[47]   W.Y. Lu, C.W. Luo, S.T. Chen, Y.H. Kuan, S.F. Yang, and H.Y. Sun, "Comparison of medical comorbidity between patients with normal-tension glaucoma and primary open-angle glaucoma: A population-based study in Taiwan", *Healthcare (Basel),* vol. 9, no. 11, p. 1509, 2021.
[http://dx.doi.org/10.3390/healthcare9111509] [PMID: 34828558]

[48]   R. Caruana, Y. Lou, J. Gehrke, P. Koch, M. Sturm, and N. Elhadad, "Intelligible models for healthcare: Predicting pneumonia risk and hospital 30-day readmission", In: *Proceedings of the 21th ACM SIGKDD International Conference on Knowledge Discovery and Data Mining* Sydney NSW Australia, 2015.
[http://dx.doi.org/10.1145/2783258.2788613]

[49]   A. Weinberg, and F. Creed, "Stress and psychiatric disorder in healthcare professionals and hospital staff", *Lancet,* vol. 355, no. 9203, pp. 533-537, 2000.
[http://dx.doi.org/10.1016/S0140-6736(99)07366-3] [PMID: 10683003]

[50]   K.B. DeSalvo, V.S. Fan, M.B. McDonell, and S.D. Fihn, "Predicting mortality and healthcare utilization with a single question", *Health Serv. Res.,* vol. 40, no. 4, pp. 1234-1246, 2005.
[http://dx.doi.org/10.1111/j.1475-6773.2005.00404.x] [PMID: 16033502]

[51]   Y. Kobayashi, M. Oe, T. Ishida, M. Matsuoka, H. Chiba, and N. Uchimura, "Workplace violence and its effects on burnout and secondary traumatic stress among mental healthcare nurses in Japan", *Int. J. Environ. Res. Public Health,* vol. 17, no. 8, p. 2747, 2020.
[http://dx.doi.org/10.3390/ijerph17082747] [PMID: 32316142]

[52]   J.I. Silverberg, and E.L. Simpson, "Association between severe eczema in children and multiple comorbid conditions and increased healthcare utilization", *Pediatr. Allergy Immunol.,* vol. 24, no. 5, pp. 476-486, 2013.
[http://dx.doi.org/10.1111/pai.12095] [PMID: 23773154]

[53]   J.V. Cook, H.O. Dickinson, and M.P. Eccles, "Response rates in postal surveys of healthcare professionals between 1996 and 2005: An observational study", *BMC Health Serv. Res.,* vol. 9, no. 1, p. 160, 2009.
[http://dx.doi.org/10.1186/1472-6963-9-160] [PMID: 19751504]

[54]   E.C.H. Lim, R.C.S. Seet, K.H. Lee, E.P.V. Wilder-Smith, B.Y.S. Chuah, and B.K.C. Ong, "Headaches and the N95 face-mask amongst healthcare providers", *Acta Neurol. Scand.,* vol. 113, no. 3, pp. 199-202, 2006.

[http://dx.doi.org/10.1111/j.1600-0404.2005.00560.x] [PMID: 16441251]

[55] C. Renzi, S. Tabolli, A. Ianni, C. Di Pietro, and P. Puddu, "Burnout and job satisfaction comparing healthcare staff of a dermatological hospital and a general hospital", *J. Eur. Acad. Dermatol. Venereol.,* vol. 19, no. 2, pp. 153-157, 2005.
[http://dx.doi.org/10.1111/j.1468-3083.2005.01029.x] [PMID: 15752281]

[56] E. Choi, M.T. Bahadori, J. Sun, J. Kulas, A. Schuetz, and W. Stewart, "Retain: An interpretable predictive model for healthcare using reverse time attention mechanism", *Advances in neural information processing systems,* p. 29, 2016.

[57] L.E. Durso, and I.H. Meyer, "Patterns and predictors of disclosure of sexual orientation to healthcare providers among lesbians, gay men, and bisexuals", *Sex. Res. Soc. Policy,* vol. 10, no. 1, pp. 35-42, 2013.
[http://dx.doi.org/10.1007/s13178-012-0105-2] [PMID: 23463442]

[58] C.W.C. Tam, E.P.F. Pang, L.C.W. Lam, and H.F.K. Chiu, "Severe acute respiratory syndrome (SARS) in Hong Kong in 2003: stress and psychological impact among frontline healthcare workers", *Psychol. Med.,* vol. 34, no. 7, pp. 1197-1204, 2004.
[http://dx.doi.org/10.1017/S0033291704002247] [PMID: 15697046]

[59] C.B. Agborsangaya, D. Lau, M. Lahtinen, T. Cooke, and J.A. Johnson, "Health-related quality of life and healthcare utilization in multimorbidity: Results of a cross-sectional survey", *Qual. Life Res.,* vol. 22, no. 4, pp. 791-799, 2013.
[http://dx.doi.org/10.1007/s11136-012-0214-7] [PMID: 22684529]

[60] R. Booy, P. Habibi, S. Nadel, C. de Munter, J. Britto, A. Morrison, and M. Levin, "Reduction in case fatality rate from meningococcal disease associated with improved healthcare delivery", *Arch. Dis. Child.,* vol. 85, no. 5, pp. 386-390, 2001.
[http://dx.doi.org/10.1136/adc.85.5.386] [PMID: 11668100]

[61] A.Y. Naser, E.Z. Dahmash, R. Al-Rousan, H. Alwafi, H.M. Alrawashdeh, I. Ghoul, A. Abidine, M.A. Bokhary, H.T. AL-Hadithi, D. Ali, R. Abuthawabeh, G.M. Abdelwahab, Y.J. Alhartani, H. Al Muhaisen, A. Dagash, and H.S. Alyami, "Mental health status of the general population, healthcare professionals, and university students during 2019 coronavirus disease outbreak in Jordan: A cross-sectional study", *Brain Behav.,* vol. 10, no. 8, p. e01730, 2020.
[http://dx.doi.org/10.1002/brb3.1730] [PMID: 32578943]

CHAPTER 4

Unsupervised Algorithms

Abstract: The broad term "health care" refers to a system that focuses on improving medical services to meet the needs of patients. Patients, doctors, vendors, health companies, and IT companies all work to keep and restore health records in the healthcare industry. It uses machine learning. Healthcare analysis addresses a variety of diseases, including cancer, diabetes, stroke, and others. Both the labeled value and the target value are known. Training the data for unsupervised learning is also involved. Because the label value is either unknown or absent, it is impossible to evaluate the model's performance in unsupervised learning. The chapter details different unsupervised algorithms.

Keywords: Healthcare, Unsupervised Algorithms, Unlabeled Data.

4.1. INTRODUCTION

The process by which a network can study to signify some input designs in a manner that reproduces the numerical arrangement of the total collection of input designs or patterns is called unsupervised learning. The assumption of a function to define the hidden structure from unlabeled data is a machine learning charge. It is learning algorithms that lack labels to monitor learning and training. The algorithm accepts data and characteristics specific to each observation as inputs but not the desired output. Typically, unsupervised learning is used to divide the images into two sets or clusters based on inherent characteristics like color, size, shape, and so on. Because there is no external source of information for the network, it is referred to as either an adaptive learning algorithm or a self-organizing algorithm. It is contingent on the internal mechanism and local facts. The system receives the training figures and input patterns, which it organizes into categories or clusters. At the stage of the input layer, the system receives a group of training patterns or data. The output layer's nodes compete to adjust the network association weights, with the winner being the node with the highest value. The majority of algorithms for clustering and association make use of unsupervised learning.

A novel strategy [1] for unsupervised component condition identification is presented in this study. For modelling, it uses test cycle data of machine components under various faulty and healthy conditions. A test cycle is performed on any machine tool component without engaging the workpiece and outside machining times. It ensures that the requirements for generating and acquiring data are comparable. The test cycles' used to train the model and the model used to make predictions are the same. While the process of measuring and modeling remains the same for each machine component, each component undergoes its independent analysis. The method is shown to be effective for machine axes in this study. The test cycle's results in healthy and various faulty states are gathered for each axis. Similarly, a rotatory axis is rotated from its starting position to its limit of outward movement and then back to its starting position. There are four segments in each trajectory direction: a constant velocity segment, an acceleration ramp with a transient response, and a deceleration ramp with a quick response until the vehicle comes to a complete stop. It recreates the operating conditions necessary for detecting and quantifying anomalies. The test cycles are carried out with the standard process dynamics and velocities of the machine components that are currently in use. In addition, the test cycles are repeated multiple times to enable the detection of outliers in the recordings and reduce sample variation. The resulting data set is divided into test and training sets. Test cycle data of machine axes under unknown conditions are used to evaluate their health status during a prediction model deployment. The aggregated feature sets can train a model to learn similarities and differences between feature set samples. It predicts a time series sample of an unidentified machine condition. The time series is divided into the defined ROIs. After selecting and calculating the model's retained features, the model scalar normalizes the resulting characteristics and applies the trained HDBSCAN model to the unknown feature set. Fig. (**1**) Solution approach for both model training and prediction of test cycle samples.

This work [2] first shows that the unsupervised learning paradigm can also be used to classify images of HEp-2 cells. A deep convolutional autoencoder with an encoding-decoding method for feature extraction is proposed. It can identify the two components of the network: the encoder, which gradually reduces the input's spatial size, and the decoder, which gradually expands the input's spatial scope while decreasing its depth. As we progress within the network until we reach the space of the latent representations, the input image is systematically down-sampled before the decoding or up-sampling begins. It has the outcome that the organization loses the spatial data of the picture in many layers. This distortion complicates the reconstruction process. It employs two approaches utilized in the segmentation issues. The encoder's maximum pooling process entails storing the positions of the selected activations. The unpooling process in the decoder will only consist of setting all remaining values to zero and placing the activations at the stored posts. It obtained the outcomes by using the SNPHEp-2 dataset. There are five types of cells in the SNPHEp-2 dataset-homogeneous cells, coarse and fine speckles, cells with nuclei, and cells with the centromere. This dataset has two levels of fluorescence intensity: powers, both positive and negative. It used all 40 different cell samples to extract the images. Twenty of the forty specimens were utilized for the training sets, while the remaining twenty were used for the testing sets. There are separate 905 and 979 cell pictures for the preparation and testing sets. Fig. (**2**) denotes the same.

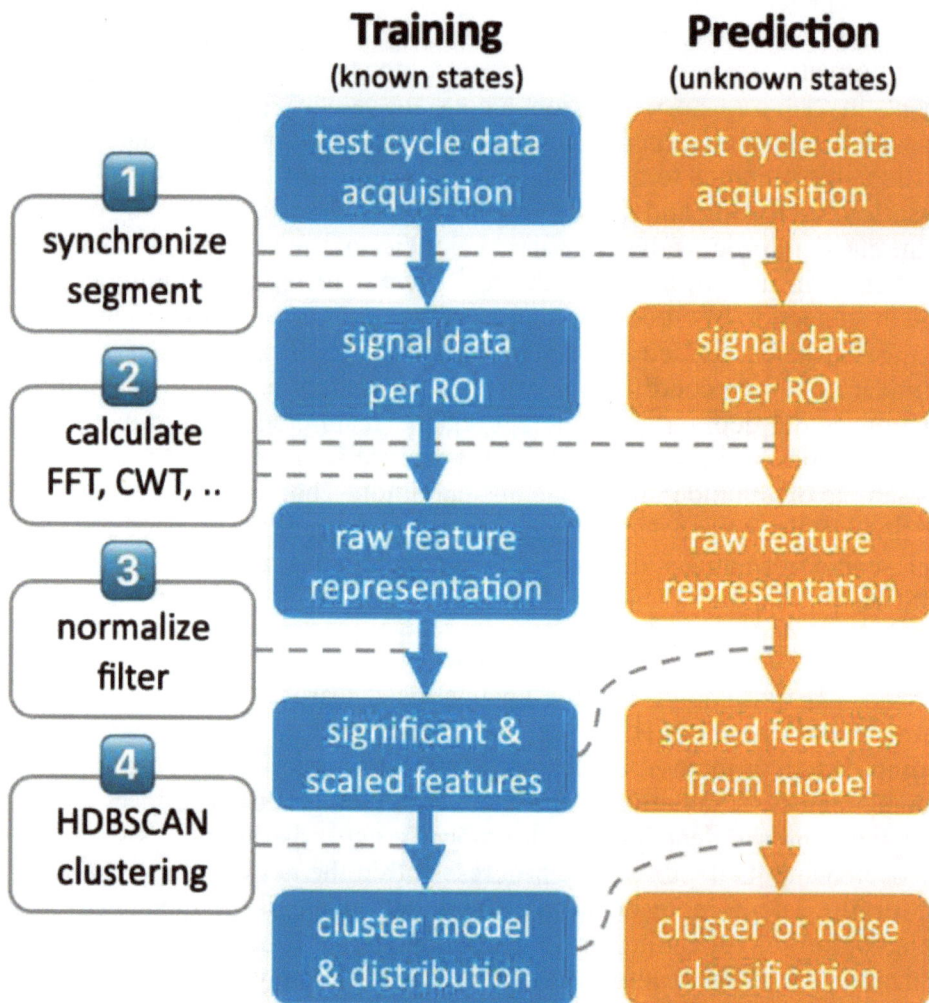

Fig. (1). Solution approach for both model training and prediction of test cycle samples [1].

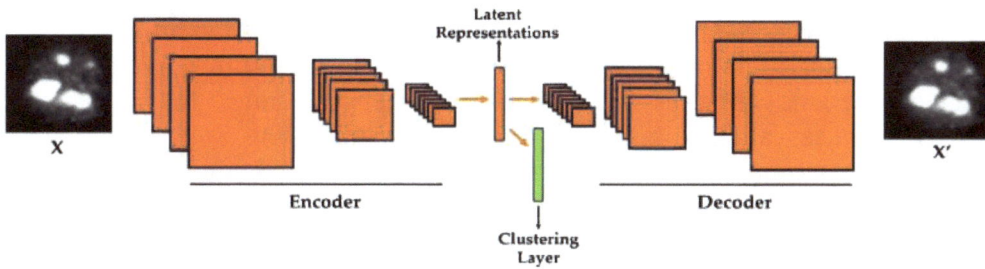

Fig. (2). Proposed framework [2].

It is an unsupervised method [3] for annotating medical data. It has performed morphological and syntactic analyses of the EMR's textual data as sentences. Word embeddings were trained using Word2Vec and Node2Vec techniques on a corpus of syntactic trees. It added the most similar ones to the initial tree for each word as new nodes on the same level. The similarity metric used was the cosine distance. After these modifications to the initial parsed trees, it merged them into a single tree. A labeling module operates the medical knowledge base to label groups. The language-specific Wikidata-based knowledge base is set once before being labelled. It uses morphological and syllabary analyzers. It can glean information about sentence structure. This procedure guarantees the structural meaning of groups with similar semantic constructions. It uses pos-tags supplied by a morphological analyzer to ensure that similar words have the same part of speech. Syntactic relations link semantically dependent nodes. Phrases frequently found in the received syntactic trees had similar meanings but were expressed in different words. Word embedding prediction is then made by using the trained model's weights. A Node2Vec approach is used to introduce a CBOW model. Five thousand Russian sentences with time constructions served as the subject of experiments. Corrections were taken from an anonymous set of EMR histories of patients with acute coronary syndrome who were observed at the Almazov National Medical Research Centre (Almazov Centre) between 2010 and 2015. On a personal computer with 8 GB of RAM and a 1.8 GHz Dual-Core Intel Core i5 processor, labelling took an average of 6.2 minutes. It used the Python programming language to create the method's implementation. Fig. (**3**) denotes the method schema of sequential modules with EMR as input and labelled groups as output.

FL-PMI [4] uses the deep reinforcement learning (DRL) framework to label unlabeled data automatically. The data are trained with federated learning, in which the edge servers let just the parameters pass through the cloud instead of a lot of sensor data. Finally, the data for the various SHC-related processes are classified by the bidirectional long-short-term memory in FL-PMI. Each wearable device stores the data it collects at the device's edge. The person's characteristics are stored in each wearable device, which is used to learn about the data. To improve the classification module and infer high-level features from unlabeled raw data, the BiLSTM uses two hidden neural network states. DRL's interspace reward law uses an auto-labeling module to support the SHC and train the unlabeled data from each wearable device. The FL-based edge learning model receives the local parameter, which then updates the global model before pushing it to wearable devices. Each wearable device's local parameters are sent to the server, which use federated averaging and the regional model's weights to update the global model. After that, the edge server uses the estimated average to update the model, creating the worldwide model. It will push this newly updated model to each wearable device for the subsequent training session. FL-PMI increases learning efficiency, decreases computational costs and improves accuracy. Fig. (**4**) represents the same.

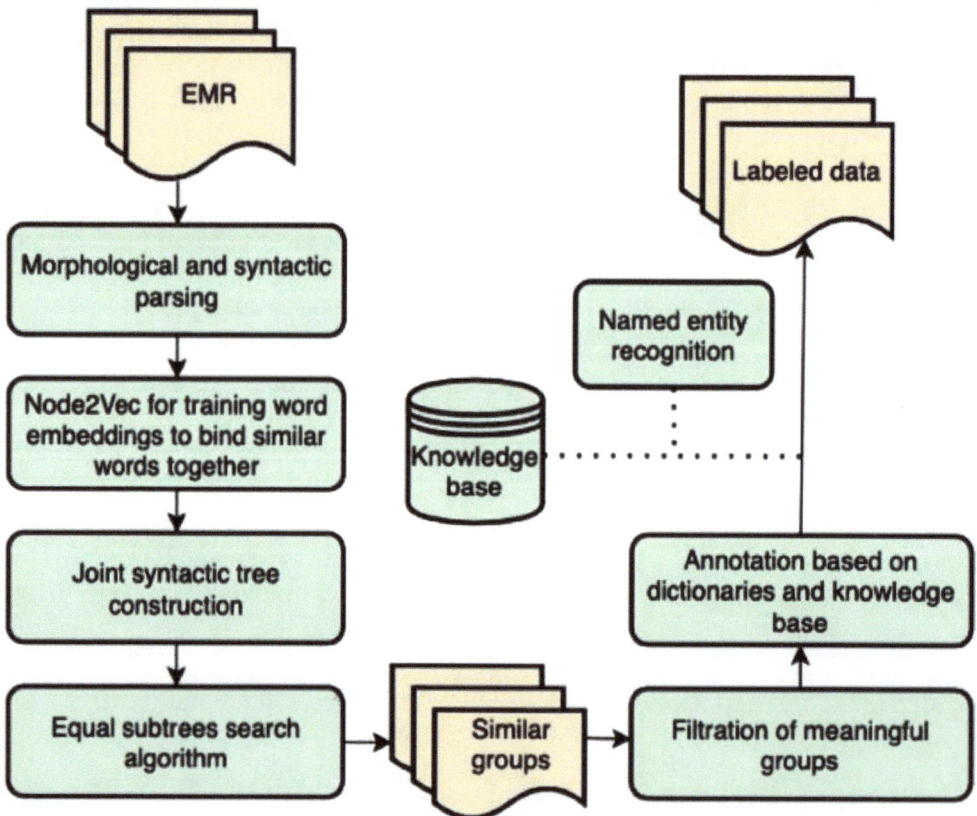

Fig. (3). Method schema of sequential modules with EMR as input and labeled groups as output [3].

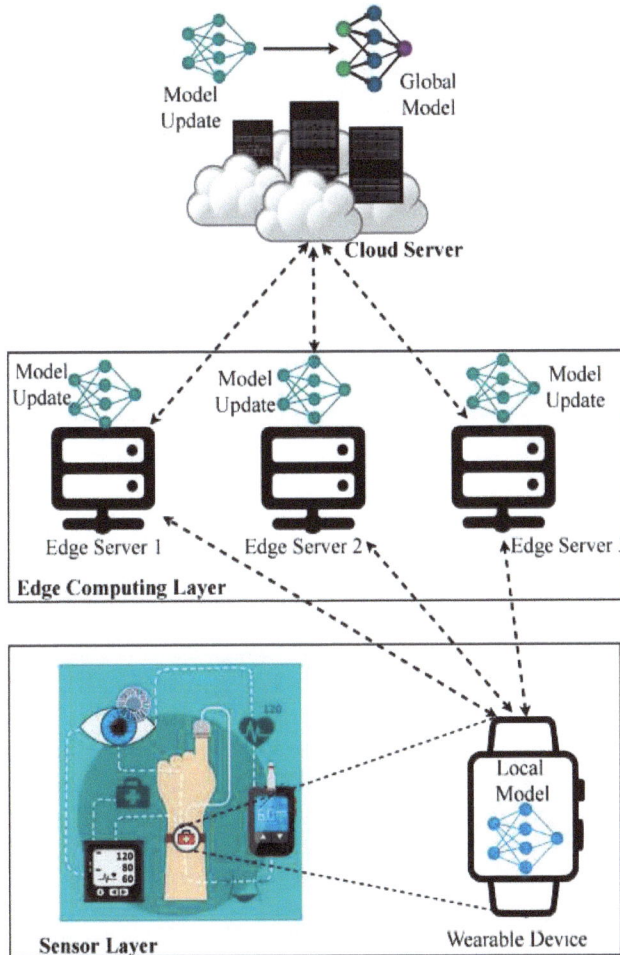

Fig. (4). Proposed Framework [4].

The proposed approach [5] aims to investigate the connection between mood states and categories of human communication derived from facial expressions, gaze distribution area and density, and rapid eye movements, which are referred to as saccades. For unsupervised clustering and data visualization, it utilized self-organizing maps. The 20 m-tall partitions installed in the room separated the sections for the experimenter as an observer and the subject. It connected a measurement instrument to the laptop computers. The experimenter kept an eye on the progress of the protocols and the subject's responses. The issue sat in a chair at the back of the room. It viewed a 50-inch monitor 3 meters across the table. On the table, the facial measurement instrument was set up. The monitor displayed a video intended for interlocutor communication. The study kept the room silent to allow the subjects to participate in the experiment in a relaxed state. The blinds on the windows were closed. It used an air conditioner to maintain the room's constant temperature and humidity. An emitter and stereo camera with 0.5–1.0 deg angular resolution and 60 Hz data sampling make up the faceLAB five apparatus. The included application programming produces heatmap results determined from look focus thickness and the number of saccades, characterized as rapid eye developments between obsession focus. The sheets from the Profile of Mood States, Second Edition, were used to measure the psychological information of the various subjects. Volunteer sampling was used to select 20 male and female university students for the benchmark dataset. Fig. (**5**) represents the same.

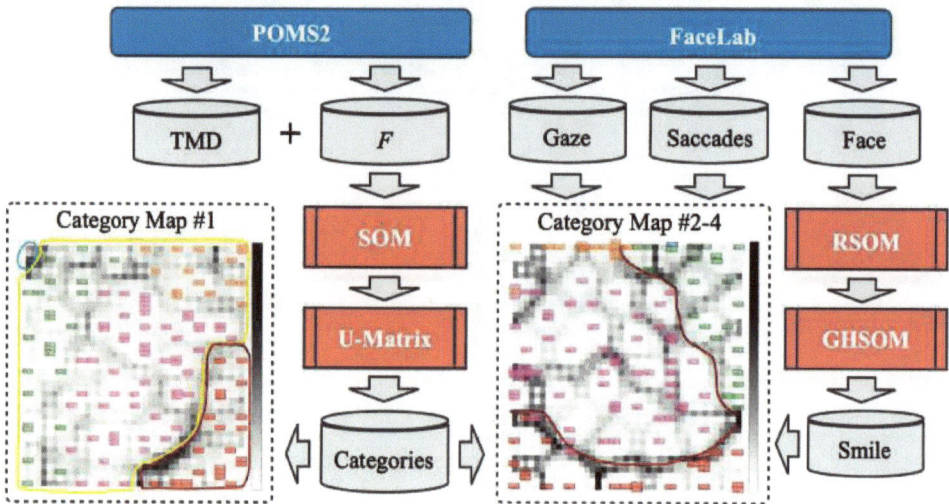

Fig. (5). Structure and data flow of the proposed method [5].

An intelligent home visual analysis system [6] assists analysts in recognizing and comprehending unusual resident behaviors and making intelligent health information predictions. The system uses a variety of characteristics derived from the daily activities recorded by sensor devices in an innovative home environment and an appropriate unsupervised anomaly detection algorithm to identify unusual behavior patterns among the residents of this environment. The data set includes information about an adult living in a smart home that was gathered by various sensors. The system looks at 30 activities performed by residents and groups them according to the methods described above. It chooses which actions can be used to calculate anomalies by filtering them based on their features. The Gantt Chart depicts the beginning and duration of daily activities performed by residents.

The Sehaa system [7] identifies the most prevalent health conditions and symptoms. The system's design and methodology are universally applicable. Using a Twitter streaming API and a set of predetermined parameters, it captures and downloads public tweet messages from Saudi Arabia. These parameters are the language (Arabic), location, and a set of search keywords that represent health symptoms and diseases. The acquired data are cleaned and pre-processed in the pre-processing module to ensure their readiness for the learning, classification, and prediction phases. It separates the dataset into testing datasets and training datasets. Arabic does not have a lexicon or libraries that it can use for machine learning. It used a filter based on keywords to gather the tweets. It ensured that it generated tweets from Saudi Arabia by filtering them according to their geographical location. The stream listener extracted the tweets from within the defined bounding box. It incorporated the two filters described above into the stream listener utilizing a Python function written with the Tweepy library. The goal of classification in machine learning is to use the rules created during the learning or training phase to predict a category, class, or label for a given set of input data. The class boundaries are well-defined in the training data, and the label values are already known. It learns how to predict the labels for the data that it will provide in the future. The classifier uses the labeled data to generate the classification rules during the learning phase. Fig. (6) represents the same.

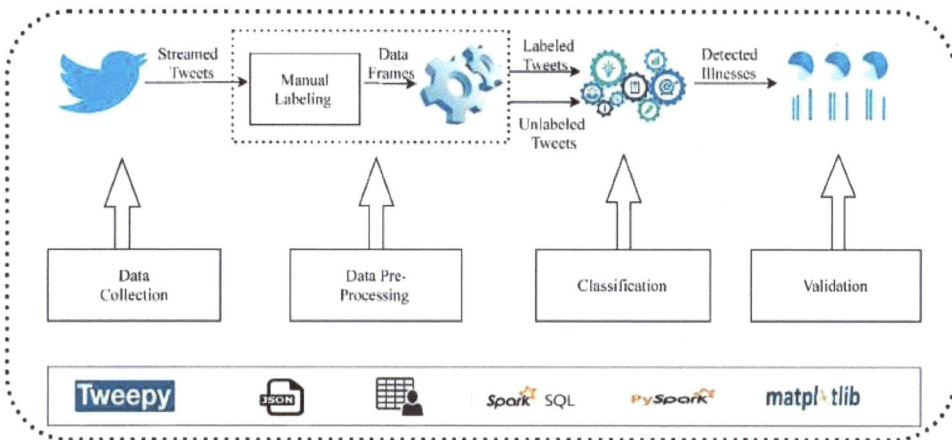

Fig. (6). Proposed Architecture [7].

It is [8] made up of various tools that meet the specific requirements of particular applications and the requirements of the domain. The framework's tools put the needs of the customer first and ensure that the needs of the customer come first. Participatory design is the first essential tool for designing the framework. It refers to stakeholder's active participation. During designing the framework, patients should exercise active patient care because feedback from patients can enhance the system as a whole and fill in any gaps that may be present. As a result, the patient's feedback is crucial. When patients draft the recommender framework, they remember well-being-related issues, not deals and promoting by drug organizations, because these frameworks can turn into their associates assisting them with defeating medical problems that are influential for them. The most requested part is to estimate a current system to permit the enormous scope investment of patients and specialists. Without the direct intervention of doctors, these tools may aid in treatment. The main issue with recommender systems is maintaining data privacy and security with HRS. Communication that is adequate and appropriate is the third tool to incorporate. The recommender system's goal should be addressed by data visualization, as should the ability to comprehend patients, doctors, and their intentions. The RBM is an artificial neural network that learns a probability distribution over a set of inputs and is generative stochastic. There is a visible layer and a hidden layer to this two-layer neural network—the discrete ratings of 10,000 patients from 500 hospitals in this healthcare dataset range from 1 to 5. Fig. (**7**) represents the same.

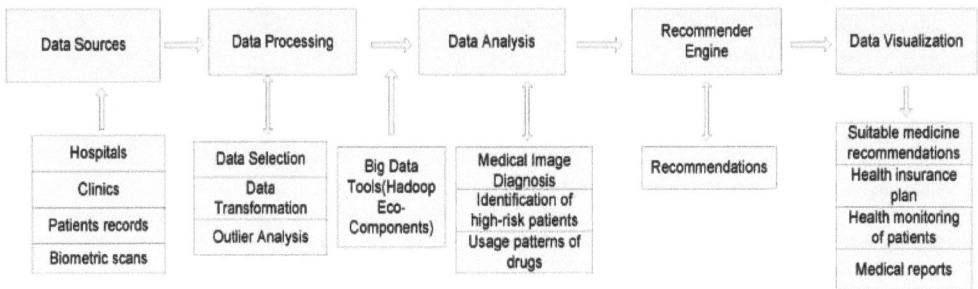

Fig. (7). Proposed framework [8].

The selected sensor kit and a home WiFi router must be installed as part of the AAL system [9]. It ensures that all sensors receive the best signal. The WiFi router is positioned in the center of the house. The "point of passage" of the house, typically the main corridor, is where the motion sensor is installed. The entryway sensor is conveyed at the main entrance of the home. According to the pilot installations, a full deployment typically takes 45 to 60 minutes. The CC3220 System on Chip from Texas Instruments serves as all device's microcontrollers and network processors. This device is optimized for low-power operation and is a Wi-Fi-certified product that provides IoT networking security, device identity, and keys. With industry-standard, optimized BSD sockets, the certified stack uses IPv4 and IPv6 protocols and is protected by SSL/TLS. The MQTT communication protocol, a lightweight and data-independent protocol, sends data from the sensors to the local server. MQTT supports a variety of Quality Service levels and relies on a broker for data exchange between publishers and subscribers. Under the direction of the local health authority, general practitioners in Italy's Emilia-Romagna region recruited participants for this study. Fig. (**8**) represents the same.

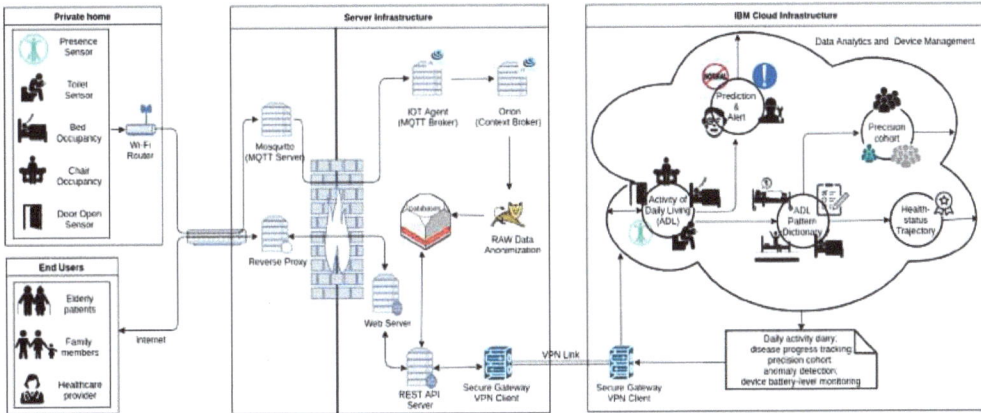

Fig. (8). Proposed framework [9].

The work [10] describes the method used to create the deep learning-based complex human activity identification. It includes orientation invariance methods and the theoretical concept of the proposed deep-stacked autoencoder. Due to signal degradation or signal variation generated during each subject's activities, raw signal sensor data collected using smartphones and other wearable devices are corrupted by noise and missing values. Filtering techniques are necessary to get rid of low-frequency data, correct sensor dimension geometric bias, and improve the correlation between each data point. The autoencoder algorithm is suggested for complex human activity identification with acceleration sensor data. The deep-stacked autoencoder technique is simple to develop and use. A generative feature learning technique known as deep autoencoder-based deep learning produces copies of the input values as outputs. The input, encoding, decoding, and output layers make up the deep autoencoder. The encoding layer transforms the smartphone device's sensor streams into hidden features. The decoding layer then reconstructs the transform input features to approximate values to reduce reconstruction errors. The sparse autoencoder is an unsupervised deep learning technique that uses the sparsity term. It models the loss function and sets some active units to zero to learn over-complete feature representation from raw sensor data. During dataset collection, ten subjects engaged in thirteen activities while attaching Samsung Galaxy S2 smartphones to their wrists and pockets. Jogging, walking, standing, sitting, biking, ascending, and descending stairs are all three-minute activities. In addition, each student engaged in various other activities, including eating, typing, writing, smoking, drinking coffee, and delivering three to five-minute talks. Fig. (**9**) represents the same.

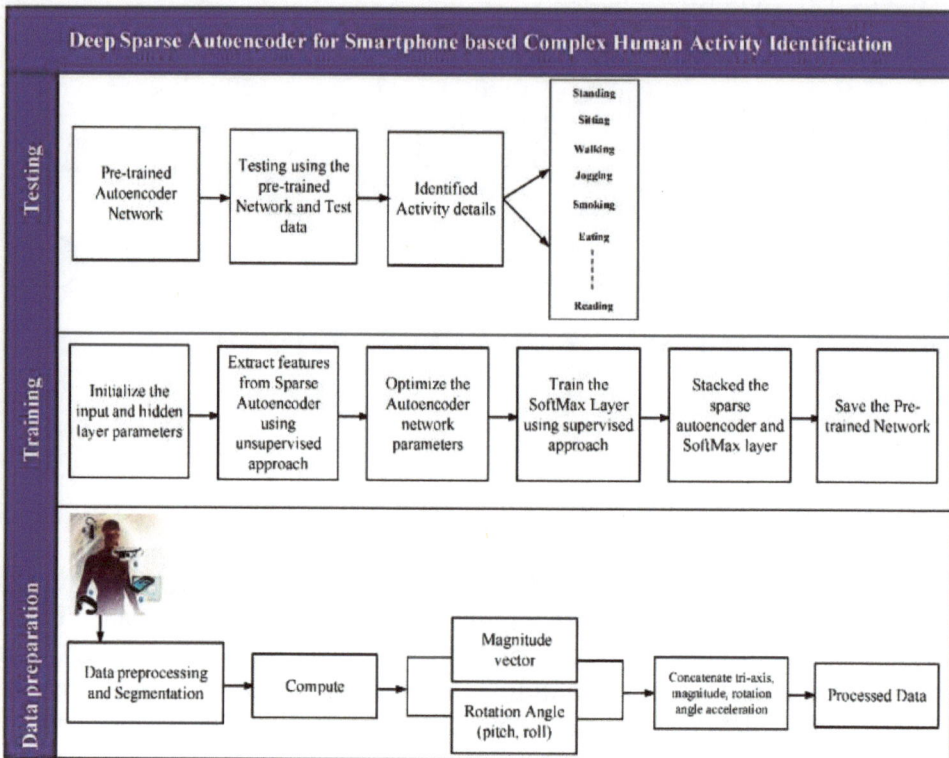

Fig. (9). Proposed framework [10].

A substantial healthcare database [11] containing patient-level self-reported outcomes following knee replacement surgery is the subject of this investigation. The study employs cluster analysis on an important, nationally representative dataset routinely collected from all participating UK-based NHS patients undergoing knee replacement surgery. To identify patient pain patterns and subgroups of patients with distinct outcomes based on their pain characteristics, a model based on unsupervised machine learning techniques like k-means and hierarchical clustering is proposed. Every patient with a knee replacement is asked to fill out a questionnaire with 12 questions about their knee pain and functional ability over the past four weeks. A Likert scale of 0 to 4 is used to score the responses. Patient's OKS responses are gathered from them six months after and within four weeks of their knee replacement. From the PROMs database,

It extracted OKS records about knee replacement for 2012–2016. The analysis included 126,064 complete-case records of knee replacement patients. It utilized the OKS that patients reported six months after surgery.

The deep model [12] can combine feature representation and learning into a single model, simulating human thought processes. A modified version of convolutional deep belief networks is utilized for large-scale data sets as an efficient training strategy. A DBN is assumed to be a neural network with numerous hidden layers. A conditional Gaussian distribution is utilized for pair-wise training between the input layer and hidden layer nodes. It performs layer-wise preparation between the information layer, the closest hidden layer, and other contiguous secret layers. Increasing the number of hidden layers can produce various feature representations of the original features. It can adjust the network parameters in a supervised manner after the network has been trained to create multiple feature representations. Two data sets are used to test the proposed algorithm. The first data set from an electronic medical record is a clinical set (D1). It documents senior doctor's treatment plans, symptoms, and personal and disease history. The information was physically input and recorded with common findings of ICD10 by certificated clinical specialists. Nine hundred-eight hypertension patient records are included in the second data set (D2), retrieved from HIS. Each document contains 167 features, including 22 laboratory indicators, 16 common indexes, 129 symptoms from inspection, auscultation and olfaction, inquiry and palpation, and other methods.

Unsupervised work [13] is used for both representation learning and anomaly detection. There are two main steps: portrayal, education, and discovery. It uses a Variational Recurrent Autoencoder as its learning model. The model reads an input time series with timesteps. The model is compelled to reconstruct the initial input due to the corruption at the input level. A bidirectional long short-term memory organization parametrizes the encoder. It processes the info time series and produces a succession of stowed-away states in the two headings. The encoder's final hidden states during the forward and backward passes. The Variational Bi-LSTM Autoencoder model's representations serve as the basis for the anomaly detection process. The representation learning model teaches itself how to map input data sequences with various patterns into various parts of the space. It employs three distinct approaches. Unsupervised clustering is applied to the latent representations in the approximate posterior mean area as part of the clustering-based detection strategy to locate the clusters that best describe the data's normal and abnormal classes. The algorithms for clustering were set to create two groups, one for each category. The results of these algorithms are matched with the standard and abnormal classes by choosing the cluster with the most data points to be the normal one. It implemented the models using the

TensorFlow backend and the Keras deep learning library. A variant of Adam, the AMS-Grad optimizer, was used for training. On a computer with an i7 8th generation processor and 16GB of DDR4 RAM, training was carried out on an NVIDIA GTX 1080TI graphics processing unit with 11GB of memory. The dataset is the ECG5000, which was given to the UCR Time Series Classification archive by Eamonn Keogh and Yanping Chen. It is accessible to the general public.

4.2. CLUSTERING

The unlabeled dataset is grouped using a machine-learning technique called clustering [14] or cluster analysis. It accomplishes this by locating similar patterns in the unlabeled dataset, such as behavior, shape, size, and color, and dividing them according to whether similar ways are present. It is an unaided learning technique. Thus, no oversight is given to the calculation, and it manages the unlabeled dataset. After applying this bunching strategy, each group or gathering is furnished with a bunch ID. An ML system can use this id to simplify the processing of large and complex datasets. When analyzing statistical data, the clustering method is frequently employed.

A novel machine learning-based approach [15] to maximizing medical benefits in healthcare settings is presented in this work. It is broken up into three cascading steps: mapping and clustering are used to create a need-based package, medical benefits are calculated using the packages, and data-driven analysis uses a probability distribution to estimate the amount. It analyzes transactional data using a category-based approach. The centroid for each cluster is found. The distance between each computed centroid and all records in the category is calculated. Based on these calculated distances, all categorie's documents are added to the distance between centroids; Each cluster is given to a patient. All records maintain the same values for the number of visits and amount. All the centroids go through the same procedure. The JAVA programming language is used to implement the proposed approach in Eclipse. Fig. (**10**) represents the same.

The central idea of the proposed architecture [16] is that clustering can be used to share content. CCN and NV form the basis of the architecture. Hash functions identify users with a common interest and are then organized into clusters using the proposed multifactor algorithm. Fuzzy optimization, which helps optimize clustering and other cellular network parameters, is used to optimize the clustering algorithm. It is the responsibility of the cluster head (CH) in each cluster to multicast the necessary information to its members. All content requests from any given set pass through the CH after clustering and D2D communication

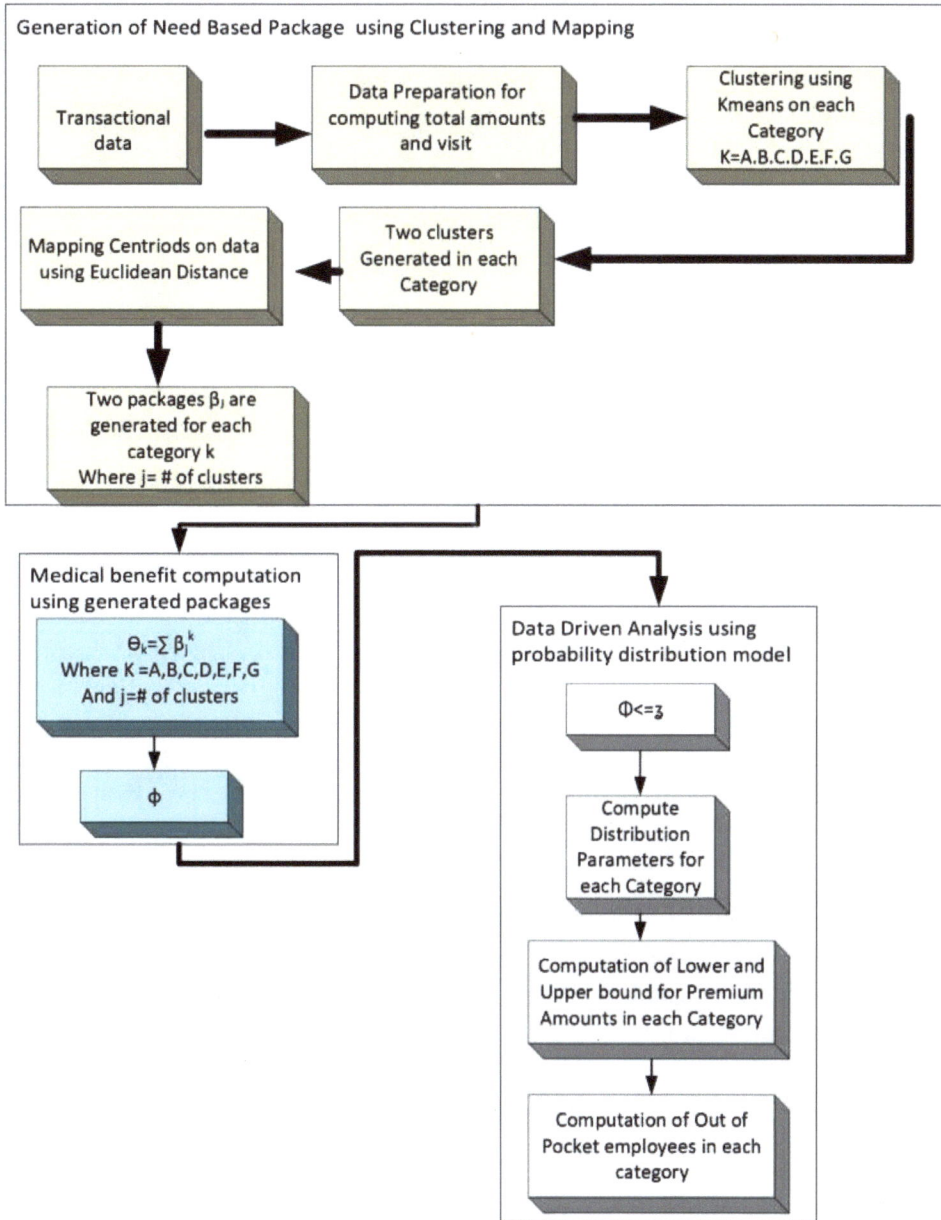

Fig. (10). Proposed Method [15].

serves users through the CH. Virtualization of networks and Content-Centric Networking are two components of the proposed architecture. Without the information of the host that holds that content, a mobile user requests certain content. The caching server is yet another significant component of the proposed architecture. It is an essential network component because it caches popular content and reduces transmission duplication. The social ties between various user groups are represented by the first layer, which is referred to as the social layer. The mobile devices that model communication in different clusters represented by a CH are represented by the physical layer. It demonstrates the infrastructure that supports communication and content delivery. Hash functions carry out the mapping between the given data and a particular length hash. Once users who want the same content are found, clustering begins. There are three main steps to the user clustering process:

- Determination of proper grouping measurements.
- Distinguishing proof of the gadgets reasonable for being a CH.
- Partnering the bunch of individuals with their separate CHs.

Each frame is used to choose CHs. During a single frame, the nodes remain in the same position. However, because the distribution and placement of users change for the subsequent frame, each simulation represents a distinct distribution of users. The algorithm creates clusters by compiling data on the clustering metrics following initialization. CHs announce the members of its collection. It is presumed that the CH can simultaneously identify multiple users. All members listen to the CH's broadcasts and become attached to the one that serves them best, considering distance and channel conditions. The discovery signals are received by users who are close to one another. This signal contains information such as the device or user ID and its link characteristics with the user. Devices decode it. There is a weight assigned to each factor. It used MATLAB to create the simulation platform. Fig. (**11**) represents the same.

There are two stages to the proposed procedure [17]. The setup phase is where cluster head selection and cluster formation occur, while the steady-state phase is where data transmission occurs. The node with the highest probability is chosen as the head of the cluster. At first, the optimal number of members and groups is determined. It solicits nominations for the position of cluster head. Each network node sends out a message to its neighbors. The base station saves all of the data it collects. When a node in the network recognizes an event, it sends data to the cluster head, which then sends the data to the base station. The cluster head and nodes use reinforcement learning to determine the most energy-efficient route for data transmission to the base station. It reduces network traffic and prevents the early death of cluster heads. The sink estimates the new position of the node and assigns it as a member node to a new cluster whenever a member of the node leaves the cluster region. The proposed algorithm's performance is evaluated using MATLAB. Fig. (**12**) represents the same.

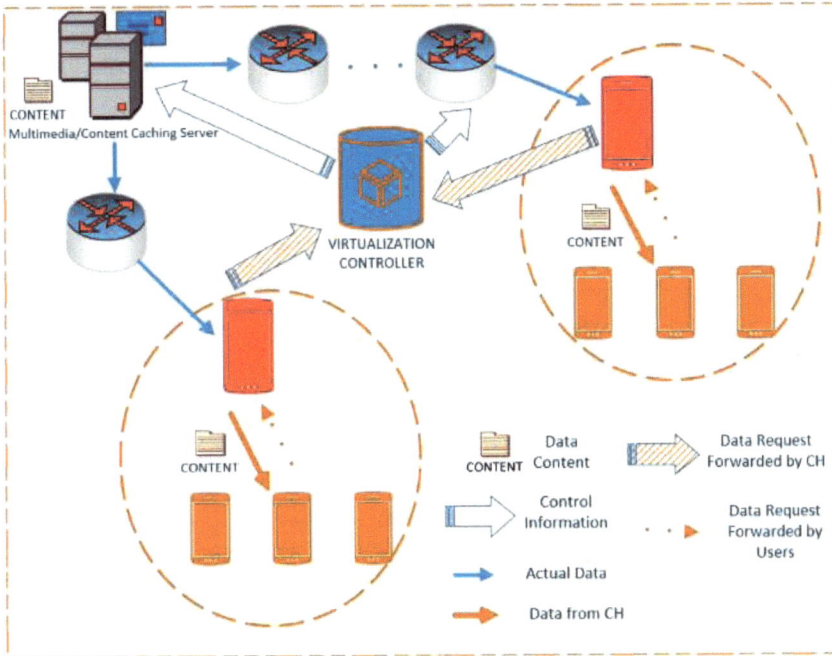

Fig. (11). Proposed Architecture [16].

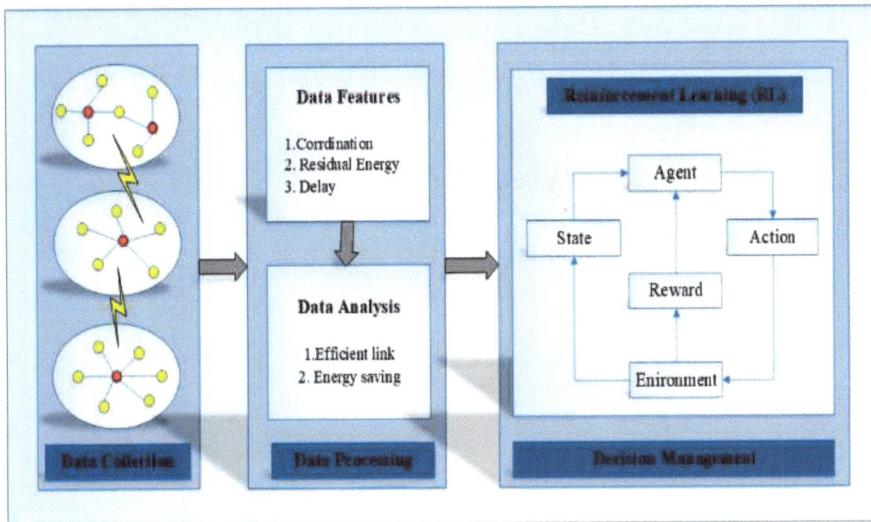

Fig. (12). Data processing framework [17].

Healthcare systems record each diabetic patient's examinations and their dates. There are three significant steps in discovering knowledge [18] - data preparation, learning new information, and evaluating the outcomes that lead to knowledge discovery depending on the data preparation steps. The extracted knowledge is considered during the results evaluation step. Medical professionals assessed the results following medical guidelines, and the evaluation index is used following the applied data mining technique. The experiments were carried out on a computer with 8 GB of RAM and a 3 GHz Dual-Core Intel Core i7 processor. It used the Java programming language to implement the data mining methods. Fig. (**13**) represents the same.

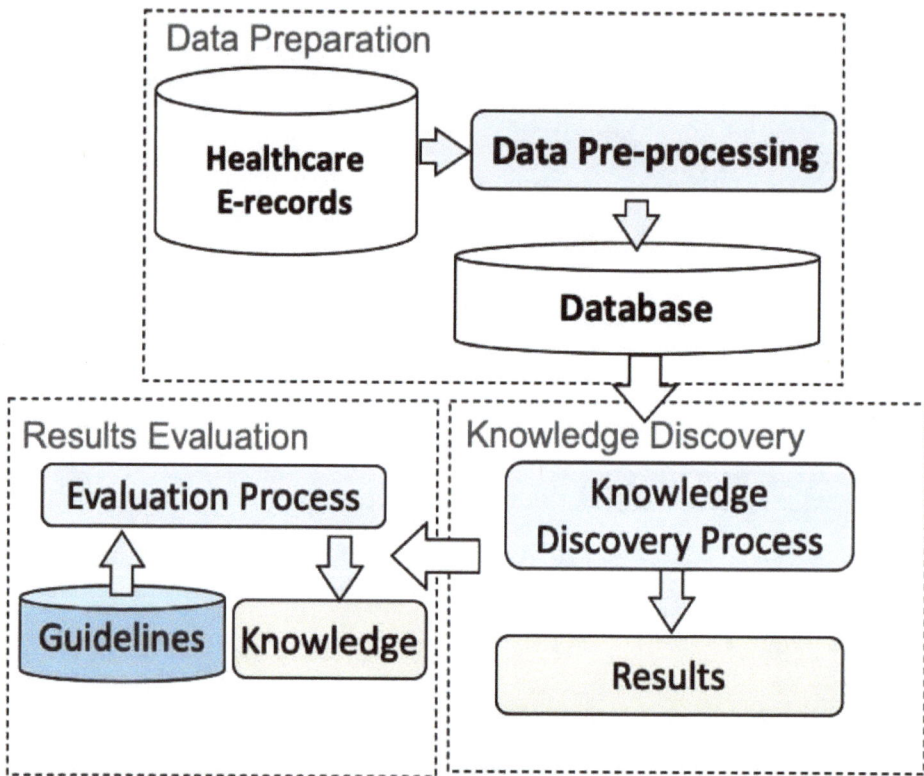

Fig. (13). Discovering knowledge from healthcare data [18].

4.3. DRAWBACKS

When patients have yet to receive adequate training, specimen collection alone does not provide the same diagnostic performance as healthcare professionals.

According to the Cochrane COVID-19 Diagnostic Test Accuracy Group, rapid point of care (POC) molecular or antigenic assays does not provide comparable diagnostic performance to routine, laboratory-based tests. Another potential limitation is insufficient quality assurance throughout the entire POC testing process.

One of the most crucial downsides of chest X-beam examination is their inability to perceive Coronavirus in its beginning stages because of an absence of responsiveness while performing GGO recognition. On the other hand, well-trained deep learning models can focus on details that the human eye misses, potentially reversing this view. Unsupervised learning has been used in various ways with RNNs, including the LSTM and GRUs approaches. Its primary drawbacks are its computational complexity of unsupervised learning and its inability to provide precise data sorting information.

CONCLUSION

The ability of both supervised and unsupervised learning algorithms to acquire knowledge from large data sets has been demonstrated to be very promising. An algorithm's ability to generalize knowledge from available data with the target or labeled cases to predict new (unlabeled) issues is reflected in supervised learning. The process of grouping data into clusters using automated methods or algorithms on data that has not been classified or categorized is referred to as unsupervised learning. Algorithms must, in this case, "learn" the underlying relationships or characteristics from the available data and group cases with similar characteristics or features. The learning is referred to as "semi-supervised" when only a small amount of labeled data is available. These algorithms can solve many health-related problems by analyzing the datasets.

REFERENCES

[1]   T. Gittler, S. Scholze, A. Rupenyan, and K. Wegener, "Machine tool component health identification with unsupervised learning", *J. Manuf. Mater. Process,* vol. 4, no. 3, p. 86, 2020.
[http://dx.doi.org/10.3390/jmmp4030086]

[2]   C. Vununu, S.H. Lee, and K.R. Kwon, "A strictly unsupervised deep learning method for hep-2 cell image classification", *Sensors,* vol. 20, no. 9, p. 2717, 2020.
[http://dx.doi.org/10.3390/s20092717] [PMID: 32397567]

[3]   V. Koshman, A. Funkner, and S. Kovalchuk, "An unsupervised approach to structuring and analyzing repetitive semantic structures in free text of electronic medical records", *J. Pers. Med.,* vol. 12, no. 1, p. 25, 2022.
[http://dx.doi.org/10.3390/jpm12010025] [PMID: 35055340]

[4]   K.S. Arikumar, S.B. Prathiba, M. Alazab, T.R. Gadekallu, S. Pandya, J.M. Khan, and R.S. Moorthy, "FL-PMI: Federated learning-based person movement identification through wearable devices in smart healthcare systems", *Sensors,* vol. 22, no. 4, p. 1377, 2022.

[http://dx.doi.org/10.3390/s22041377] [PMID: 35214282]

[5]   H. Madokoro, S. Nix, and K. Sato, "Visualization and semantic labeling of mood states based on time-series features of eye gaze and facial expressions by unsupervised learning", *Healthcare,* vol. 10, no. 8, p. 1493, 2022.
[http://dx.doi.org/10.3390/healthcare10081493] [PMID: 36011150]

[6]   Z. Liao, L. Kong, X. Wang, Y. Zhao, F. Zhou, Z. Liao, and X. Fan, "A visual analytics approach for detecting and understanding anomalous resident behaviors in smart healthcare", *Appl. Sci.,* vol. 7, no. 3, p. 254, 2017.
[http://dx.doi.org/10.3390/app7030254]

[7]   S. Alotaibi, R. Mehmood, I. Katib, O. Rana, and A. Albeshri, "Sehaa: A big data analytics tool for healthcare symptoms and diseases detection using twitter, apache spark, and machine learning", *Appl. Sci.,* vol. 10, no. 4, p. 1398, 2020.
[http://dx.doi.org/10.3390/app10041398]

[8]   A.K. Sahoo, C. Pradhan, R.K. Barik, and H. Dubey, "DeepReco: Deep learning based health recommender system using collaborative filtering", *Comput.,* vol. 7, no. 2, p. 25, 2019.
[http://dx.doi.org/10.3390/computation7020025]

[9]   R. Hu, B. Michel, D. Russo, N. Mora, G. Matrella, P. Ciampolini, F. Cocchi, E. Montanari, S. Nunziata, and T. Brunschwiler, "An unsupervised behavioral modeling and alerting system based on passive sensing for elderly care", *Future Internet,* vol. 13, no. 1, p. 6, 2020.
[http://dx.doi.org/10.3390/fi13010006]

[10]   U.R. Alo, H.F. Nweke, Y.W. Teh, and G. Murtaza, "Smartphone motion sensor-based complex human activity identification using deep stacked autoencoder algorithm for enhanced smart healthcare system", *Sensors,* vol. 20, no. 21, p. 6300, 2020.
[http://dx.doi.org/10.3390/s20216300] [PMID: 33167424]

[11]   S. Khalid, A. Judge, and R. Pinedo-Villanueva, An unsupervised learning model for pattern recognition in routinely collected healthcare data.*Nuffield Dept. of Orthopaedics, Rheumatology & Musculoskeletal Sciences* University of Oxford: Oxford, U.K., 2018.

[12]   Z. Liang, G. Zhang, J.X. Huang, and Q.V. Hu, "Deep learning for healthcare decision making with EMRs", In: *IEEE International Conference on Bioinformatics and Biomedicine (BIBM)* Belfast: UK, 2014.
[http://dx.doi.org/10.1109/BIBM.2014.6999219]

[13]   J. Pereira, and M. Silveira, Learning representations from healthcare time series data for unsupervised anomaly detection.*IEEE International Conference on Big Data and Smart Computing (BigComp)* Kyoto: Japan, 2019.
[http://dx.doi.org/10.1109/BIGCOMP.2019.8679157]

[14]   E.H. Ruspini, "A new approach to clustering", *Inf. Control,* vol. 15, no. 1, pp. 22-32, 1969.
[http://dx.doi.org/10.1016/S0019-9958(69)90591-9]

[15]   I. Matloob, S.A. Khan, F. Hussain, W.H. Butt, R. Rukaiya, and F. Khalique, "Need-based and optimized health insurance package using clustering algorithm", *Appl. Sci.,* vol. 11, no. 18, p. 8478, 2021.
[http://dx.doi.org/10.3390/app11188478]

[16]   S. Aslam, F. Alam, S.F. Hasan, and M. Rashid, "A novel weighted clustering algorithm supported by a distributed architecture for D2D enabled content-centric networks", *Sensors,* vol. 20, no. 19, p. 5509, 2020.
[http://dx.doi.org/10.3390/s20195509] [PMID: 32993039]

[17]   A. Ahad, M. Tahir, M.A. Sheikh, K.I. Ahmed, and A. Mughees, "An intelligent clustering-based routing protocol (CRP-GR) for 5G-based smart healthcare using game theory and reinforcement learning", *Appl. Sci.,* vol. 11, no. 21, p. 9993, 2021.
[http://dx.doi.org/10.3390/app11219993]

[18]   N.A. Mahoto, A. Shaikh, M.S. Al Reshan, M.A. Memon, and A. Sulaiman, "Knowledge discovery from healthcare electronic records for sustainable environment", *Sustainability,* vol. 13, no. 16, p. 8900, 2021.
[http://dx.doi.org/10.3390/su13168900]

CHAPTER 5

Role of Internet-of-Things During Covid-19

Abstract: In December 2019, the severe acute respiratory syndrome coronavirus 2 (SARS-CoV-2) infection that caused pneumonia spread to Wuhan City, Hubei Province, China. Fever, dry cough, and fatigue are typical clinical manifestations of COVID-19, frequently accompanied by pulmonary involvement. SARS-CoV-2 is highly contagious, making most people in the general population susceptible to infection. One of the most popular technologies, the Internet of Things (IoT), has much potential for combating the coronavirus outbreak. It has transformed real-world objects into sophisticated virtual ones. The Internet of Things (IoT) aims to connect everything in our world and assist users in controlling the objects in their immediate vicinity and keeping them informed of their current state. IoT devices sense the environment without human or machine interaction and send the gathered data to the Internet cloud. Tens of millions of devices are connected *via* the Internet of Things (IoT), and the number of connected devices is rapidly increasing.

The chapter aims to highlight the role of IoT devices in detecting Covid-19. It details the different architectures of the system. Various domains, like the role of machines in healthcare, transportation, entertainment, retailing, and education, are detailed. It addresses challenges - awareness, accessibility, human power crisis, affordability, and accountability. Some of the future directions managed including edge architecture, cryptography, blockchain, machine learning, digital twin, unified network integration, context-aware accessibility, edge and fog computing, and sensor and actuator integration are summarized.

Keywords: Coronavirus 2, Covid-19, Detection, IoT, Prevention, SARS-CoV-2.

5.1. INTRODUCTION

Due to its significance in numerous applications in education, industry, and commerce, Internet of Things research looks promising. The process of connecting machines, equipment, software and things in our environment is what the Internet is all about. Instead of thinking of the Internet as a collection of connected computing devices, it is now thought of as a collection of related things in a person's living space, like machines, transportation, goods, business storage, and home appliances, among other things. The living space contains more objects than the entire human population. An item in the Internet of Things [1] should have a unique address for each component. The technology known as radio-frequency identification (RFID) is used for communication. There should be a way for IoT [2] to determine its users are and their rights and restrictions. Fig. (1) portrays the applications of IoT.

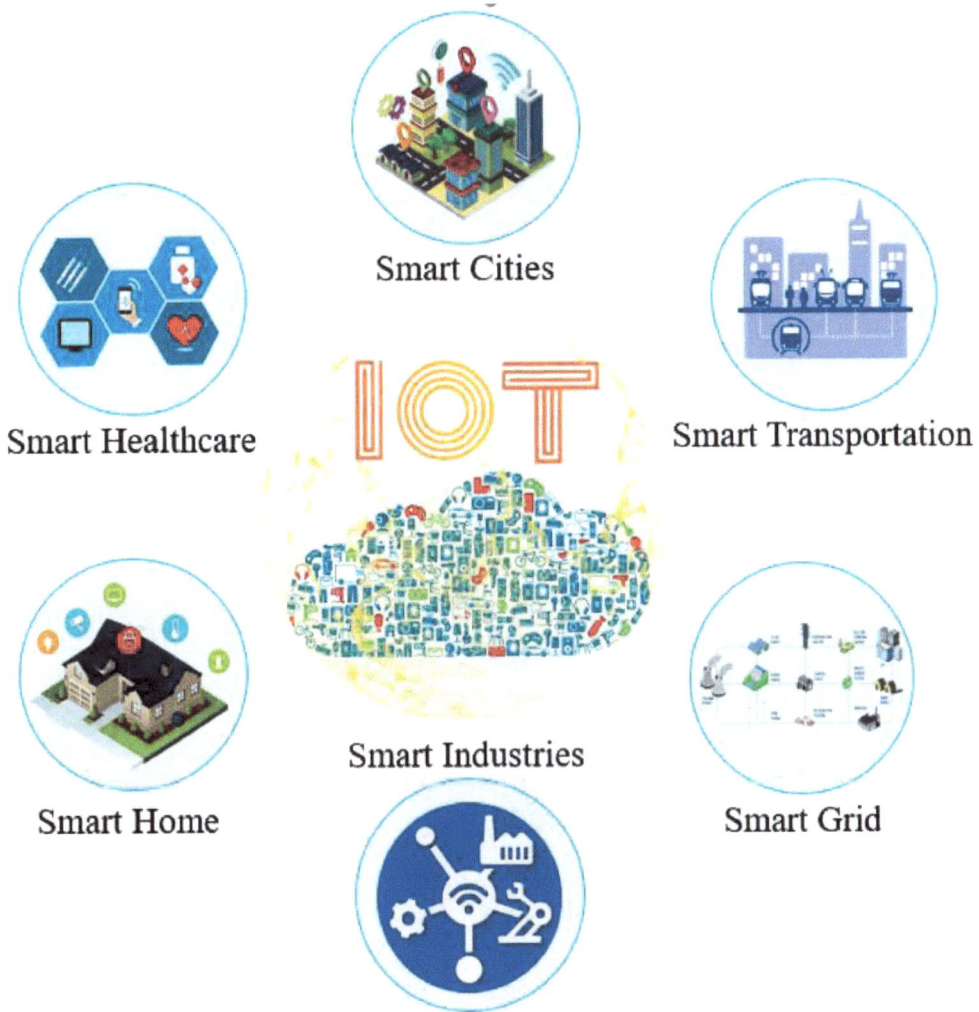

Fig. (1). IoT-based applications [3].

5.2. ARCHITECTURE

The term "Internet of Things" (IoT) [4] refers to a system of devices that are connected, have computing power (smart objects), can be identified, and can transfer data over a network without the need for human interaction. To be incorporated into everyday objects, IoT [5, 6] requires a few components. The incorporation of silicon components into metallic or fabric materials has the potential to broaden the field of component miniaturization and integration. Fig. (**2**) represents the 3-tier architecture of IoT.

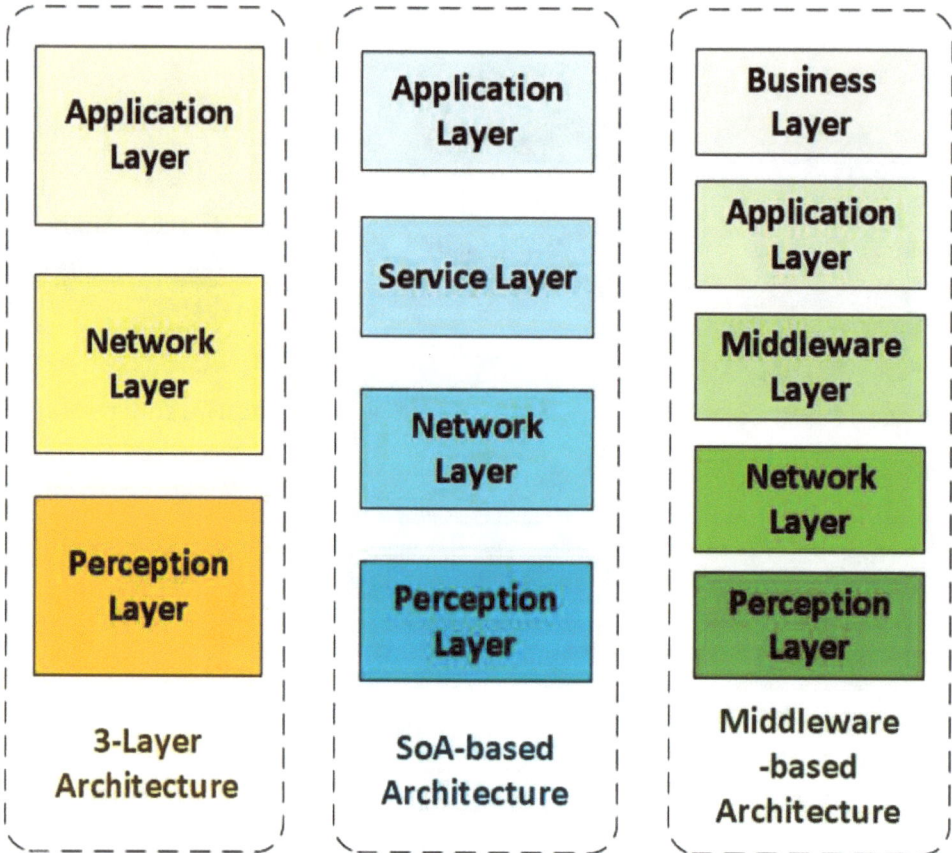

Fig. (2). - 3-tier Architecture [7].

The perception layer collects and processes information to interact with the environment and represents the physical level of objects. This level has things that can communicate with the outside world. The data provided by the perception level must be transported to the application layer by the network layer. It includes all of the protocols and technologies that enable this connection. The software required to provide a particular service is all contained in the application layer. Databases, analysis software, *etc.*, that are used to store, aggregate, filter, and process the data from previous levels at this level are in use. Fig. (**2**) portrays the same.

The component-model-based service-oriented architecture (SoA) can be designed to connect various functional units of applications through interfaces and protocols. It can coordinate services and reuse software and hardware components with SoA. By adding a new layer between the application layer and the network layer, known as the service layer, which provides services to support the application layer, It can easily integrate SoA into the IoT architecture.

Software or service programming, known as middleware, can be an abstraction between IoT applications and technologies. Middleware hides the specifics of various technologies and provides standard interfaces so that developers can concentrate on developing applications without worrying about whether applications and infrastructures are compatible.

Given the aging of the global population, the study [8] of systems and architectures for ambient assisted living (AAL) is undoubtedly a topic of great relevance. The XBee module implements the ZigBee networking protocol and the IEEE 802.15.4 radio. It is used to carry out wireless communication. The physical and medium access control layers for low data-rate wireless personal area networks are outlined in the IEEE 802.15.4 standard. Based on 802.15.4, ZigBee is a low-cost, low-power wireless mesh networking standard. XBee sends signals from the iAQ Sensor to the iAQ Gateway base station. Outdoor Radio Frequency line-of-sight ranges up to 4000 ft, and RF data rates up to 250,000 bps are supported by the modules, which operate in the 2.4 GHz frequency band. The iAQ system is an automatic indoor air quality monitoring system that gives the user, like the building manager, real-time information about a variety of environmental parameters, like the temperature of the air, the relative humidity, the concentrations of carbon monoxide, carbon dioxide (CO_2), and luminosity. The iAQ Sensor system is used to monitor the parameters. It gathers data and sends it to the iAQ Gateway system, which stores it in a MySQL database using web services made with Hypertext Preprocessor. The end user can access the data through the PHP-based web portal iAQ Web. After logging in, the end user can access the iAQ Web and all environmental parameter information. The system assists the user in conducting precise and in-depth analyses of air quality behavior. Fig. (**3**) portrays the same.

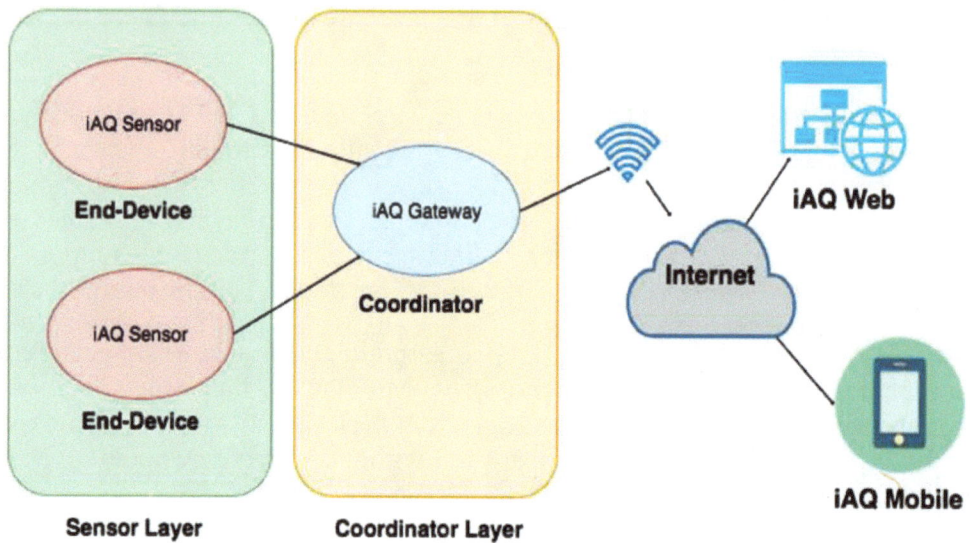

Fig. (3). WSN architecture [8].

The edge nodes [9] only have a limited amount of storage and processing power. Edge nodes offer low latency and bandwidth consumption and act as a centralized server for real-time response to inquiries. Edge nodes contain participant's signature keys and access control mechanisms. The sensed data are first gathered at a gateway for pre-processing and filtering. The optimal number of components is then determined using the broken stick rule and principal component analysis. Smart contracts respond, control, and generate alerts following the conditions by adhering to DIM's defined threshold limit values. The managers can inquire through the user interface, which is managed by a decentralized application for remote monitoring. Miner's nodes with a large storage capacity are in charge of creating new blocks, verifying proof-of-work, and storing smart contracts for autonomous decision-making in the core network. It implemented digital signatures and immutable hash functions to guarantee the integrity of the data in the core network. In the PoW mechanism, a miner node collects all pending transactions and iteratively hashes the collected data and their hashes after hashing them in the Merkle tree. This iterative hashing process continues until the transaction hash equals or falls below a specified target value that serves as a threshold. Windows 10 was used to run all of the simulation tests on a 3.90 GHz Intel Core i5 processor. Fig. (**4**) portrays the same.

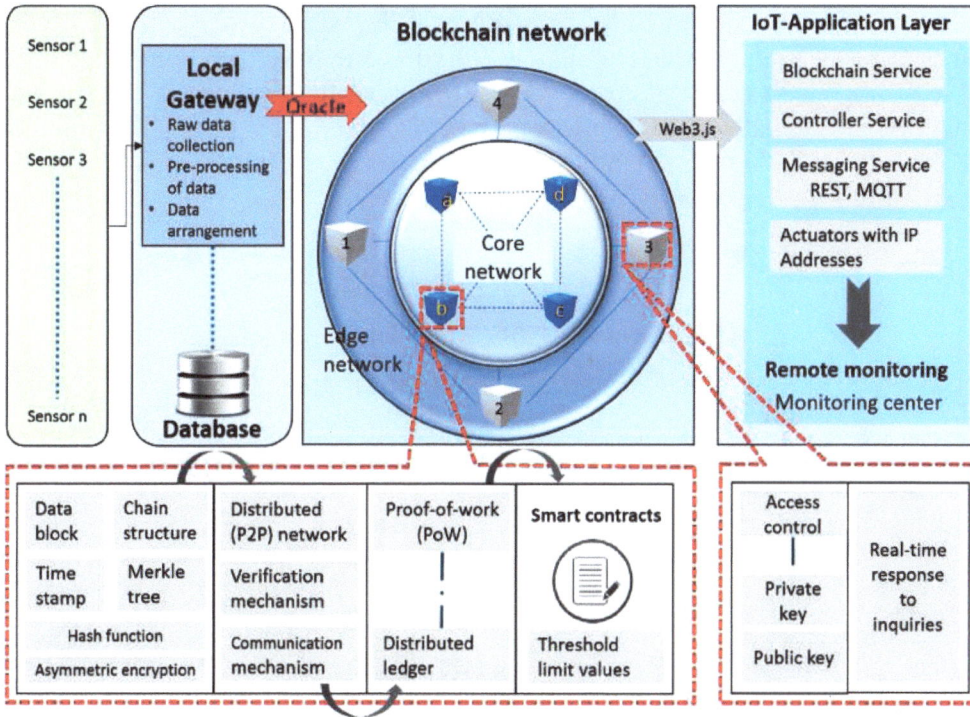

Fig. (4). - Proposed Architecture [9].

Three subsystems make up the system's architecture [10]. There are two wearable sensor hubs regarding each matter: the Health Node for measuring physiological parameters and the Safe Node for environmental monitoring. The Wellbeing Hub includes:

- A BLE module is empowering WBAN correspondence.
- A PPG sensor for pulse checking.
- An internal heat level sensor.

The Safe Node has four environmental sensors to measure CO_2, UV, ambient temperature, and relative humidity. Two wireless modules in the Safe Node are LoRa for transmission in the LPWAN and BLE for communication within the WBAN. The Safe Node's BLE receives sensor data from the Health Node in the WBAN. This data will be sent *via* the LoRa network to a remote gateway. The transmission range limits BLE's ability to transmit data at a high rate and low power consumption. LoRa can transmit data over a significant distance with reduced data rates and increased power consumption. The gateway comprises a single Raspberry Pi, an Internet connection, and a LoRa module. The Safe Node sends data to the Pi connected to the LoRa module, which processes and stores it in a local MySQL database. The data is stored in the MySQL cloud database by the IoT cloud server after receiving it from the IoT gateway. The primary component of the gateway is the Raspberry Pi Model 3 B. With 2 GB of memory and 25 GB of disk space, Ubuntu 16.04.5 powers the cloud server. Fig. (**5**) portrays the same.

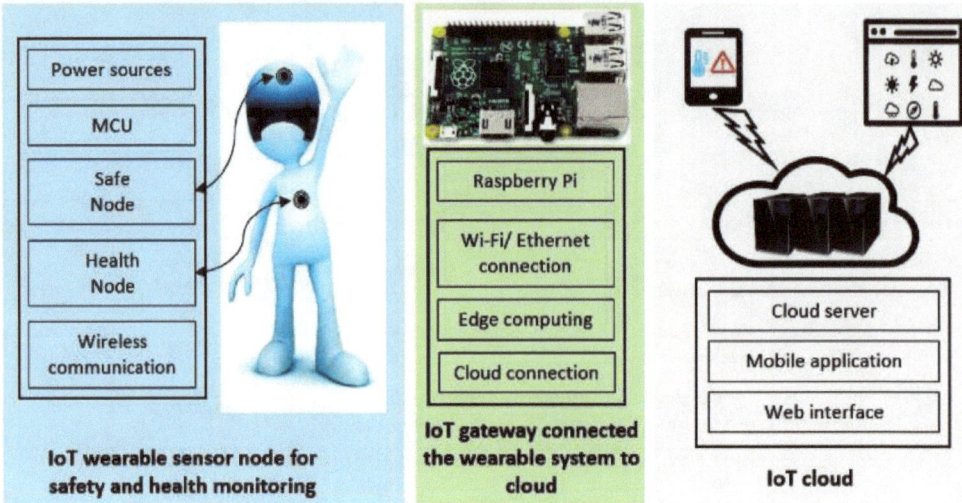

Fig. (5). - System Framework [10].

Data from multiple on-body and environmental sensors can be collected using the proposed architecture [11] to process and extract useful information about a patient's current state and the environment in which they live. Continuous data about vital signs is gathered by biomedical sensors, whose samples should be preserved. When compared to biomedical sensors, environmental sensors, on the other hand, obtain information less frequently. Preparing sensor node signals for storage, analysis, and presentation is part of the data acquisition layer. This system architecture collects data measurements on a remote server in the Cloud and a developed relational database. It utilizes social datasets. It is likewise conceivable to store the information in records or use NoSQL datasets that can, similarly to a social data set, live on a nearby server in the Cloud. SDN introduces a control plane to manage the actual transmission of user data and a data plane to implement logical network functions. An Application Programming Interface known as the southbound API serves as the interface between the two planes, while the northbound API is used by applications to access the control plane. The

SDN controller manages the control plane and defines network logic functions based on data plane status. Fig. (6) portrays the same.

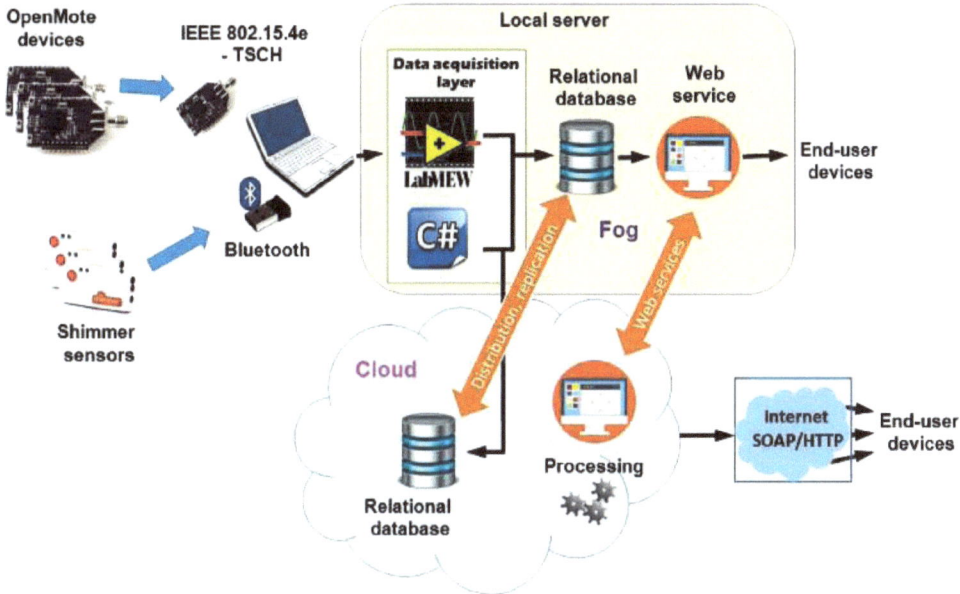

Fig. (6). - System Architecture [11].

This work [12] presents the AirPlus constant indoor ecological quality checking framework, which integrates a few benefits when contrasted with different frameworks, like versatility, adaptability, seclusion, simple establishment, and design, as well as portable figuring programming for information counseling and warnings. AirPlus supports data consulting and notifications on both the web and mobile devices. It utilizes web services. The monitored data is stored in a Microsoft SQL Server database. Using ASP.NET and Swift, a web portal called AirPlusWeb and an iOS mobile application called AirPlusMobile were developed for data consulting. The acquisition module is based on open-source technologies that offer modularity, scalability, low cost, and simple installation, among other benefits. The AirPlus consists of a microcontroller that supports Wi-Fi, a PM, temperature, humidity, and formaldehyde sensor module connected *via* the serial interface, and an ESP8266. Within the 2.4 GHz band, radio transmission is supported by the IEEE 802.11 standard. Two sections comprise the acquisition module - a PLANTOWER-developed PMS5003ST sensor and a microcontroller. The NodeM ESP8266 module, manufactured by WEMOS Electronics in China, incorporates 32 Mb of additional memory and the ESP8266 system on a chip. The module can be powered by 4-9 V DC thanks to its USB-TTL serial converter, CH340G, and micro-USB port. Digital 10 GPIOs, PWM functionality, I2C, SPI communication, 1-Wire, and one analog input are all included in the NodeM. The end user can use this hotspot to set up the Wi-Fi network to which the AirPlus will be connected. This functionality provides a significant advantage. The owner can easily install the system. The PMS5003ST is a sensor with multiple functions that can also measure temperature and humidity, and particle and formaldehyde concentration. This sensor can calculate the number of suspended particles in the air to provide particle concentration levels. This sensor generates scattering by utilizing a laser unit to radiate airborne suspended particles. Using.NET web services. The collected data are uploaded to the SQL Server database. Fig. (7) portrays the same.

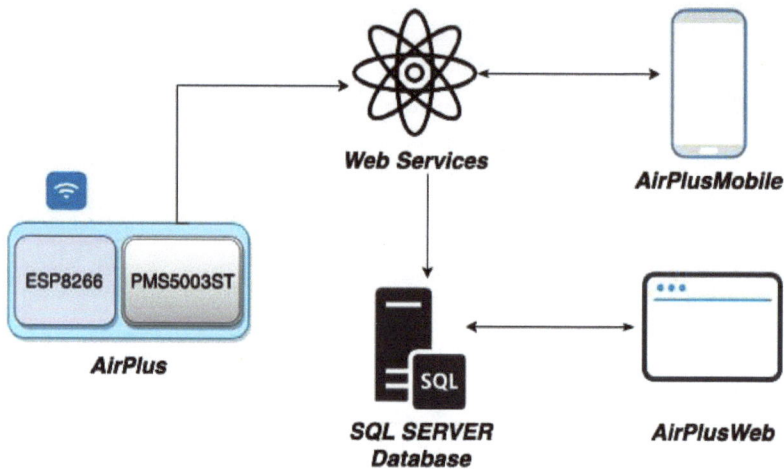

Fig. (7). - System Architecture [12].

iAirBot [13] is an Internet of Things-based assistive robot for monitoring indoor air quality. Social networks are used to automatically send alerts and communicate with building occupants. The caregiver can use the information to plan interventions for improved living environments quickly. The central node, also known as the concentrator, is referred to as the iAirNode Gateway, and it includes a WSN in the sensor node. The iAirNode Sensor, which receives data on air quality and transmits it to the iAirNode Gateway system, is used for parameter monitoring. The iAirBot computer is connected to the iAirNode Gateway *via* a USB interface. The iAirBot is in charge of the Facebook social network interface for sharing the web services-monitored data. The Facebook API software development kit (SDK) is implemented by these web services, which it developed in ASP.NET. Access to the page where the monitored data is published is made possible by this API. Sun Small Programmable Object Technology, or Sun SPOT, is the name of the platform that it used to build the sensor network. These sensor node's responsibility is to acquire data and transmit it *via* radio communication to the base station. The IEEE 802.15.4 standard determines the entrance control layers for remote correspondence in confidential regions. To browse, locate, and track individuals in indoor environments, the iAirBot includes a Kinect camera. Fig. (**8**) portrays the same.

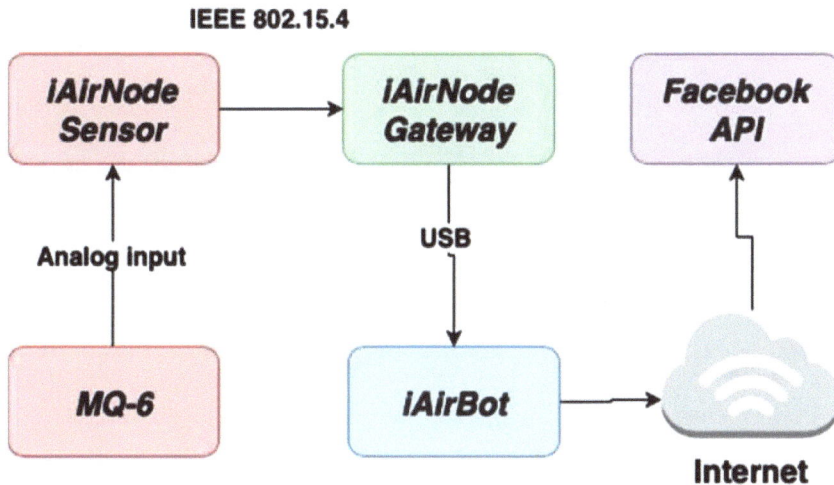

Fig. (8). - Monitoring Architecture [13].

5.3. ROLE OF IOT IN COVID-19

During the COVID-19 pandemic [15], one of the most critical industries that benefited from IoT-inspired solutions was healthcare. The respiratory system is affected by the SARS-CoV-2 virus, which causes COVID-19 [16, 17]. Through the Internet of Medical Things (IoMT), these sensors can track and monitor patient's breathing conditions and continuously inform the involved doctors of the patient's respiratory condition. It also saves time because the concerned doctors can easily make appropriate recommendations from a distance. Contact tracing has proven to be effective for protecting personal information and keeping people safe during the COVID-19 pandemic. Triax Proximity Trace is one example of a wearable light IoT device that uses contact tracing to combat social distance by alerting users when they get too close to one another. Without needing mobile phones or downloads, enterprise departments can distribute wearable devices that ensure safety regulations. Bluetooth technology transmits tags without requiring a user's location to be tracked. Fig. (**9**) portrays the importance of IoT during COVID-19. Fig. (**10**) portrays IoT applications.

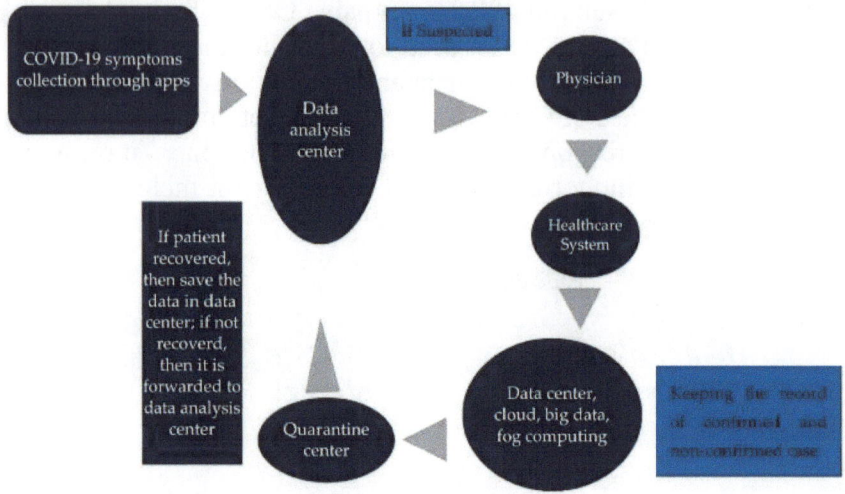

Fig. (9). IOT healthcare system during COVID-19 [14].

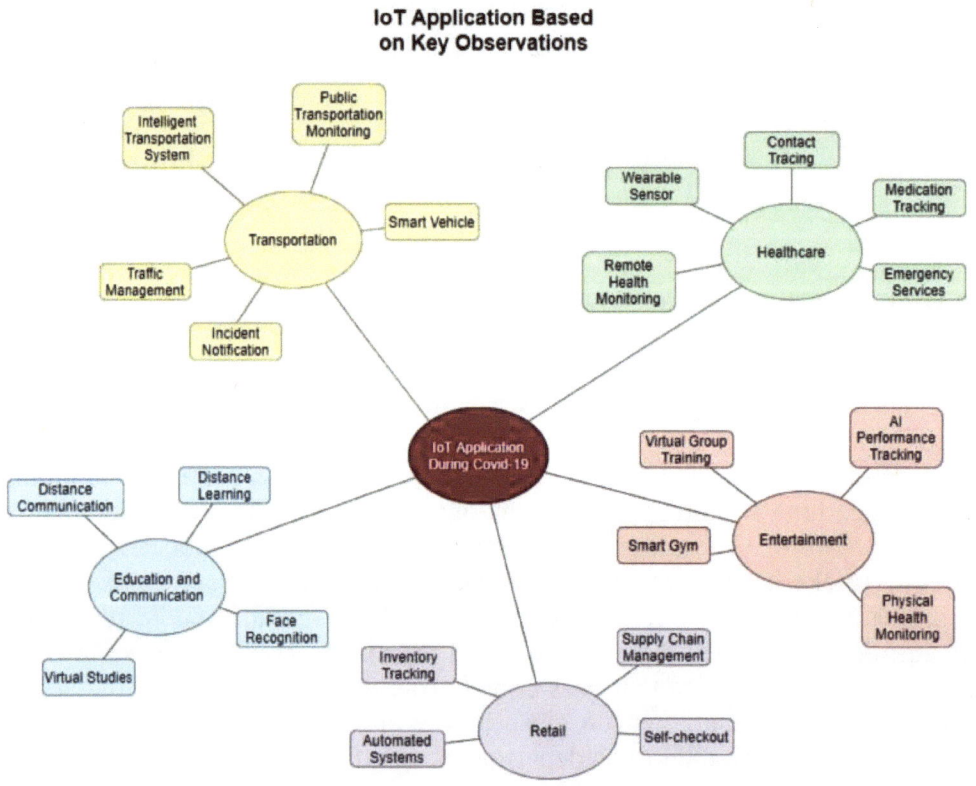

Fig. (10). IOT healthcare system during COVID-19 [18].

5.3.1. IoT – Healthcare

The extended, healthcare-specific version of the Internet of Things (IoT) is known as the Internet of Medical Things (IoMT). It could use it to create a medical platform to assist patients in receiving appropriate home healthcare and a comprehensive disease management database for healthcare organizations in the current crisis. Diagnostic and medical supplies (including protective masks, thermometers, medications, and POC COVID-19 [19] kits for infection diagnosis and monitoring) could be obtained by individuals with mild symptoms. The IoMT platform allowed patients to upload their health status *via* the internet regularly. It could move its data to local emergency clinics, the Middle for Infectious Prevention, and state and nearby well-being departments. People could dynamically monitor their disease status and receive the appropriate medical care without spreading the virus by using the IoMT platform. The government would be able to watch the spread of diseases effectively, appropriately distribute supplies, and implement emergency strategies with this systemic database, which would also help alle*via*te the pressures brought on by a lack of medical devices. Fig. (**11**) portrays the medical ecosystem.

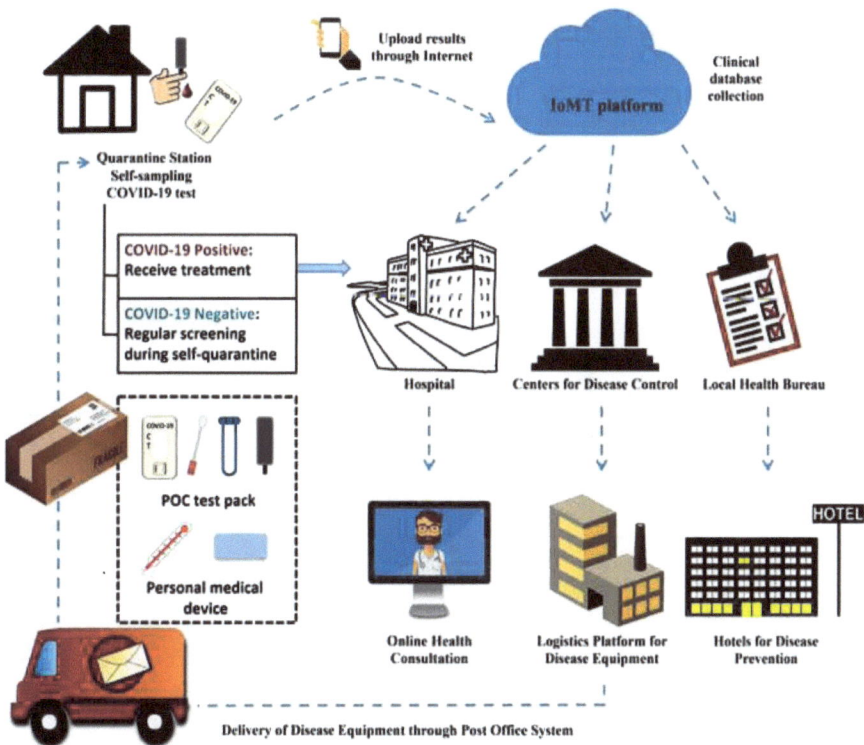

Fig. (11). - Medical Ecosystem [20].

The study [21] used a custom MLP block to fine-tune the COVID-19 detection pipeline using the Vision Transformer model and our dataset. A Patch Encoder layer in the initial portion of the network transforms the input image into multiple flattened patches. Multiple Multi-layer Perceptron blocks and multi-headed self-attention layers make up the Transformer encoder. The self-attention layer of ViT enables global information integration throughout the entire picture. ViT learns to encode the patches' relative positions to recreate the training data's visual structure. Since each image pixel serves as the input, self-attention has a quadratic cost because it requires each pixel to pay attention to every other pixel. Before each block, Layer Norm is used to cut down on training time and boost generalization performance. Twenty-three transformer encoder layers are stacked on top of each other in this initial stage. The MLP block is made up of two sets of batch normalization and dense layers that go through the flattened output of the final transformer encoder. One hundred twenty neurons are activated using a Gaussian error linear unit (GELU) in the first dense layer. To train our model for multi-class and binary classification, it uses the NovoGrad optimizer and a categorical cross-entropy loss function. It involved TensorFlow 2.4 structure in a Python 3.8 virtual climate. A 4.1 TFLOPS Tesla K80 served as the graphics processing unit in the training pipeline. There was 24 GB of RAM available online. It used Jupyter notepads to lead the tests. Fig. (**12**) portrays the same.

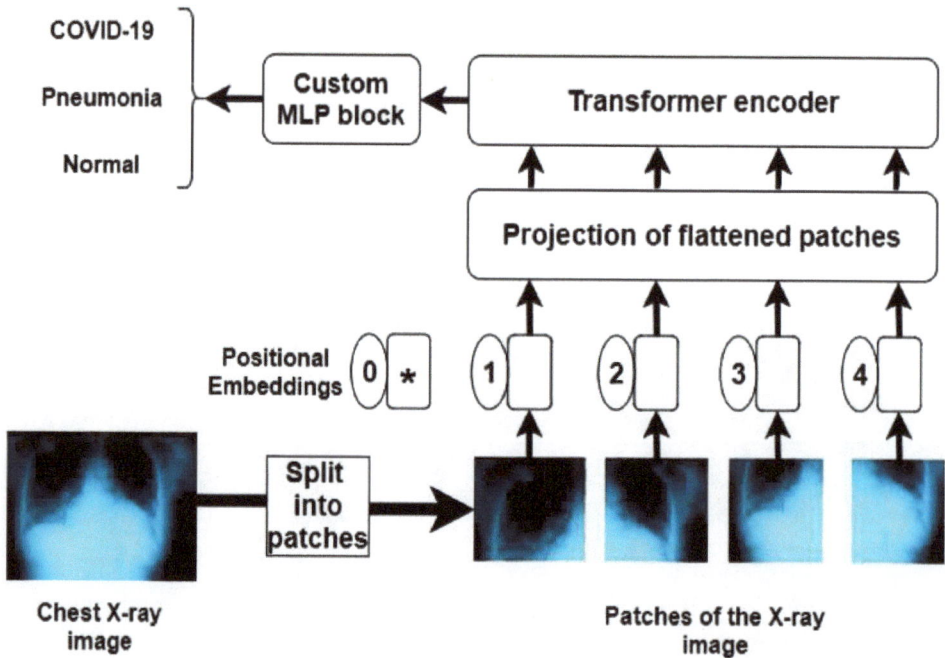

Fig. (12). Proposed ViT model for COVID-19 detection [21].

The compilation and transmission of symptom data, a quarantine center, a review repository, and a mobile application for doctors to use for visualization are the five key modules that make up the system [22]. Each module is connected to the others *via* a cloud platform. The visualization module is added to show the result to the right doctors or people who care for them. Through a collection of body-worn sensors, the data accumulation module aims to collect real-time symptoms data. Cough and acoustic classifications for various ages can be used to identify symptoms using voice-inspired devices with aerodynamics and multiple techniques. Heartbeat and movement-focused sensors have been used to detect fatigue. It can utilize a picture-based grouping strategy to analyze a sensitive throat. Finally, oxygen-based sensors can be used to determine respiration rates. It can also use ad-hoc networks of mobile applications to collect data with a 28-day travel history. A quarantine center gathers patients in a healthcare facility who have been quarantined or separated. In the proposed paradigm, the various components cooperate with the fog computing node in a coordinated manner. At first, IoT data are gathered randomly from sensors placed in an individual's body-area network. The parametric data are sent to the linked Raspberry Pi based on the collected data. The fog device has 2 GB of LPDDR2 SDRAM and an ARM Cortex-A53 quadcore CPU running at 2.1 GHz. The Apache HTTP server version 2.4.34 and the Raspbian Stretch operating system are included. Based on the IEEE 802.15.4 data communication standard, the ZigBee protocol is used to send the data. On the data it collects, the fog node runs local computations in real-time and alerts doctors of potentially harmful ambient factors that could impact healthcare. The fog computing node connects to cloud services *via* HTTP RESTful APIs. Using the HTTP POST protocol, it uploads input data and downloads the results. The widely available and simple-to-implement IEEE 802.11 WiFi protocol is used for data transfer. Besides, Microsoft Organization Screen 3.4 is utilized to follow network transmission capacity use. The 1vCPU, 2 GB RAM, 3 GB SSD, and Windows Server 2016 of Amazon EC2 cloud are used for cloud-based data processing. Fig. (**13**) portrays the same.

A study [23] defines four distinct architectural roles for the devices. A beaconing tag is a relatively straightforward device that should be tracked while consuming as little energy as possible to maximize battery life. It should keep beaconing tags from being recharged or changing their batteries for years. A device set up to monitor and send messages based on the presence, absence, or change in the position of a beaconing tag is known as a proximity detector. It implements the entire stack, including the contact tracing app's model. The proximity detector needs resources to scan the advertising channels and carry out mesh operations frequently. A hand-off hub advances messages received from different hubs over the publicizing conveyor. The Bluetooth mesh standard serves the same function as a standard relay. The gateway node provides an interface to the contact tracing server, a generic mesh node that stores pertinent data and performs advanced computations on proximity data. Fig. (**14**) portrays the same.

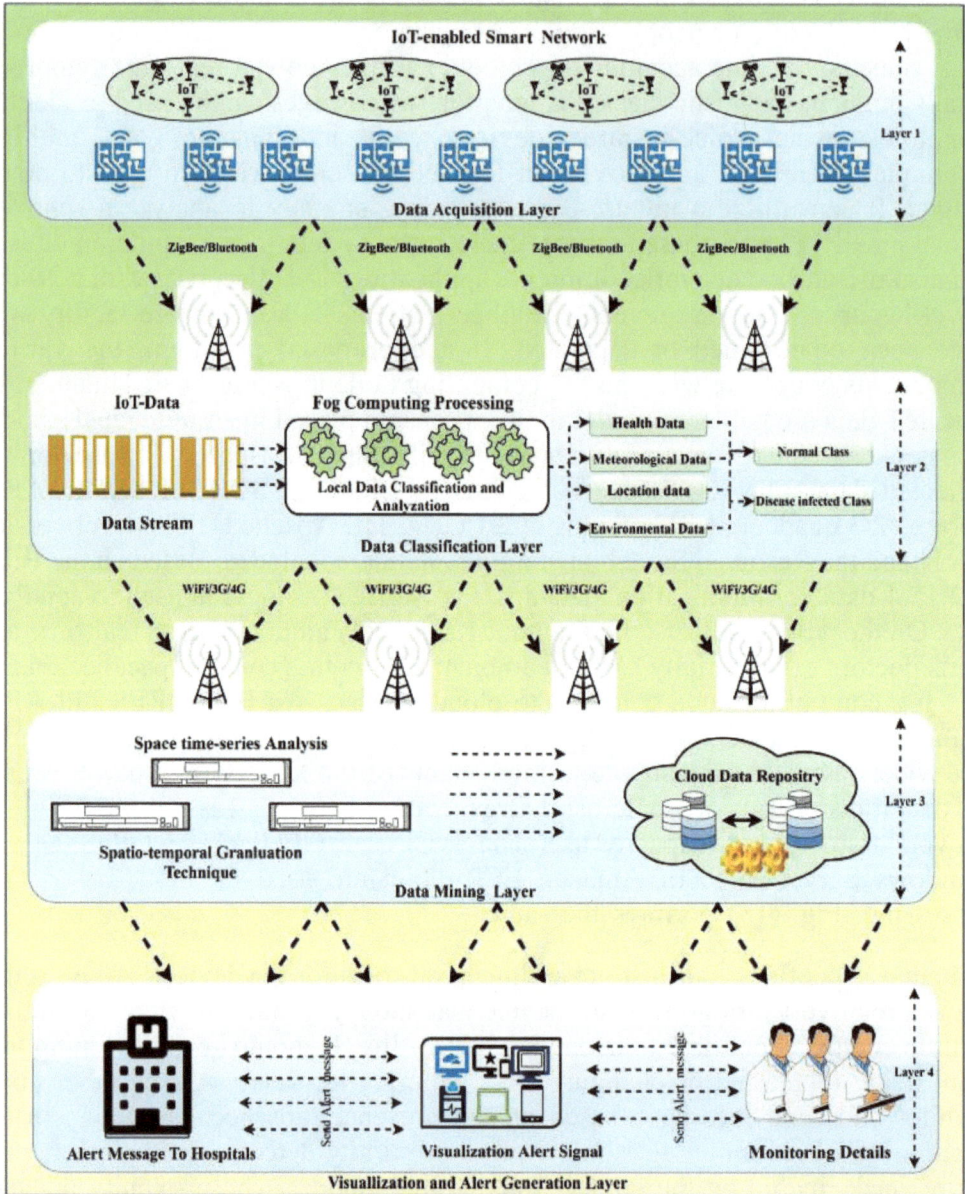

Fig. (13). Layered architecture of proposed model [22].

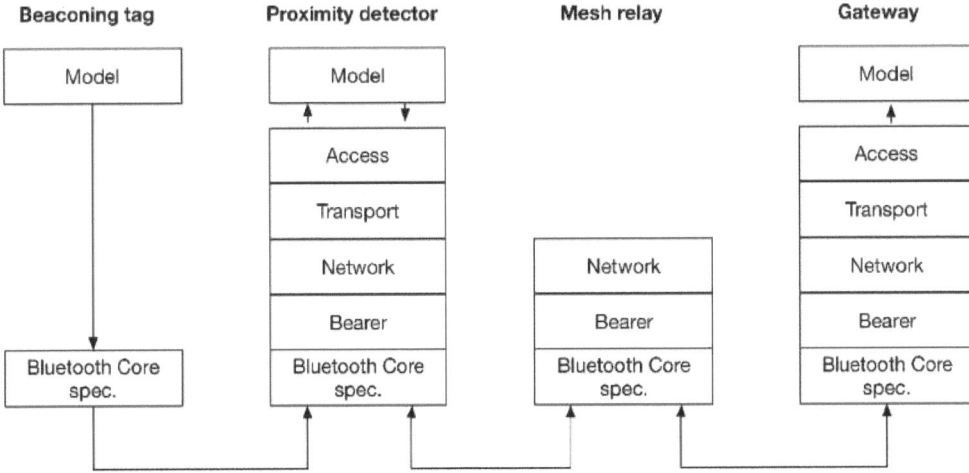

Fig. (14). System Architecture [23].

The work [24] creates a substantial X-ray image dataset. Numerous X-ray images were meticulously gathered from publicly accessible datasets. It produced the dataset by combining five distinct open-source repositories. Experienced radiologists examined these images and eliminated any that lacked convincing COVID-19 evidence. 15,153 X-ray images representing three diseases make up the dataset. Ten thousand one hundred ninety-two regular patient X-rays, 3616 COVID-19 X-rays, and 1345 pneumonia X-rays were taken. It enhances the training process. The input images are subjected to a variety of pre-processing techniques. It used a more enhanced image, contrast enhancement, and image normalization methods to resize all of the images in the dataset to the dimension of 224 x 224. All the procedures were trained and tested on the machine with an Intel Core i7 3.5 GHz processor, 16 GB of RAM, and an integrated 2 GB NVIDIA graphics card. It implemented pre-processing image algorithms, data augmentation tasks, and deep learning models with Anaconda3 (Python 3.7). Fig. (15) portrays the same.

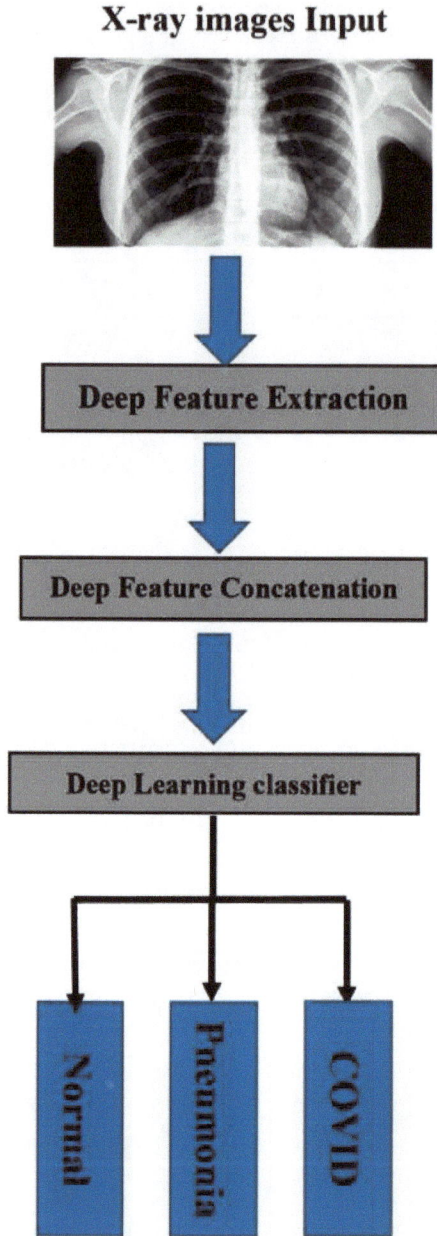

Fig. (15). Proposed model [24].

The review [25] aimed to assess the readiness of Jordanian bleeding edge specialists for the demolishing situation. The cross-sectional structure is based on a questionnaire. It found 571 doctors who were sent to missions that deal with COVID-19 patients directly. Specialists, residents, and general practitioners made up the sample. The questionnaire aimed to assess preparedness based on the knowledge of virus transmission and protective measures, compliance with guidelines, and psychological effects on doctors. It was online and completed with Google Forms. We gathered information about three main aspects of preparedness. The University of Jordan's institutional review board committee approved the study's questionnaire and design. It contacted five hundred seventy-one physicians *via* email and phone. The questionnaire and consent form were completed by 308 physicians, resulting in a response rate of 53.9 percent.

A sensor fusion algorithm is used in the proposed approach [26] to identify face masks and infected suspects in the early stages of infection—algorithms for sensor fusion, deep neural networks, and the system's hardware and software. To enhance the information, it combines sensory inputs from various channels. It is utilized in biomedical devices, robotics, and autonomous automobiles. In COVID-19 patients, the most common symptoms are fever and low oxygen levels. Now is the time to talk about self-isolation and the possibility of needing medical attention. Asymptomatic individuals are not identified by the proposed method. The method doesn't prove infection. It predicts who might have COVID; tracing and testing can benefit from this early on. The simple mail transfer protocol (SMTP) was installed on the Raspberry Pi. The SMTP server sends an alert email containing vital health information and the suspect's GPS location to a healthcare provider. Links, text, and files can be transferred between devices using the Pushbullet server. Android alerts are sent by this server that is not urgent but requires immediate attention. The Pushbullet server sends messages and notifications to a device that has been registered with its ID. It uses platforms such as OpenCV and TensorFlow are utilized in image processing. It used the RFMD dataset for testing and training, which contains 1930 pictures without masks and 2165 pictures with covers. The MLX 90614 sensor detects body temperature. The SparkFun sensor detects the heart rate and oxygen levels in the blood. The GPS signal is identified by an LM80 sensor associated with a USB port. The Raspberry Pi and Arduino incorporate the SparkFun and MLX 90614 biosensors. The biometric sensors are connected using the I2C protocol. For face mask recognition and real-time video streaming, the spy camera is installed in the camera slot of the Raspberry Pi. Fig. (**16**) portrays the same.

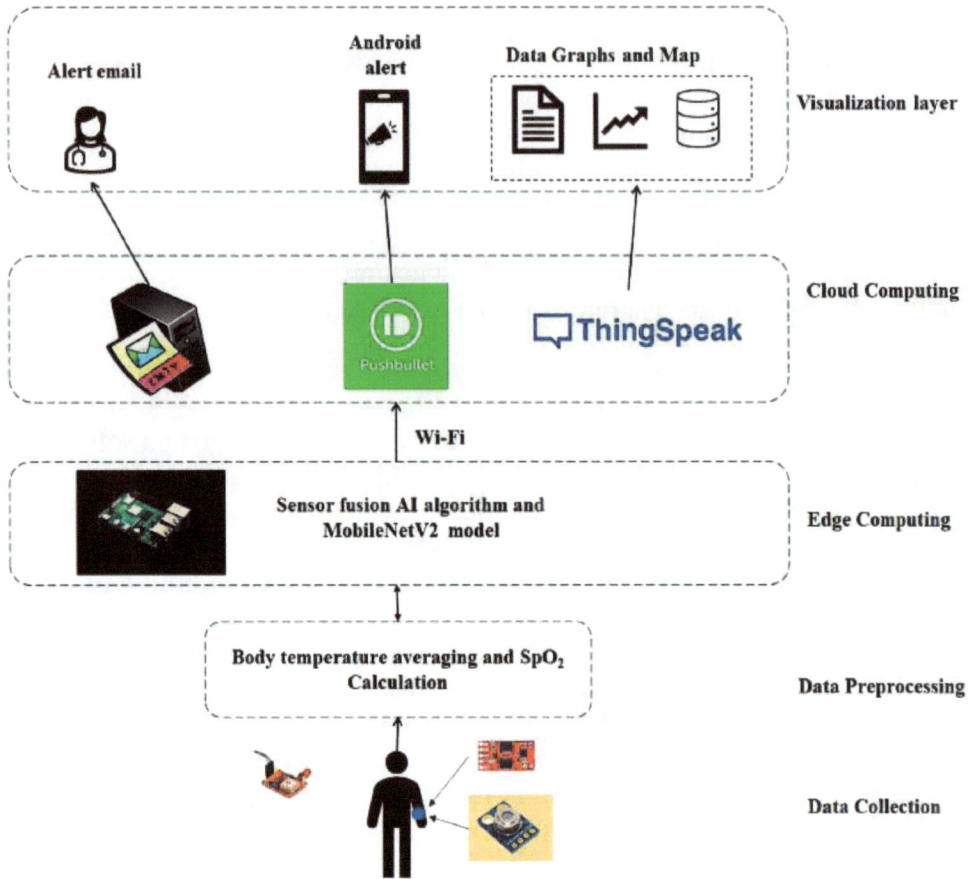

Fig. (16). Proposed IIoT device [26].

The proposed model [27] incorporates two primary profound learning parts, the principal part is GAN, and the next part is the profound exchange model. The COVID-19 X-ray Images dataset is utilized to fine-tune each deep transfer model. Deep learning models, in their own right, are referred to as "generative adversarial networks." The generator is the first network, while the discriminator is the second. The discriminator network consists of five convolutional layers. It includes four leaky ReLU, and three batch normalization layers. The generator network in this study has five transposed convolutional layers, four ReLU layers, four batch normalization layers, and a Tanh Layer at the model's end. All convolutional and transposed convolutional layers used the window size of 4 by 4 pixels. Each layer had 64 filters. It used a program called MATLAB to code the model that was presented. It involved CPU-specific development. It produced all results on a computer server with 96 GB of RAM and an Intel Xeon processor running at 2 GHz. Fig. (**17**) portrays the same.

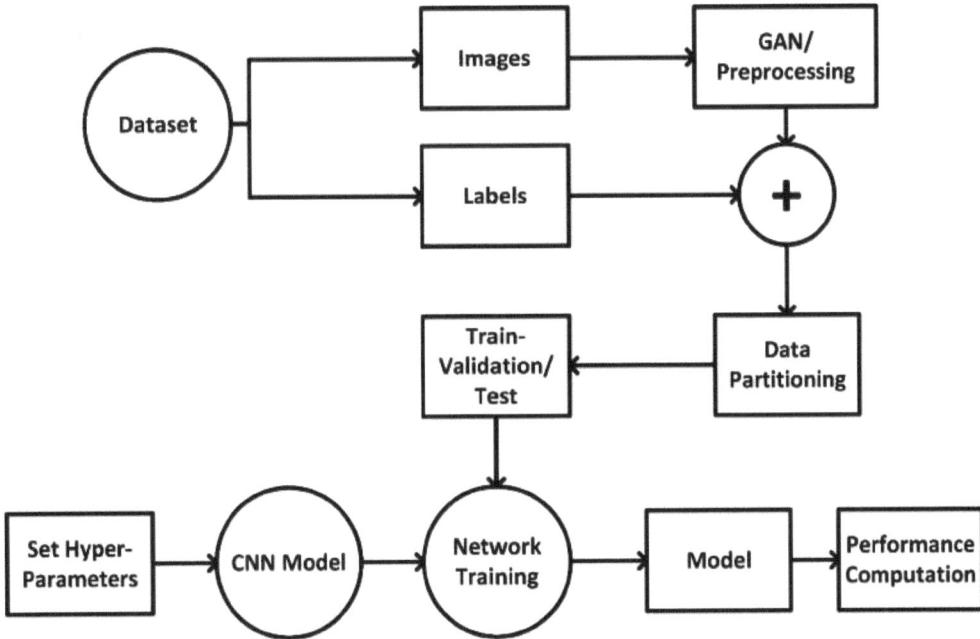

Fig. (17). Proposed GAN/deep transfer learning mode [27].

The study [14] created architectures based on three layers. It stores data in the cloud or big data thanks to the perception layer, which also makes decisions about patient data. The first layer, the Object Layer, collects and processes information between physical devices like sensors and actuators. These physical objects are utilized for various purposes, including location querying, temperature sensing, vibration, motion, and more. The object abstraction layer is now in charge of securely transferring the data produced between the object and service management layers. The object layer creates data. A service is paired with the name and address of the requester through the Service Management Layer. Regardless of the hardware platform, it provides a service to the IoT application programmer to coordinate with the objects layer. The Application Layer provides the services upon user request and demand. In the healthcare system, the Business Layer manages the IoT's overall activities and services. The business layer attempts to construct graphs, business models, flowcharts, and other system representations based on the data it receives from the application layer. Fig. (**18**) portrays the same.

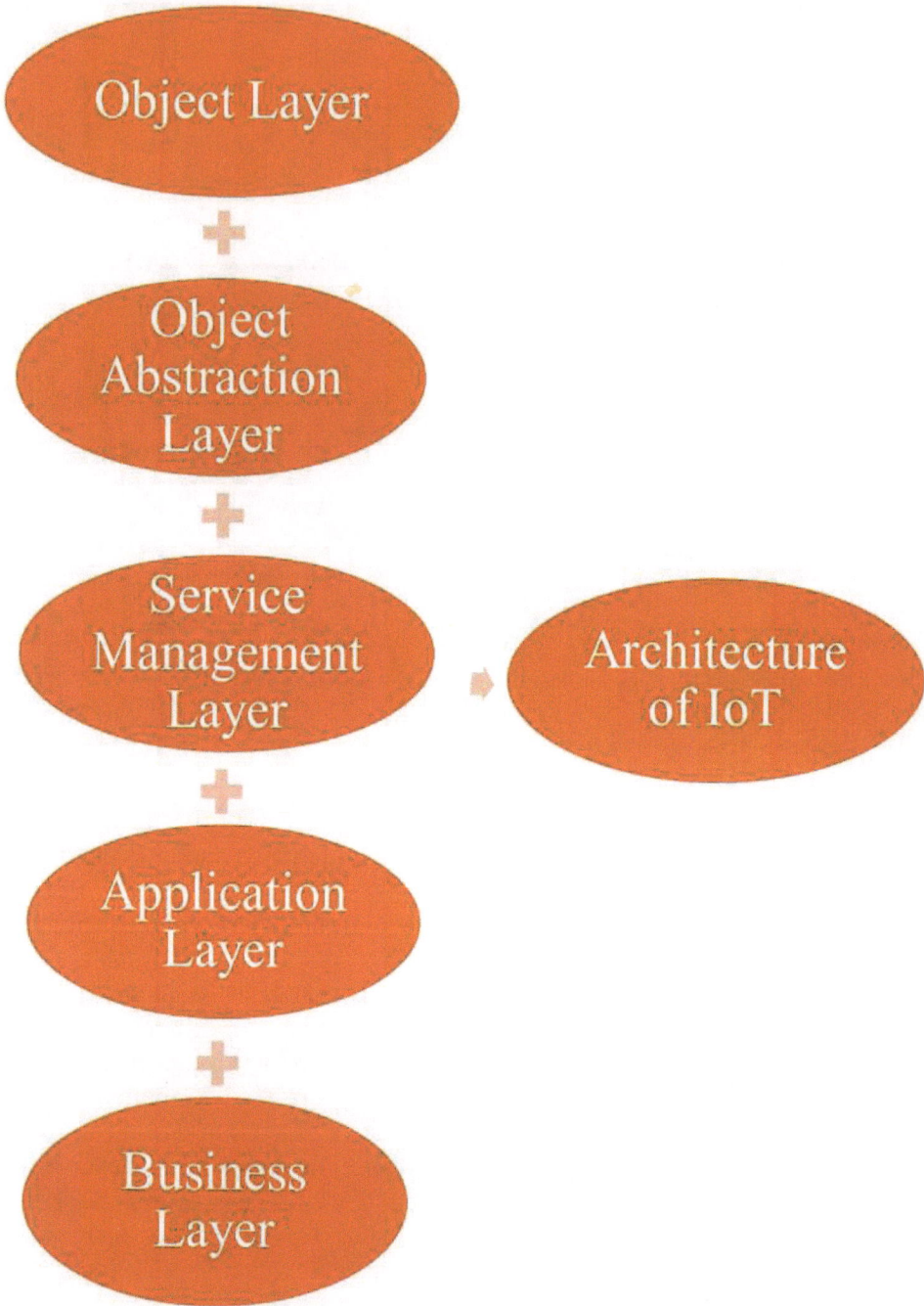

Fig. (18). IoT architecture [14].

The support, resources, and data providers contribute to the framework's implementation [28]. Various secure communication channels are used by the IoT infrastructure to communicate with the three different providers. Sensing devices that collect real-time data from individuals and submit it for processing and analysis are the data providers. Resource providers are the computing and communication devices connected to the infrastructure that enable data analysis, visualization, and decision-making. The network of caregivers and medical facilities accountable for patient's treatment and safety make up the support providers. The encouraging group of people the individual follows up once they are determined to have Coronavirus. The screening device lets doctors or professionals who supervise patients take physiological measurements, analyze their patients remotely, always know their health conditions, and figure out the necessary medical characteristics without touching them physically. Suppose the patient is infected with the Coronavirus or influenza. In that case, the smartphone app that comes with the device can remotely monitor and assess the patient's health using a combination of the sensor data. The application uses an algorithm to determine whether a patient has no symptoms or mild, moderate, or severe symptoms. It also uses each sensor reading to explain and evaluate the patient. Medical sensors are connected to the device's processor and Wi-Fi module for data processing and cloud transfer. It used Arduino in work. Fig. (**19**) portrays the same.

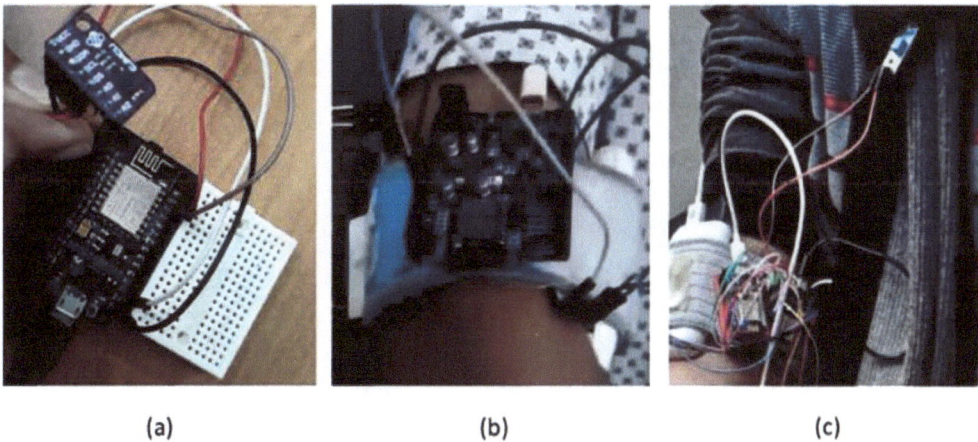

(a)   (b)   (c)

Fig. (19). Protocol Implementation [28].

There are various modules in the IoT-based Smart Screening and Disinfection Walkthrough Gate (SSDWG) [29]. It is an intelligent device with multiple sensors and is used to prevent the spread of COVID-19 carriers. When someone enters SSDWG, the temperature-checking module checks the temperature without making any contact in the initial step. A picture of the individual is taken and stored in a database with his temperature and suspected health status if the temperature is above 99 degrees Fahrenheit. The mask detection module can determine whether or not a person is wearing mask. In the meantime, the individual in charge of the entrance can divert the suspect for proper COVID-19 testing. It has two modules and can be placed at the entrance of any public place, hospital, or crowded area suspected of having COVID-19. It keeps a picture of the suspect and the person's body temperature. The sensor used to measure temperature is the MLX90614. It is a wireless infrared thermometer that does not touch the human body and can communicate wirelessly to its microcontroller. An image processing module takes a photo with an unusually high body temperature. It extracts the data from the image. They combined lesion detection techniques with pathological pattern mining. The second module of SSDWG is responsible for identifying individuals passing through it who are donning masks.VGG-16, MobileNetV2, Inception V3, ResNet-50, and a Convolutional Neural Network are the five pre-trained deep learning models. They divide the various types of face masks into two categories. An input layer, an output layer, and multiple hidden layers make up CNN's architecture. Convolutional layers, pooling layers, fully connected layers, and normalization layers are typically hidden layers (ReLU). Images with and without a face mask have an input size of 224 by 224 pixels and three RGB channels for this network's input. It utilizes an enormous dataset comprising 149,806 pictures. Fig. (**20**) portrays the same.

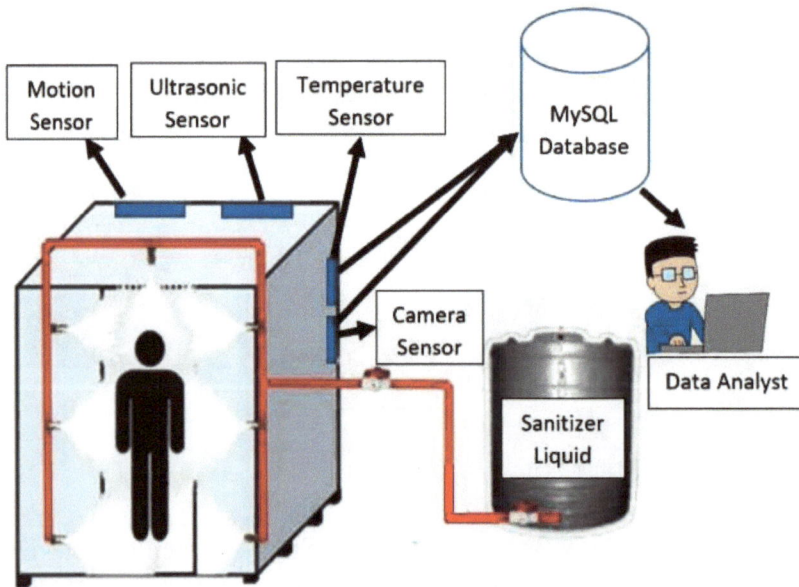

Fig. (20). Smart Screening and Disinfection Walkthrough Gate (SSDWG) [29].

Potential patients request a sample, a UAV is sent out, and the selection is collected in five steps [30]. The likely patient initiates a request for a COVID-19 self-test kit. An immediate consultation or questionnaire is required to determine whether the patient is qualified to receive the equipment. Either *via* AI-based automated questionnaires or a video call with the medical expert's panel in the UAV dispatch section, a service initiation request is sent to the UAV dispatch department once a patient is eligible for the service. Before being sent to the patient, the staff in the dispatch department makes sure that the UAV, sample collection box, and self-testing kits are clean. In the second step, AI obtains patient location information from the dispatch team or the patient database in hospital records. The route-optimizing algorithms determine the most efficient and shortest route for returning the sample to the hospital and delivering the kits to the patient. The UAV receives the optimized path GPS coordinates in the third step. A sealed box attached to the UAV contains a self-testing kit. The patient gets the equipment in the fourth step, and the UAV hands over the box with all information. The fifth step asks for permission to return to the depot or collect additional samples based on its battery status and holding capacity, particularly if AI informs it of a nearby UAV whose battery is dying. Fig. (**21**) portrays the same.

The MEMS accelerometer [31] is responsible for acquiring acceleration, which the RSC model utilizes for activity recognition. From the recognition stage, the TTH is automatically adjusted and compared to the Tbody for a body temperature check. The ambient sensor gathers indoor statistics. An alert message is sent if the temperature rises continuously for a predetermined time. Through Bluetooth or Wi-Fi, the cloud-stored data are sent to the LCD screen for the user and other shared devices. The wearable device M5stickC, outfitted with the user, is coupled with all the sensors. The IDE can program the M5stickC, a development platform with 4 MB of flash memory and a 95 mA-3.7 V Lipo battery. This board contains the MEMS 3-pivot accelerometer MPU6886. M5stickC is connected to the thermal body sensor MLX90614 *via* I2C serial communication. MQTT broker is used to send the data to the cloud. Fig. (**22**) portrays the same.

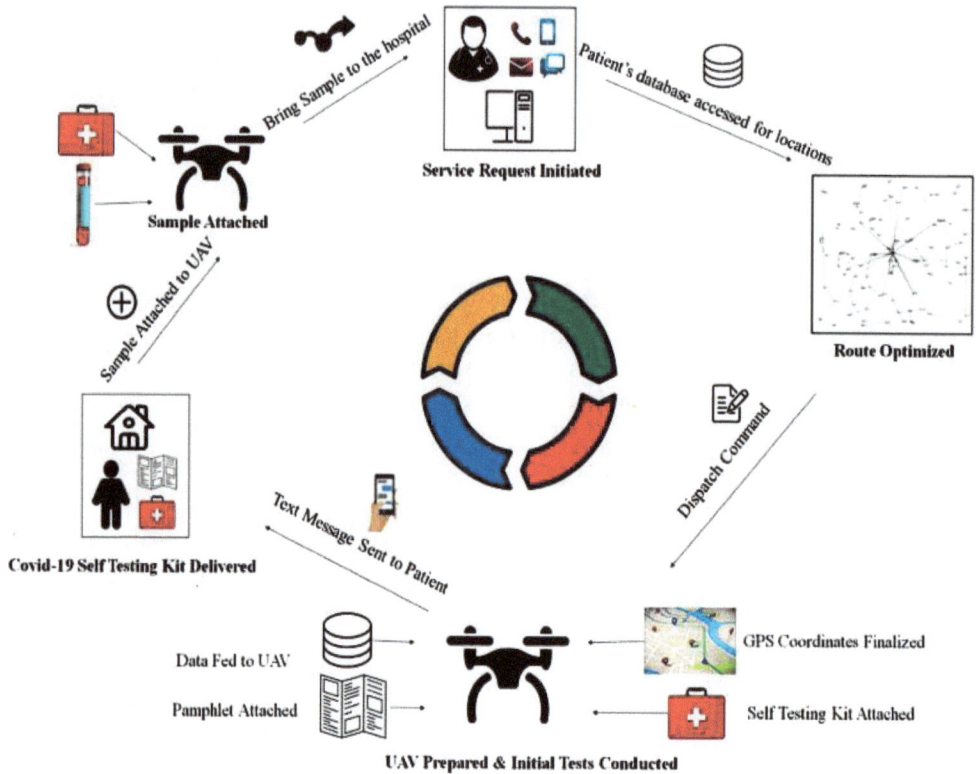

Fig. (21). Framework designed for route optimization of UAVs for the delivery of COVID-19 self-testing kits [30].

The system [32] makes possible early detection, continuous monitoring for suspected cases, and patient isolation for both suspected and confirmed cases. There are three main parts to the framework. This side's proposed system relies on a lightweight mobile application that continuously monitors the patient's condition. It must scan the QR code before anyone can enter. Usually, healthy cases can pass, but suspected cases must follow a specific route to prevent the spread of the infection. Other infected issues cannot. Keeping track of where people are going prevents both suspected and confirmed cases from spreading the diseases. Using the LoRa network, the data gathered by sensors is sent to the closest fog node. A test platform was the Network Simulation version 2 (NS2.35). A patient's status and data are gathered from various sources. It, including their medical history, wearable devices, scan results, *etc.*, are saved in the cloud, continuously updated in the patient's electronic health record (EHR), and sent to the analytics module to see if the potential risk is higher than a predetermined threshold. Notifications are sent to the patient and the doctor when a problem is found. The COVID-19 dataset, gathered from various parts of the world, can be found in References and is accessible to the general public. There are 622 cases in it. Fig. (**23**) represents the same.

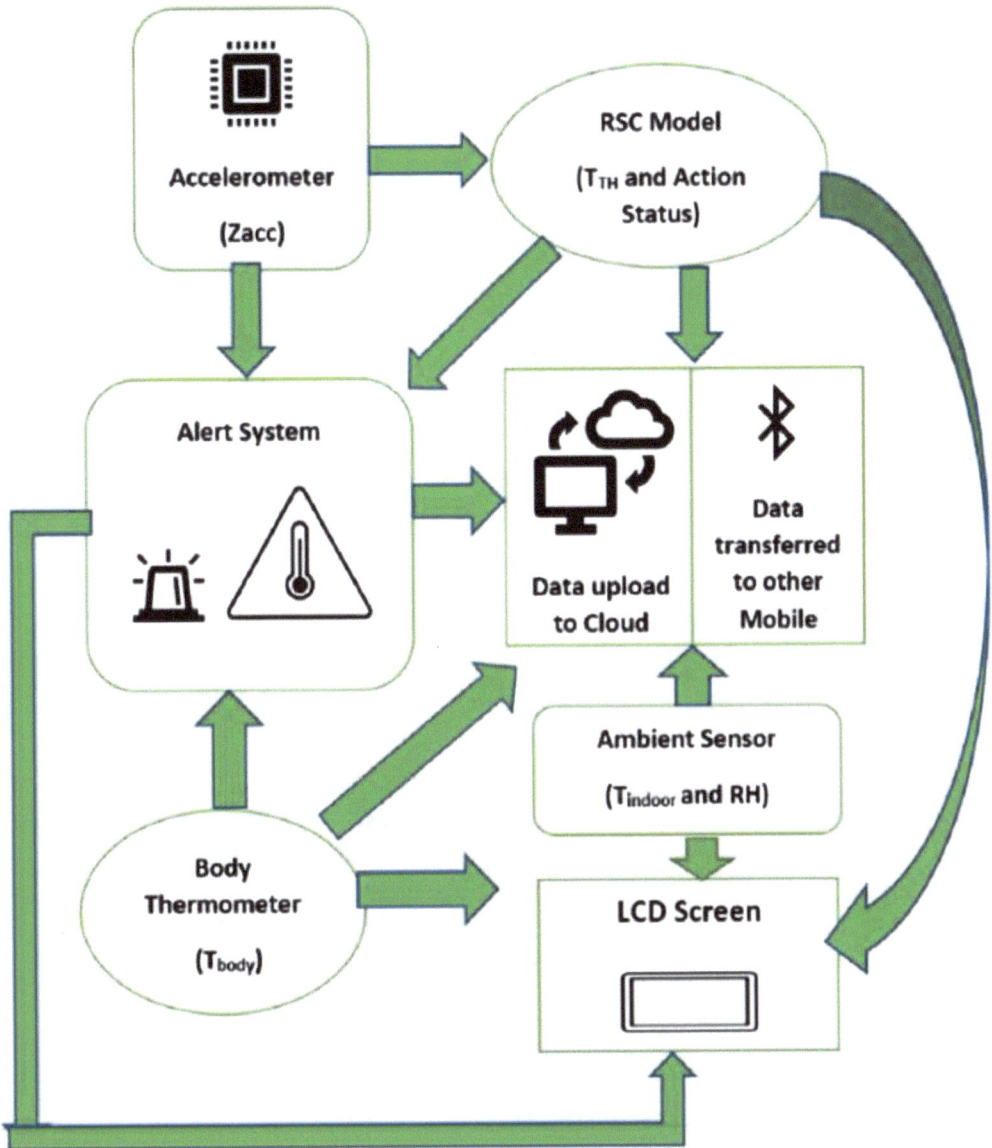

Fig. (22). System model [31].

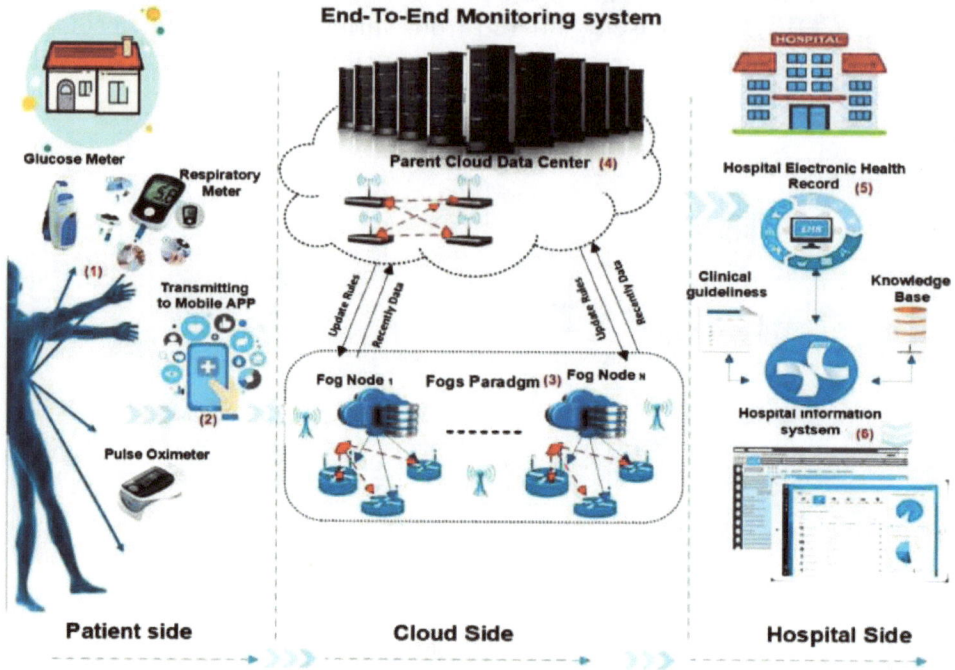

Fig. (23). Proposed Framework [32].

5.3.2. Role of IOT-Transportation in Covid-19

COVID-19 threatens this substantial anticipated growth and has already slowed this market's expansion. The COVID-19 pandemic has resulted in severe setbacks for freight and passenger transport. There has been a significant drop in the number of trips made by public transportation. There has also been a substantial drop in the number of people using subways. Road transportation continued to operate, but with fewer routes. The European Road Freight Rate Benchmark Q1 2020 report reveals that these alterations have increased the volatility of freight charges. Before COVID-19, the automotive industry was already in a recession. This recession has experienced yet another dip due to the pandemic, which is anticipated to delay the recovery until 2025. The current economic downturn has slowed the adoption of autonomous driving and advanced driver assistance systems in automobiles. Fig. **(24)** portrays IoT Adoption in Transportation.

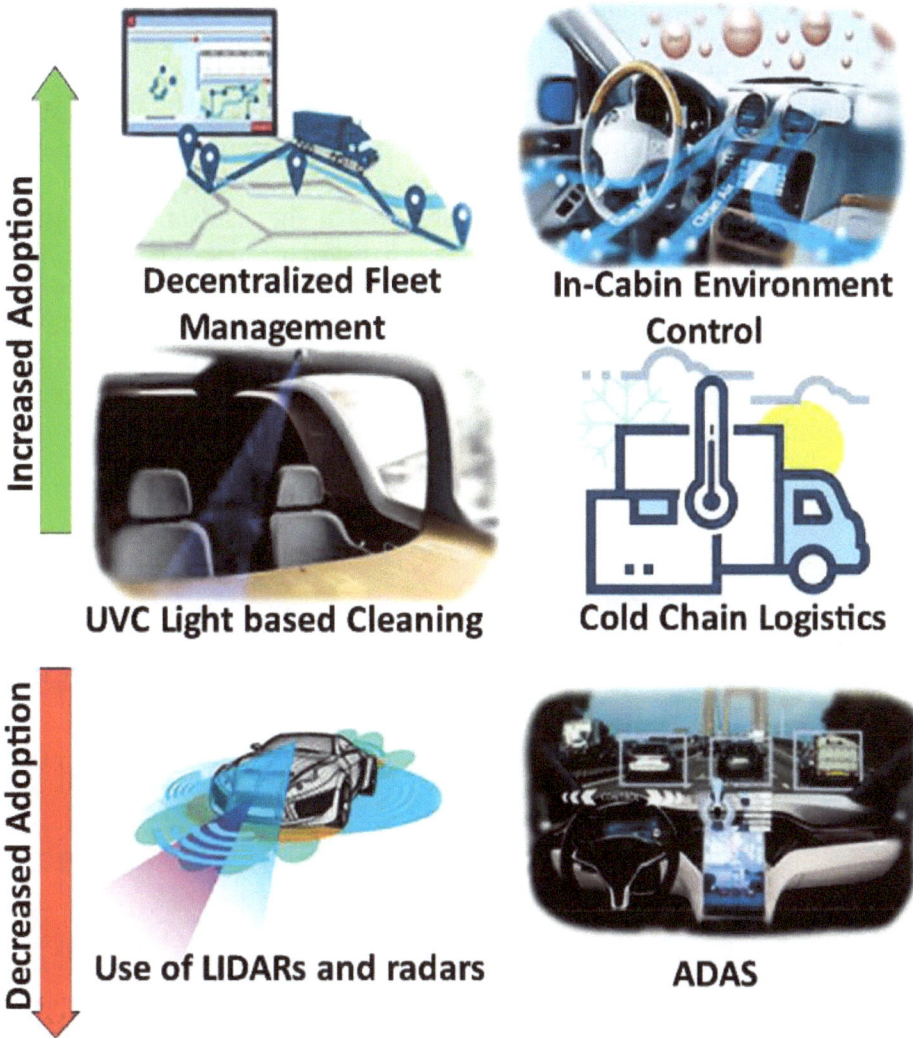

Fig. (24). IoT Adoption in Transportation [33].

The proposed system's methodology [34] consists of two main steps. The first step is a face-matching model using deep learning and standard machine learning methods. A face detector based on computer vision was constructed using the generated dataset, OpenCV, Python with TensorFlow, and TensorFlow. It used deep learning and computer vision techniques to determine whether the individual was wearing a face mask. It uses a hybrid deep CNN classifier to classify facial features into relevant segments. Instead of using photos from a database, CNN collects pictures of people wearing face masks. Based on facial expressions, content, and spatial information, the images of people wearing face masks are differentiated from those of other people's photos. Its framework makes real-time use of Raspberry Pi's capabilities, like live imaging. It used the Medical Mask datasets from Kaggle and Witkowski to expand the model's training datasets. The Kaggle dataset contains numerous people with faces obscured to safeguard their security and essential XML documents that portray their namelessness insurance gadgets. There are a total of 678 photographs in the dataset. It uses Natural masking settings in PySearch to expand the PyImage dataset. There are two distinct groups of 1376 photos in the dataset. People without masks can be detected and alerted using the app and any IP cameras connected to the system through network extenders. If administrators believe that a user needs to be correctly identified in the camera, they can send notifications to that user. Fig. (**25**) represents a Hardware communication module for face mask detection.

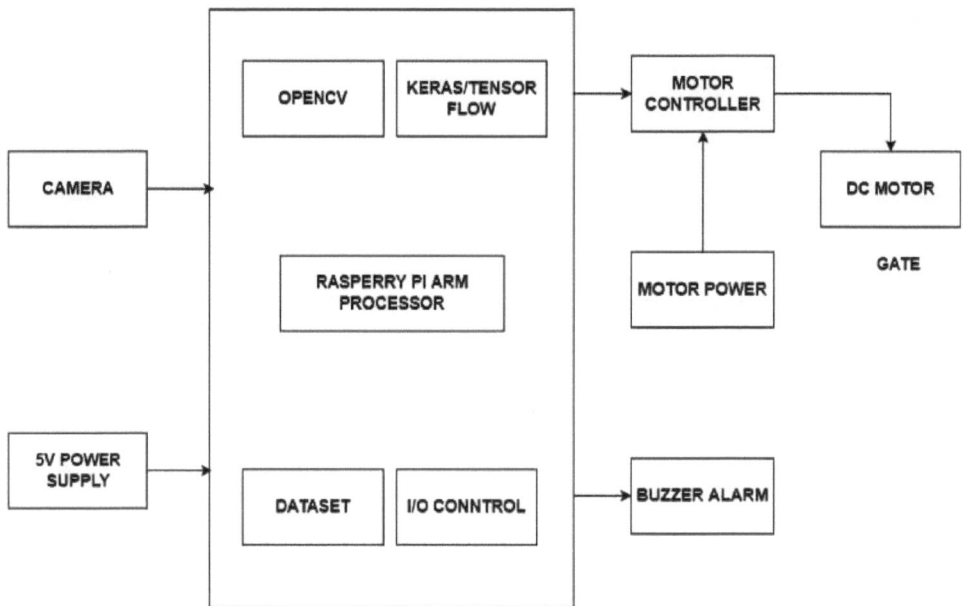

Fig. (25). Hardware communication module for face mask detection [34].

Twitter [35] is the social media platform chosen because of its high popularity. With this product, qualified academic researchers can gain significantly elevated access to endpoints for studying Twitter conversations. It used to learn more about traveler's needs and expectations and obtained feedback from various transportation providers. The Python programming language, version 3.9, was used to gather data from Twitter. Pre-processing the data is the first step toward an accurate sentiment analysis. The collected data go through several phases during this process, such as getting rid of words or characters that aren't needed, filtering out the same tweets, and so on. It used the Python programming language to carry out every one of the steps outlined below for the tweet's pre-processing in this paper. It initially filtered out the non-English tweets in the collected datasets. For the 2019 and 2020 datasets, the database search produced 17,702 and 16,789 tweets, respectively. It performed additional cleaning to remove retweets, mentions, hashtags, numbers, webpage links, whitespace, punctuation marks, and other special characters from each tweet in both datasets. By removing characters that it could not evaluate in terms of sentiment, this filtering process improved the relevance of each tweet. Throughout the study's data collection period, 539,375 posts were collected and processed. Fig. (**26**) portrays Methodology flowchart.

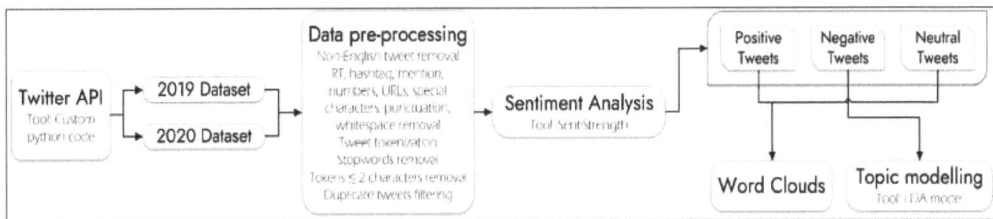

Fig. (26). Methodology flowchart [35].

5.3.3. Role of IOT-Entertainment During Covid-19

Savvy home administrations are another age of customer administration. They improve consumer's quality of life by providing security, comfort, entertainment, assisted living, efficient home management, and the support of the Internet of Things (IoT) technology. Even though more smart home services are becoming available, more is needed to know why people continue to use them and how the spread of intelligent devices and services in the home affects people's well-being. Several business interests have pushed the growth of the smart home market. IoT innovative home products and services present a substantial appeal with great potential for today's mobile carriers and cable TV businesses, which are experiencing stagnation from traditional market models. Technology giants like Google, Microsoft, Apple, Amazon, AT&T, and others have developed strategies to monetize the smart home market. They also know that innovative home services provide an opportunity to collect extensive customer data. However, people's well-being and quality of life are affected by the technology they use and continue to use for an extended period.

The architecture's [36] primary components are the effective persistence of various parts and the mechanism for interacting with the outside world. The Application Management and Client interface module is the foundation of the proposed architecture for SSGs in the healthcare industry. The executive module has four sub-parts. The first part is the game composition. It uses natural language processing to generate game episodes with their respective goals and winning criteria from game requirements and player-specific goals. The player management module, the second component, tracks player records, registration, and removal in the event of a penalty. Players can use the RESTful API to request to participate in the game. The player is added to the player log once it is approved. The final part is active management, where the primary goal is to decide what to do based on the game's episodes, winning criteria, goals, and penalties. These settings are obtained from the game composition module. The second pillar of the architecture, data management, is exposed to the action data, penalty log, device sensing data, and player score and penalty history by these four layers. Fig. (**27**) represents the same.

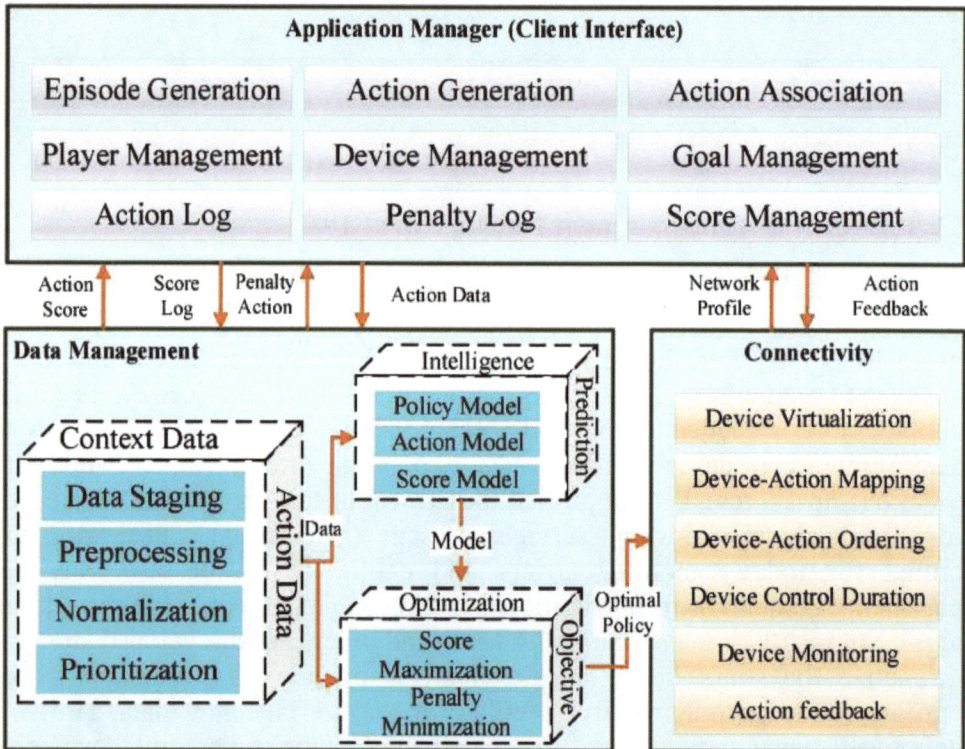

Fig. (27). Conceptual Model [36].

5.3.4. Role of IOT-Retail

The Coronavirus pandemic has caused unforeseeable worldwide ramifications for the market, customers, and public activity. The lockdown policy, which was the only thing it could do to stop the pandemic, made it harder for people to move around, making it harder for businesses to do their business and changed the habits of customers who, in a panic, started buying stocks. Common consumption patterns have been distorted, and market anomalies have emerged due to panic among consumers and businesses. The supply chain is not sufficiently adaptable to market shocks and cannot deal with them. According to retailers, delivery costs, errors, and delays are on the rise. Suppliers face significant delays and costs due to the need for safe transportation, which necessitates completing numerous safety procedures and approvals that take considerable time. At the same time, more and more businesses and employees are working from home, and more and more people are ordering products online and making electronic purchases. Input delivery is limited for many companies, especially raw materials from COVID-19-affected areas. In times of shock, many actors in the supply chain, most of whom are small and medium-sized businesses (SMEs), cannot contribute to the chain's sustainability. They leave the chains and withdraw, jeopardizing all other participant's *via*bility. Fig. (**28**) represents Internet of Things (IoT) based supply chain.

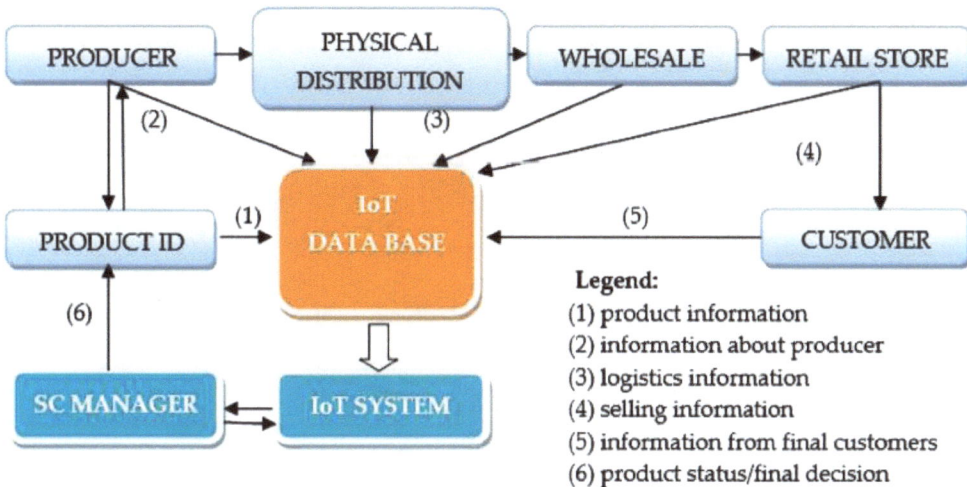

Fig. (28). Internet of Things (IoT) based supply chain [37].

A Google Forms-based online survey was used to collect data for the current study [38] from Indian consumers over two months in February and March 2021.

It uses snowball sampling. Consumers were invited to participate in the survey *via* email and by posting invitations on well-known websites. A method known as snowball sampling involves participants in a study or test recruiting additional participants. It is used when participants need help in searching. Primary data sources are asked to suggest different potential primary data sources for the research using this sampling strategy. The initial distribution of a questionnaire required likely respondents to complete it and forward it to a known respondent. The survey questionnaire had three sections. It included questions about respondent's demographic profiles and reasons for buying groceries online in the first section. The attributes related to the variables that influence consumer adaptation to technology in online grocery shopping are included in the second section of the questionnaire. Customer's perceptions of risk and level of trust in online shopping technologies are the focus of the third section of the survey. The first questionnaire was evaluated by a panel of three marketing academics, who looked at its content validity, item meaning clarity, and the connections between discovered variables and the research goals. With 45 respondents, it evaluated the questionnaire's reliability. Analysts got 479 reactions, and in the wake of altering, 443 were viewed as appropriate for use in this review, barring 36 responses that were deficient or unscrupulously replied. SPSS 22 was used to organize, tabulate, and analyze the collected data systematically. Fig. (**29**) represents the same.

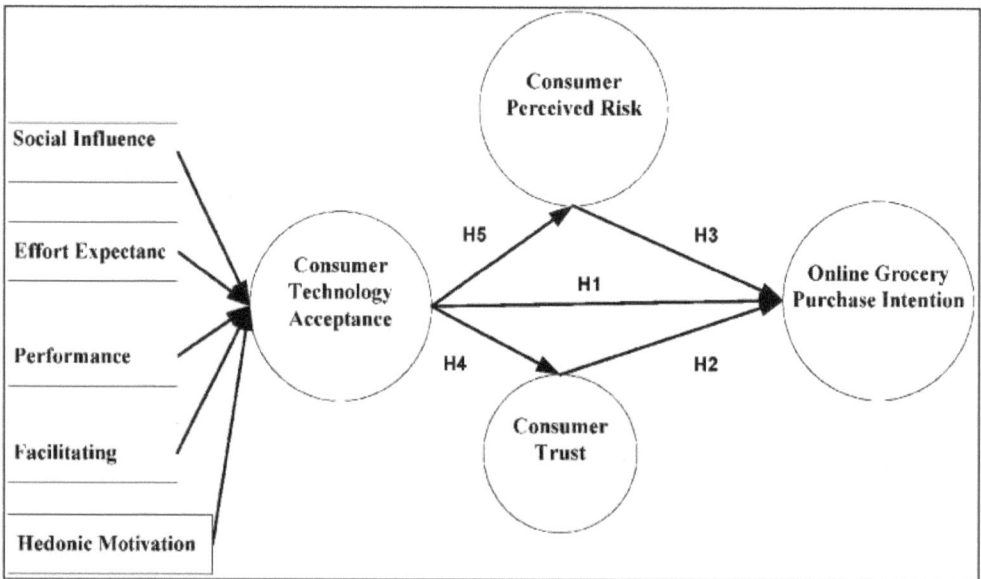

Fig. (29). Conceptual Framework [38].

This system [39] is a cooperative construction among organizations and outside players of government and local area, with a data stream that is suitable and proficiently applied in production network risk the executives. When disaster strikes or in uncertainty, supply chain management shifts its pace. The public, businesses, and governments receive the media and make their own decisions or plans for action after a typical disaster. Fig. (**30**) represents the same.

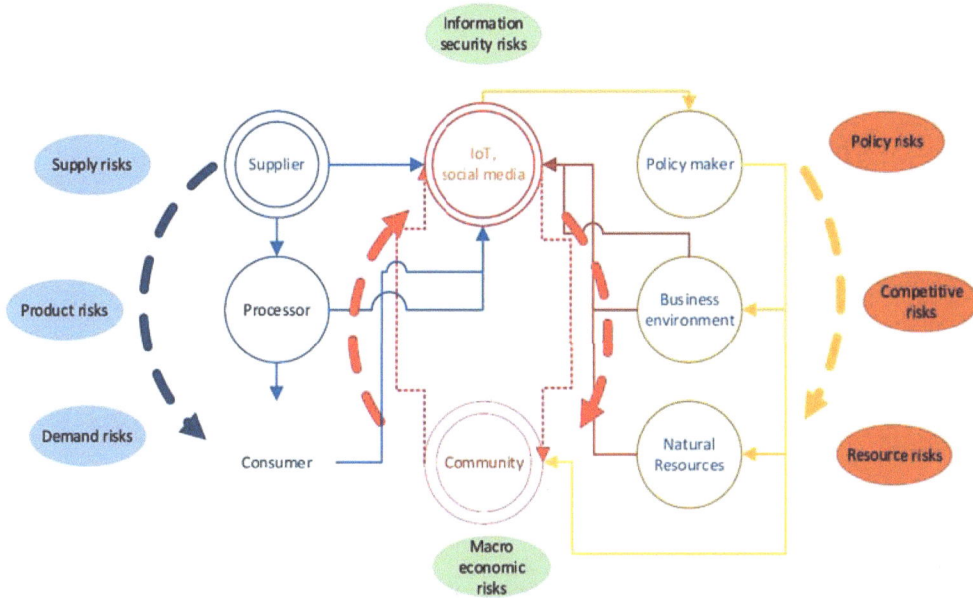

Fig. (30). IoT-based supply risk chain management and information flow [39].

The study [40] was carried out within nine months of the first COVID-19 case in the WB region. The ability to respond to demands during a pandemic, the degree of development of an information and communications network, and good connectivity between FSC participants are all examples of infrastructure. Respondent's opinions on the ability to identify critical points and monitor product flow, as well as their satisfaction with the information exchange, are included in FSC consistency and transparency. The workforce consists of the response's perspectives on the benefits of working from home, employee contentment with their skillset, and infection, isolation, and social distance. A decrease in investment, an increase in transaction costs, and a reduction in inventory costs are considered operating costs. The total quantity of food, the quantity of food that was available, and the implementation of preventive measures in the food industry that directly impact where food is placed were used as measures of food safety and security. The high costs of per diems, lodging, quarantine, reduced transport efficiency, and rising physical distribution costs contribute to the food price. Due to limited mobility and transportation, energy consumption is defined as oil, gas emissions, and fuel consumption. The respondent's attitudes toward avoiding traditional stores, the rate of growth of e-commerce, and the decline in the demand for long-lasting products are examples of consumer needs. 277 FSC managers received the questionnaire *via* email. Fig. (**31**) portrays the same.

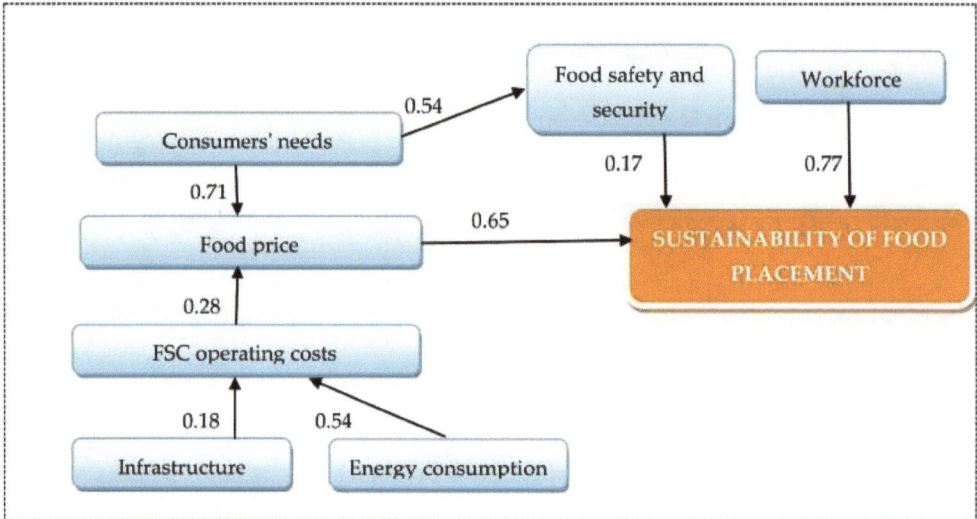

Fig. (31). Structural Model [40].

5.3.5. Role of IOT-Education During Covid-19

The Internet of Things, or IoT, is changing many aspects of our daily lives. In contrast to previous innovations, IoT technologies encourage intelligent and autonomous solutions and are widespread. IoT advancements are a significant strategic technology trend. The new learning model was seen as having a conceptual framework in the form of ubiquitous sensors and the capacity to connect the physical and machine worlds. The ability to connect billions of objects and devices to the existing Internet infrastructure utilizing Machine-t--Machine (M2M) communication and the ability to embed sensors into any object are the concepts that underpin this significant paradigm shift. The physical world as a whole is rapidly becoming online. The Internet of Things (IoT) is a global physical network that allows devices, objects, and things to communicate or interact with the internal and external environment by connecting to the Internet infrastructure. The Internet of Things (IoT) is making it possible for anyone to connect to a network anywhere, at any time, and with any network or service to intelligently identify, track, and manage things. It is an extension and expansion of an Internet-based network that expands human-to-human, human-to-thing, and things-to-thing communication. Higher education institutions, particularly universities, are being asked to digitize their content and activities and adapt their methods to enable academics and researchers to work effectively in a digital environment. A well-designed physical campus that fully integrates technology is essential to build the brand of a digital university by improving the student experience and providing the appropriate settings and facilities for teaching, learning, and research. It encourages, and supports lifelong learning. The technology that facilitates collaborative research and education, and knowledge is essential for a digital university.

The OBNiSE IoT architecture [41] for MEIoT 2D-CACSET consists of configurations and parts that let devices at various system levels communicate and send information. There are two types of users: participants and educators. The web system is kept in a cloud system at the OBNiSE facilities and can only be accessed by educators. The Mindstorms EV3 mobile robot's coordinates are displayed in real-time as the web system establishes a connection with the Raspberry Pi. Participant's access to the training web is restricted as part of the primary system. It is only permitted to display up to ten robot movements simultaneously. MIT 2D-CACSET is an Internet of Things (IoT) device that combines a Raspberry Pi for robot control, a Bluetooth module, an encoder, an ultrawideband tag, an UWB anchor, and UWB listener modules. The MIT 2D-CACSET uses Wi-Fi to establish communication between the training website and the LEGO Mindstorms EV3 mobile robot to capture and execute the robot's coordinates. In the OBNiSE IoT architecture, the EV3IA serves as an edge device and has two primary functions- manage user-created kinematics through the GUI and notify its positioning data. Fig. (**32**) represents the same.

5.4. ROLE OF CLOUD

The cloud computing environment is a system made up of applications, IT infrastructure, and network services. Thanks to virtualization technology, it uses resources that it can share in a data center. It is now a complete package offering the platform, hardware, software, and infrastructure service. These service models are now referred to as the types of services provided. The size, type of services, location, type of users, and security of a cloud can all be factors. The technology of virtualization is used to put the environment into action. It gives users access to features that simplify business operations and cut costs. Since more and more schools and universities are switching to online courses, Blackboard's teams have taken several preventative infrastructure measures to help manage significantly increased traffic during this pandemic. Blackboard provides services through CC. The massive shift toward remote work and learning is supported by the public cloud and the technologies that make it possible. Over the next few quarters, the value of several environmental stocks, including Zoom, will rise. The cloud-based suite of communication tools offered by RingCentral, Inc. saw a 34% growth in sales to $902 million. Thirty-five labs and businesses are participating in the launch. It provides a wide range of services, including website hosting. It offers a platform for application development and online software. CCE has a substantial infrastructure as a distributed service-oriented paradigm with multiple operating systems, multiple domains, and multiple users. It usually has more protection against threats and weaknesses like DDoS and EDoS attacks.

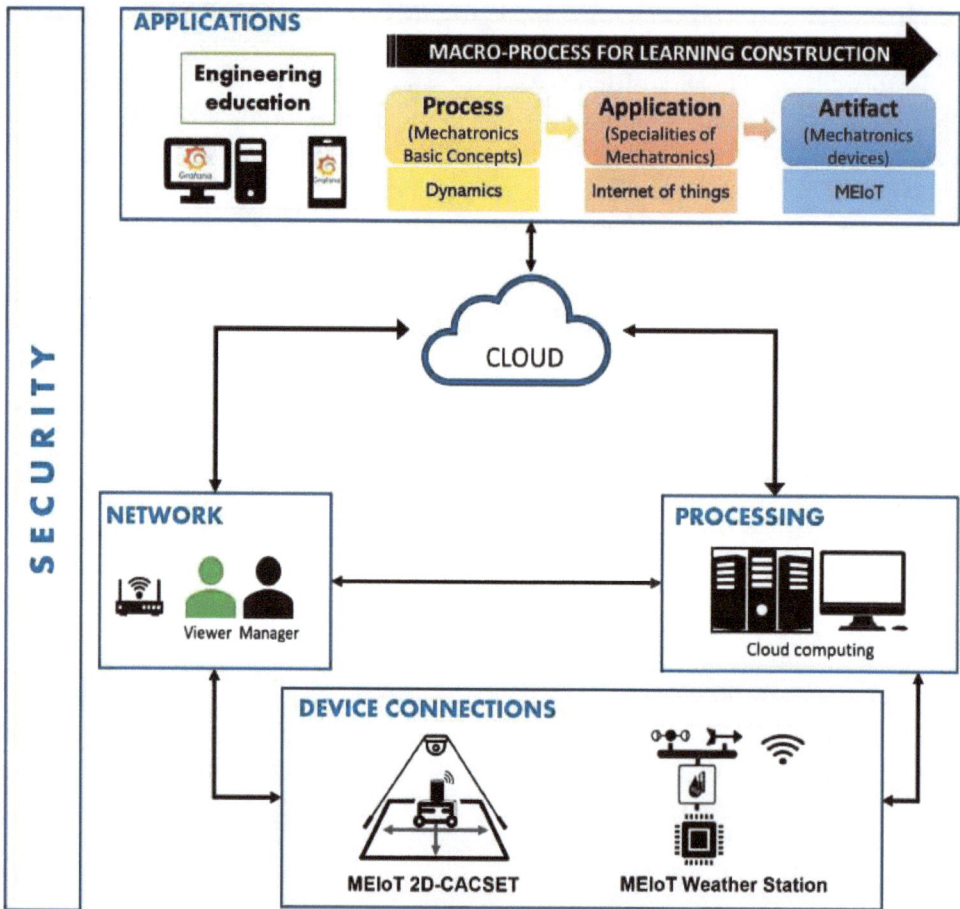

Fig. (32). OBNiSE architecture [41].

The software aims to shorten the COVID-19 transmission chain and reduce the outbreak. Through intelligent cloud connectivity, these systems are designed to detect, alert, and provide information to specific government agencies involved in the fight against this pandemic and the community, including application users. The server will function as the mainframe for data storage, analysis, and alert notification to all users following their roles and responsibilities. The first function is that the data that users enter into the application will be saved on the server so that potential COVID19 positive patients can be found and studied in the future. The second function is to make it easier for authorities to locate patients who are in quarantine at the time by serving as a tracking device. Last, a feature that monitors the people near users will require Bluetooth. Fig. (**33**) portrays the Architecture of cloud based smart health.

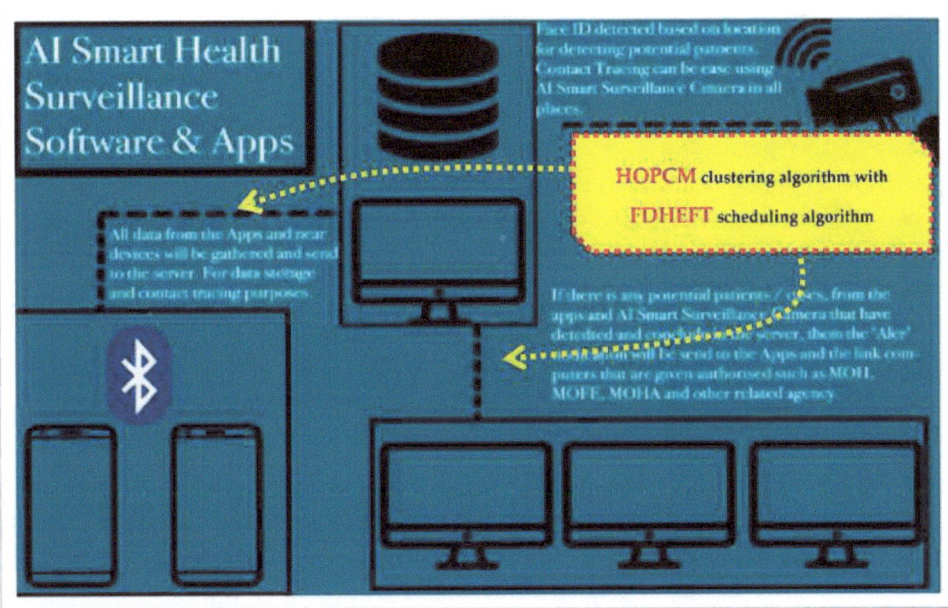

Fig. (33). Architecture of cloud based smart health [42].

Through the development and successful 72-hour deployment of the Honghu Hybrid System (HHS) [43] for COVID-19 in the city of Honghu in Hubei, China, the purpose of this study was to demonstrate how new medical informatics technologies may enable effective pandemic control. Cloud-based hardware effectively mitigated issues like a lack of local technical support, the inaccessibility of experts and physical hardware due to transportation restrictions, rapidly shifting functionality requirements, and connections with multiple sources across various platforms. The system gathered structured electronic medical record data from nine hospitals daily from the WeChat platform. It is one of the largest mobile social network apps in China. It has more than 1 billion monthly active users, real-time information about symptoms and personal contact history, and daily reported case diagnosis data from one public health information system, a third-party antibody lab, and a polymerase chain reaction lab. It developed a novel mini program for the WeChat platform software development kit for symptom reporting and spatial data collection by utilizing the nine hospitals' existing health information systems.

The suggestion [44] provides research opportunities and the foundation for additional practical applications. The dataset utilized for this situation study is the Our Reality in Information by Hannah Ritchie. The ML models are designed to accurately forecast the number of new cases and possible end dates of the pandemic. It suggests a structure for using these models in cloud data centers. Government hospitals and private health centers continuously transmit their positive patient count in a cloud-based environment. The population density, average and median age, weather, health facilities, *etc.*, are also to be incorporated to improve the prediction's accuracy. It utilized three instances of single-core Azure B1s virtual machines with 1 gigabyte of RAM, SSD storage, and 64-bit Microsoft Windows Server 20164 for this case study. To predict various metrics, such as the anticipated number of facilities to manage patients and hospitals, we deployed multiple analysis tasks in an ensemble learning fashion using the HealthFog framework and FogBus. According to our analysis, the daily cost of tracking patients, amortized CPU usage, and cloud execution is only 1.2 USD per day.

The Honghu Hybrid System (HHS) [45] was developed to monitor Covid-19 in Hubei, China, and was put into operation within seventy-two hours. Some of the HH'ss main features are syndromic surveillance on mobile devices, policy-making decision support, clinical decision support, prioritization of resources, and follow-up of discharged patients. The IoT-Fog-Cloud architecture monitors the patient's movements, allows for remote Covid-19 testing, alerts in the event of an emergency, and provides hygiene reminders. It used cameras to record the faces of people coming from their homes. The image data is saved in the cloud. Convolutional Neural Network (CNN)-enabled AI systems are used to detect faces. The preliminary testing of some portion of this pandemic is Contact Following. The process of manually tracing contacts is inefficient and time-consuming, but new technologies like smartphones and applications make it possible to locate a person's contact information.

This study [46] used quantitative methods to test hypotheses and examine item validity and reliability. The theory of UTAUT2 models was used in this study, along with a few other variables. A total of 175 people filled out this questionnaire: the university's lecturers, teachers, and students were selected randomly. It kept one dependent variable and ten independent variables. For a random sample of 175 respondents from Indonesian schools and universities, 26 lecturers (15%), 57 university students (33%), and 92 teachers participated. The gender distribution was 70 percent male and 30 percent female, with an average age of 35. It will invite lecturers, teachers, and university students to contribute to this study by providing the highest platform experience in the COVID-19 pandemic learning process *via* Zoom cloud meeting. It will study the value of the best solution in Indonesian education in research problems. All participants explained the purpose of this study and the procedure for filling out the questionnaire before they started filling it out. Each participant can complete the questionnaire in as little as 15 minutes on average. This study used the structural equation modeling method to evaluate the data analysis and hypothesis. This study was carried out using Smart PLS Version 3.0.

COVIDomic [47] is a multi-omics online platform that makes it easier to analyze and make sense of many health data from COVID-19 patients. The COVIDomic platform provides a comprehensive set of bioinformatic tools. It determines the coronavirus strain's origin and the disease's anticipated severity. It is made up of three parts. A web interface is the first part. This interface allows users to upload a wide range of genetic and clinicopathological data from patient cohorts. It includes details such as age, disease progression, and death causes. The platform also supports meta-transcriptomic data from the patient's pulmonary fluid. It reveals the gene regulation of the microflora during the coronavirus infection. The bioinformatic analysis and processing of the uploaded data comprise the second part. The pipeline performs several analytical protocols automatically after a dataset is uploaded. It can obtain a comprehensive overview of the species diversity of the patient's microbiome. It also includes its potential correlations with COVID-19 severity from the meta-transcriptomic data of the lung tissues. These data are also used to analyze the molecular evolution mechanisms of the pathology. A collection of tools in the third part of the platform make it possible for the user to examine the outcomes of the analyses carried out by the second part of the platform, visualize the uploaded data, and carry out additional post-analysis tasks. The interface for uploading samples and their associated metadata is simple to use. Users can upload the SARS-CoV-2 genome sequence, biochemical parameters, age, and raw data from their meta-transcriptomic samples.

This work [48] aims to improve KNN and research into IoT-cloud-based COVID - 19 detection. All seven datasets were also subjected to the eKNN classifier. A classifier's job is to divide the input data into classes in the supervised ML method known as classification. Only one group applies to each object. The neighbors are selected from a list of training things whose types are already present. Only the class of the test sample's closest neighbor is assigned. Because the k value chooses the number of neighbors that make up the class, this factor significantly impacts how well the KNN algorithm performs. The ACO-based feature selection mechanism was paired with the KNN algorithm during this second phase of implementation. There are eight features in the first dataset. There are 15 features in Dataset 2, Dataset 6, and Dataset 7. There are 18 features in datasets 3 and 4, and 19 in dataset 5. The possibility that the proposed eKNN's implementation potential will be harmed by ACO-based feature selection is investigated. Optimizing ant colonies imitates the way ants search for food. Other ants can use the shortest path provided by the pheromone trail to locate the food source. The pheromone's evaporation rate causes the decay of less traveled routes. ACO is a probabilistic method that encourages rapid solution-finding and guarantees convergence. The first dataset contained 5000 records and was obtained from Kaggle. A cross-country dataset is the second one. Age, gender, country, heart disease, COPD, diabetes, pregnancy, smoking habits, and other characteristics are present in each dataset.

Cloud and artificial intelligence [49] technologies have been incorporated into the design of this framework model [50]. The incident management system's database gathers local data on COVID-19-infected isolated seafarer's mental and physical states. To keep track of common health conditions, the seafarer can sign in to the provided application and record the parameters. A smartphone app notifies the seafarer and makes an immediate appointment with the emergency center when an onboard person experiences a sudden rise in body temperature or difficulty breathing. The incident management system always keeps track of how many people are infected on a given ship and gives the authorities on the system the daily effective infection rates.

5.5. CHALLENGES

5.5.1. Awareness

The Internet of Things (IoT) over the Wireless Body Area Network (WBAN) for healthcare purposes is one scenario for IoT devices that has attracted much research attention in recent years. The Health Internet of Things, or H-IoT, is a significant development in information systems. It substantially impacts people's health and increases their sense of worth in life. It is a complicated system involving many fields, including computer science, medical and health, and microelectronics systems. The Internet of Things is transforming the healthcare industry by redefining the devices, apps, and people related to and associated with healthcare solutions. As the integrated healthcare sector's efficiency ensures better patient care, it continually provides new tools. The Internet of Things seamlessly links all subjects and the healthcare system. One or more vital signs, such as heart rate, blood pressure, oxygen saturation, activities, or environmental parameters, such as location, temperature, humidity, and so on, can be sampled, processed, and communicated by a WBAN sensor node. By strategically placing these sensors as tiny patches on the human body or concealing them in the person's clothing, prolonged ubiquitous health monitoring is possible.

Although context awareness has been a concept for some time, technologies like wireless, mobile tools, sensors, wearable instruments, intelligent artifacts, and handheld computers are now available to support application development. Such advancements could assist the well-being of caring experts in dealing with their undertakings while expanding the nature of patient consideration. However, agent's communication is impacted by new technologies. Fig. (**34**) represents similar system architecture.

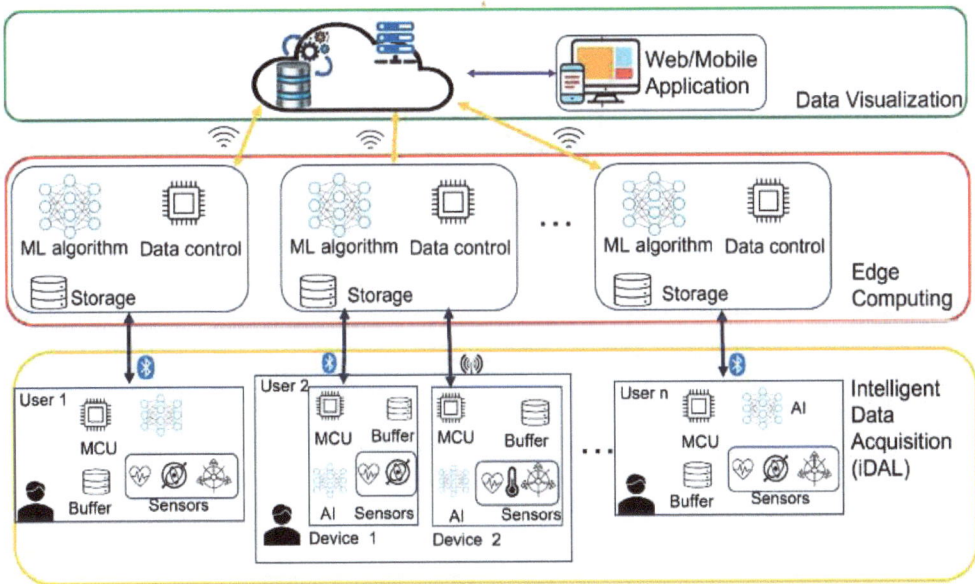

Fig. (34). Proposed Architecture [51].

A data life cycle [52] depicts the phases through which data moves in software systems. Web-based context management services provide context information management throughout the context's life cycle. There are four stages. To begin, it must gather context from a variety of sources. Physical or digital sensors could serve as the sources. Second, meaningful modeling and representation of the collected data are required. Third, to extract high-level context information from low-level raw sensor data, it must process modeled data. The consumers interested in context need to be provided with high-level and low-level context. The software component that collects sensor data requests the sensor hardware to acquire data regularly or instantly. The software component that is in charge of periodically or immediately acquiring sensor data receives data from the physical or virtual sensor. It ensures that it can present all 50 projects on a single page. The work made extensive use of abbrev*ia*tions. It allows readers to analyze and discover positive and negative patterns that we have yet to discuss explicitly.

A novel, IoT-aware innovative architecture [53] is proposed in this work for hospitals and nursing schools to use for automatic monitoring and tracking of patients, staff, and biomedical devices. An integrated RFID-WSN 6LoWPAN network with four typologies makes up the HSN. On the other hand, the primary purpose of 6LRR nodes is to track patients, nursing staff, and biomedical devices labeled with RFID Gen2 tags. The proposed SHS assumes that several 6LR are deployed in the hospital to collect data from the environment, such as temperature, pressure, and ambient light conditions. Important physiological parameters, such as heartbeat and movement, can be detected by patients wearing HT nodes. The RFID Gen2 tag's user memory stores sensed data regularly, making it possible for the environment's six LRR nodes to retrieve and deliver them to the IoT [54] Smart Gateway. The gateway acts as a 6LBR, making it possible for WSN nodes and users located far away to communicate. The received data are analyzed and stored in the database by a Monitoring Application (MA) that runs on the gateway. Network administrators can manage the environmental parameters of sensor and actuator nodes through a graphical Web interface. Doctors with specific privileges can access current and past patient data through the same interface. The medical staff can also manage this information remotely through a specialized mobile software application. Doctors can read the most recent information stored in the user memory of the RFID Gen2 tag or historical data stored in the Control DB during the daily medical inspections in hospitals to check the patient's physiological parameters. The Medical App also lets doctors add reminders of important information to the memory. A 6LRR consists of an Advanticsys XM1000 mote and a commercial off-the-shelf (COTS) RFID Gen2 Reader connected *via* the universal asynchronous receiver/transmitter (UART) communication bus. The upgraded 116-kilobyte EEPROM, 8-kilobyte RAM, and integrated temperature, humidity, and light sensors of the "TelosB"-based XM1000 are included. A 16-bit ultra-low-power TI MSP430F2618 micro-controller is included. The IEEE 802.15.4-compliant TI CC2420 transceiver with a transmission frequency of 2.4 GHz provides wireless communication capabilities. The Sensor ID Discovery Gate UHF, the chosen RFID Gen2 reader, can be easily set up and controlled by the XM1000 board *via* the UART interface.

It concentrates on the most proficient method to use semantic IoT information [55] for thinking of noteworthy information by applying for cutting-edge semantic advances. With Apache Camel and Java Message Service, ActiveMQ manages loosely coupled message delivery between IoT nodes and reasoning nodes. Utilizing Enterprise Integration Patterns and the Apache Camel integration framework, ActiveMQ is a highly configurable, scalable, and quick messaging solution for integrating various systems and components. It facilitates interoperability between sensors, reasoner nodes, and the knowledge base, as well as flexibility for data aggregation and dissemination. Using a simple MQTT protocol, IoT nodes send semantic data to the ActiveMQ message broker. Messages are sent from the message broker to the JMS queue, where they are compiled and used by subscribed reasoning nodes. The Jena reasoning framework is used to make reasoning tasks flexible to use. It can interpret most IoT data formats utilized and implements a comprehensive subset of the OWL language. The reasoning engine can operate in forward chaining, backward chaining, or a hybrid mode and supports user-defined rules. The reasoning service gathers data, uses the Jena rule reasoner and the OWL ontology to reason about it, and saves the results to the RDF database. A system that distributes data and reasoning tasks to reasoning nodes that are physically distributed and form a reasoning cluster [56]. A sequence of messages is first aggregated, then the reasoning is processed over aggregated messages with implemented rules and an OWL ontology node in the message broker. It ensures that messages from the exact vehicle are consumed and aggregated by the same reasoning. The message broker serves as an edge node for a specific area. Mobile nodes subscribe to the reasoning system upon entering the region, and IoT nodes send data to an ActiveMQ message broker *via* the MQTT protocol. There are 24 OWL classes and 12 properties in the ontology's 2,100 bytes of static knowledge. Within the same 1Gb/s sub-network, it physically distributed the Sesame RDF database and ActiveMQ broker across multiple servers. For distributed scalability tests, the reasoning cluster used eight physically distributed nodes. A distributed reasoning node server has 64 GB of main memory and 16 cores. A single reasoning node runs on a server with 32 cores and 128 GB of main memory. The data comes from 65,000 different taxi trajectories. There are 5,543,348 observations and 72,063,524 RDF triples in the dataset. Location coordinates in the form of longitude and latitude, velocity, direction, time stamp, and sender identification for each taxicab are all included in the data.

A wearable device [57] that combines image recognition and localization capabilities to automatically provide users with cultural content related to the observed artworks is the foundation of the proposed system. A museum-installed Bluetooth Low Energy infrastructure is used to obtain the localization data. It has three primary structure blocks. The wearable device and the processing center share the localization service. The initial one notifies the processing center of the current user's position. The user's observation of the artwork can be detected in real-time by the image processing algorithm. It can quickly analyze the video frames taken by the wearable vision device and quickly and reliably identify the target object. The heart of business logic is the processing center. It gets to, in the Cloud, the social items expected by the clients and adroitly gives such things on a few intelligent stages. The positioning data supplied by the localization infrastructure makes it possible for several location-aware services to run. It has three main components: the infrastructure of wireless landmarks that send localization data regularly. The service is installed on the wearable smart gateway and uses landmark data to determine where it is. The service gets the user's location and gives it to the other services at the processing center. The brilliant door is acknowledged through an installed PC, an Odroid-XU. It is a single ARM board with just 94 x 70 x 18 mm dimensions. It is powered by a 1.2 GHz Samsung Exynos5 Octa Core processor (Cortex-A15), has a PowerVR SGX544 MP3 graphics card, and has 2 GB of DDR3 RAM. An Odroid USB-cam 720p, which has a 1280 x 720 HD resolution, a USB 2.0 plug-and-play interface, and supports up to 30 frames per second, is used for image acquisition. A Raspberry Pi Model B was used to create the device that processes cultural content sent by the processing center when there are a lot of visitors. It has 512 MB of RAM and is based on the Broadcom BCM2835 system with a chip (SoC) with an ARM1176JZF-S 700 MHz processor and a VideoCore IV GPU.

The Context Awareness for the Internet of Things (CA4IOT) architecture [58] is proposed to assist users by automatically selecting sensors based on the issues or tasks. It focuses on the automated configuration of filtering, fusion, and reasoning mechanisms that can be applied to the sensor data streams collected by utilizing particular sensors. There are four layers to the architecture known as CA4IOT. The client Layer addresses the clients, and it's anything but a center layer in CA4IOT. Applications, services, and human users all qualify as users. The Data, Semantics, and Context Dissemination Layer manage users. This layer includes the publish/subscribe, request manager, and data dispatcher components. Data processing, reasoning, fusion, knowledge generation, and storage are all performed by the Processing and Reasoning Layer. The Context and Semantic Discovery Layer manages the era, configuration, and storage of context and semantic discoverers. Data collection is the responsibility of the Sensor Data Acquisition Layer. Most IoT, sensor network, and context management middleware solutions include this layer, which is referred to by various names, including wrappers, handlers, proxies, mediators, and so on. This layer retrieves sensor data into CA4IOT and communicates with hardware and software sensors.

An IoT-aware healthcare monitoring system [59] is the goal of this project. CC2451 sensor tag for ambient data collection. This Bluetooth sensor was made for developers of innovative phone applications that use wireless sensors. It has a battery that lasts for months and can collect temperature, humidity, and pressure data using an accelerometer, gyroscope, and magnetometer. The sensor meets the heart rate profile and low-energy standards. The gateway uses an XMPP account to send data to a server that also uses the xep-0326 extension.

It uses the digital twin framework. This work [60] proposes and implements an intelligent context-aware healthcare system. This framework contributes to digital healthcare and positively enhances healthcare operations. Through three phases, it uses IoT devices, AI, and data analytics to create a virtual patient replica, make it possible for healthcare professionals to work together effectively, and make it possible for patients with similar cases to work together. Processing and prediction are patient-centered. The first step is to use IoT wearable sensors to collect patient data. These sensors send data in real-time about body metrics, which are essential for keeping an eye on health and finding anomalies. It will temporarily store the transferred data in a cloud database that stores raw data. Later, a machine learning system will use this data for training and prediction. Healthcare professionals in the patient domain must intervene during the monitoring and correction phase. The results of the predictive models from the Result Database will be used by healthcare professionals who provide treatments and recommendations based on formal training and experience. The examination stage is the participation of patients with comparable cases happens in the third stage to use real situations, improve patient's DT, and upgrade the entire structure. The model will be able to compare the results of the current patient with those of other patients by obtaining data and results from digital twins of patients with similar cases. The MIT-BIH Arrhythmia Database is the foundation of the dataset used in this paper. It includes 48 half-hour excerpts from two-channel ambulatory ECG recordings on 47 subjects studied by the BIH Arrhythmia Laboratory between 1975 and 1979. Using an ADC, the playback unit was digitalized at 360 Hz per signal in real-time.

It is a privacy-aware offloading scheme based on reinforcement learning [61] to help healthcare IoT devices protect user location and usage pattern privacy. To provide emergency care and telehealth advice, it considers a healthcare IoT device that uses multiple sensors to measure and analyze healthcare data like blood pressure and electrocardiograms. The IoT device can process some computation tasks locally, offload some to the edge device, and save others from processing in the next time slot when powered by both the battery and the energy harvesting module. Each time slot in the simulations lasts one second, and the IoT device generates 30 kb of new healthcare data. It sends one-bit sensing data to the edge device. The IoT device requires 0.2 J of energy and uses 10^{-4} J to process the data locally.

There are three modules in the proposed quality-aware ECG monitoring system [62]: A module for sensing ECG signals, a module for automated signal quality evaluation, and an ECG transmission and analysis module aware of signal quality. The signal quality index is calculated in three steps—flat-line detection, abrupt baseline wander extraction, and high-frequency noise detection and extraction—to evaluate the clinical acceptability of ECG signals. There are 48 two-channel records in the MITBIHA database of noise-free and noisy ECG signals with various ECG waveform morphologies. The ECG signals are digitized with a resolution of 11 bits and a sampling rate of 360 samples per second.

5.5.2. Accesibility

The relative ease with which services, in this case, health care, can be reached from a given location is referred to as accessibility. It must consider both spatial and nonspatial factors in accessibility measures. Since supply and demand are spatially connected, spatial access is a well-suited problem for GIS to address because it emphasizes the importance of spatial separation. Numerous demographic and socioeconomic variables, such as social class, income, age, sex, and race, interact with spatial access through nonspatial factors. Fig. (**35**) portrays IoT enabled healthcare system.

The work [64] uses mixed-methods methods. It creates a composite healthcare accessibility index and a composite healthcare satisfaction (CHCS) index using objective and subjective indicators. In Quito, Ecuador's capital, a survey was conducted for five weeks in July, August, and October 2014. The sampling process consisted of two stages. The creation and selection of sampling clusters were the first steps. It first used a geographic information system to display the Quito land use/land cover map, after which it extracted residential areas. It uses a GIS tool. The study area was divided into 18 hexagons, which it then selected randomly. The interviewer's capacity in terms of time and financial resources for city travel was considered when choosing this number of hexagons. The population density within each sampling hexagon influenced the number of interviewees. Interviewers covered each hexagon by conducting door-to-door interviews in households where people were willing to participate.

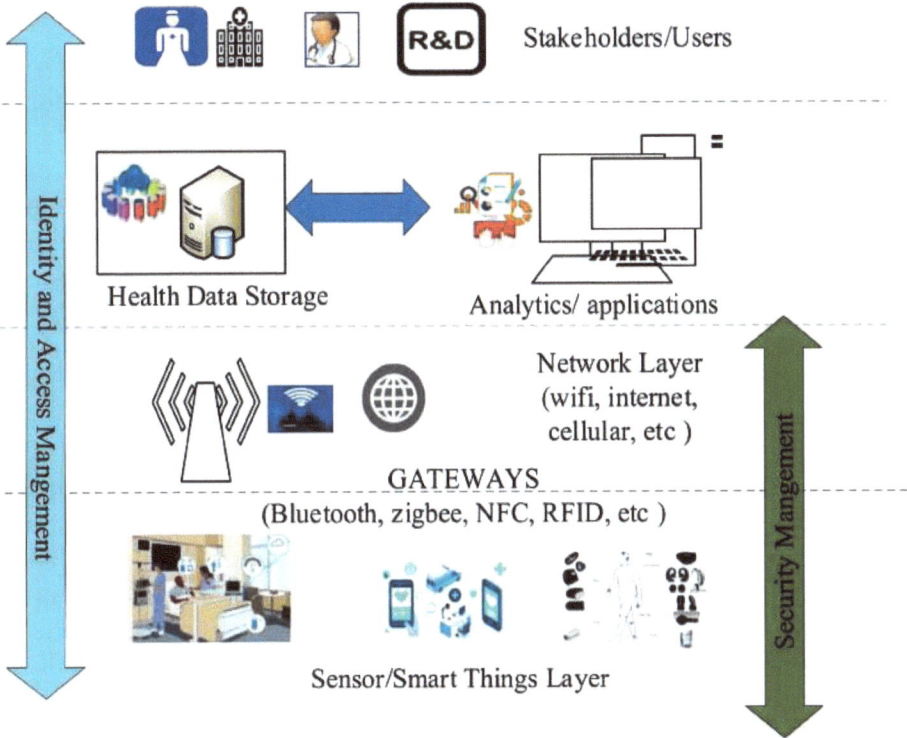

Fig. (35). IoT enabled healthcare system [63].

The work [65] uses two methods. The objective was to clarify the relationship between race and prostate cancer mortality among men. It reviewed published studies of men with prostate cancer receiving healthcare from the National Health Service in the United Kingdom, the Department of Defense or Veterans Affairs in the United States, or the Health Canada provincial/territorial healthcare system first to gain a better understanding of the existing evidence regarding equal-access healthcare systems. An impartial race-based comparison would be made possible by these equal-access systems. Second, it conducted an observational cohort analysis of race and prostate cancer mortality among men receiving care in the New England region of the Veterans Health Administration to generate new evidence on this topic. The findings are yet another report from an equal-access system. Veterans who receive health care from Veterans Affairs have lower socioeconomic statuses than the general population of the United States. Analyses were based on an extensive review of the medical records of 1270 men diagnosed with prostate cancer between 1991 and 1995. The data came from a source population of 64,545 healthcare beneficiaries at nine medical centers within the Veterans Health Administration. Through 2006, cause-specific mortality could be followed.

The 2-Step Floating Catchment Area Method serves as the foundation for the framework [66]. It estimated the resident's access to hospital beds in the US state of Florida as the study area. The following spatial datasets were relevant to this study: information from the Florida Geographic Data Library about 346 hospitals, a transportation network with 1,747,524 road segments, and a population of 11,442 block groups. The smallest geographic unit for which the Census Bureau publishes sample data regarding a population's socioeconomics and demographics is the U.S. Census, block group. The people of a census block group typically range from 600 to 3000, with 1500 being the ideal number. The block group was chosen as the basic unit of analysis because it has the most information about vehicle ownership at the best geographic level. Each block group's total number of households represents the population that could use hospital care. All houses in a block group were piled on top of the block group's centroid. It first extracted the geometric centroids of census blocks, our best understanding of population distribution, to consider the uneven distribution of households within a block group. It calculated the weighted centroids of block groups and gave each census block centroid a weight based on the number of homes in that block. It divided the households in each block group into two categories to include transportation modes in the measurement: families with and without automobiles. By dividing the length of the road segment by the speed, it calculated the car or bus travel time. The shortest route between each pair of population centroids and the hospital was determined using an algorithm.

This study [67] examined how healthcare facilities think about being accessible to people with spinal cord injuries. A code number was assigned to healthcare facilities listed in a Midwestern city's telephone directory, and then a computer generated a random list. Forty sites from this list agreed to participate in a brief, private accessibility study. Both traditional and integrated care facilities were part of the sample. One of the three experienced interviewers carried out a phone assessment. The manager took a brief oral survey on that call to determine how people felt about the clinic's accessibility. Within two weeks, assessors finished an on-location evaluation of the stopping region, access to the structure, access to the facility, entryway, diagnostic room, and washroom. One person with quadriplegia and one with paraplegia were on the survey team. The team members received instructions on how to use the survey instruments. Before collecting data for this project, the team completed nine surveys to conduct a field test of the tools and ensure their proper use.

5.5.3. Human Power Crisis

To achieve three fundamental goals—coverage, motivation, and competence—the health and educational sectors collaborate in managing the workforce for improved performance. Coverage strategies encourage outreach to vulnerable populations, appropriate worker skill mixes, and numerical adequacy. Positive work and career environments, supportive health systems, and adequate compensation are the primary components of motivational strategies. Education for the right attitudes and skills, training for continuous learning, and cultivating leadership, entrepreneurship, and innovation are all ways to improve competence. National capacity development should be the primary focus of all of these efforts. It should monitor progress and setbacks to make adjustments in the middle of the course. Fig. (**36**) represents Post-coronavirus disease-2019 (COVID-19) multi-levels health crisis.

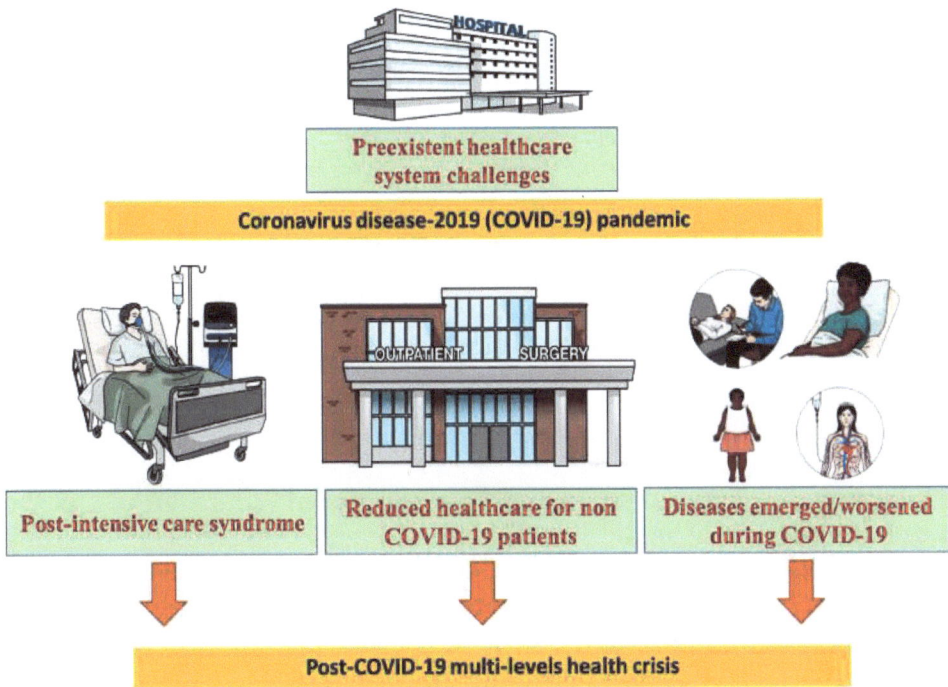

Fig. (36). Post-coronavirus disease-2019 (COVID-19) multi-levels health crisis [68].

The work [69] expects to present the division's job in general well-being emergencies in Korea. Korea has developed a system of medical resources for emergency response, including a stockpile of antiviral drugs and notification of national medical institutions in the event of public health crises. Korea operates 519 isolated beds in 16 medical facilities and has 13,000,000 doses of antiviral medications covering 26% of its population. Emerging infectious diseases, such as pandemic influenza, a*vian* influenza human infection, and severe acute respiratory syndrome, are handled by the Korea Centers for Disease Control and Prevention division of public health crisis response. Preparing for emerging infectious diseases, securing medical resources during a crisis, activating the emergency response, and strengthening public health personnel is part of its job description.

This study [70] explains how Vietnam's tourism and hospitality industries built organizational resilience to withstand the first Covid19 crisis. Additionally, qualitative research was appropriate for an in-depth examination of the effects of individual interactions, behaviors, and experiences on business operations. It selected semi-structured interviews to investigate the HR strategies employed by business managers in Vietnam during the lockdown to cope, adapt, and recover from the COVID-19 pandemic. Reviewing relevant HRM and crisis management literature was the basis for developing the interview guide. In 2020, it gathered data in May and June. Individual one-on-one interviews were conducted in Vietnamese. Audio recordings of each interview lasted between 30 and 60 minutes. The bilingual researchers transcribed and translated the interviews into English. It used the interview guide to develop the initial coding structure, and thematic analysis was used to identify themes and patterns in the data, allowing new themes and subthemes to emerge. The research team reviewed, defined, double-checked, reflected on, and discussed the identified themes and subthemes to establish a framework for interpretation and reach a consensus on the findings.

5.6. AFFORDABILITY

There are several potential advantages to the proposed Affordability Index. Both its denominator (median household income) and numerator (mean cost of insurance premiums) are dependable, credible, and generated annually. The direct connection between salaries and health care costs can be seen in this ratio of insurance premiums to wages. Incomes fall when healthcare costs rise. According to economists, total compensation (salary and benefits per employee) is ultimately a concern for employers. Only a portion of the full payment is made up of wages. Employer's health insurance "contributions" are included in total worker compensation. It could convert a more significant amount of total compensation to cash wages if the cost of health insurance decreased. The Affordability Index measures the downward pressure on wages caused by rising healthcare costs. The Moderateness File additionally has likely impediments. The index only applies to people who have insurance that their employer sponsors. It may not consider the cost of health care for people with Medicaid, Medicare, or no insurance.

Additionally, individual healthcare costs are not all covered by employer-sponsored insurance premiums. It only takes into account costs that are directly incurred. It does not account for expenses incurred indirectly, such as the time and money spent traveling to and from specialists and other specific services, the time spent administering medical treatments, and the potential loss of wages associated with doing so. Fig. (37) represents main demand-side factors affecting healthcare affordability.

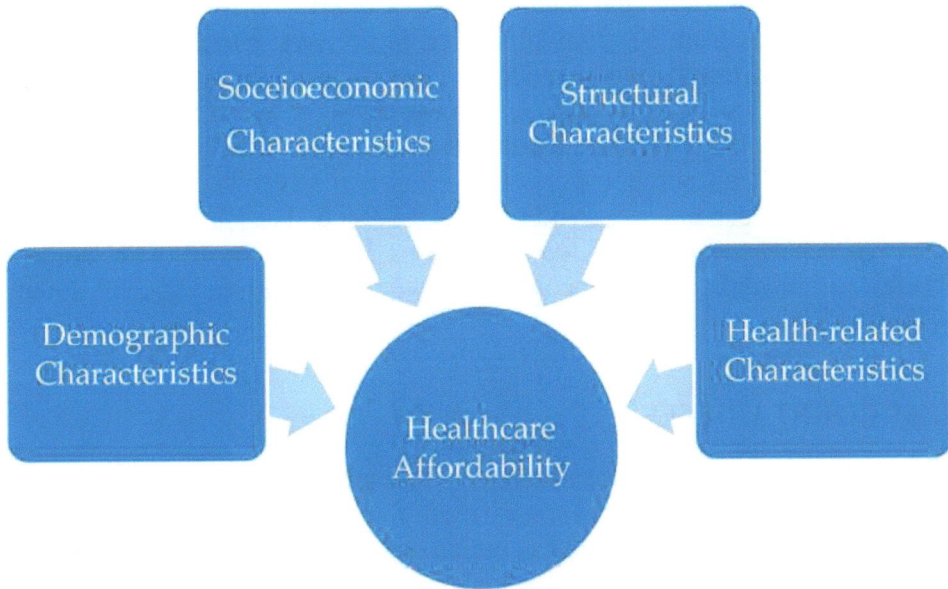

Fig. (37). Main demand-side factors affecting healthcare affordability [71].

It [72] used preferred Reporting Items for Systematic Reviews and Meta-Analyses to conduct a systematic review of the literature in this study. Articles that discussed the design, development, evaluation, and utility of smartphone-based software for healthcare workers, professionals, medical or nursing students, or patients were found using Google Scholar and MEDLINE. From 2,934 articles retrieved from PubMed, Scholar, and Medline searches, It selected 59 writings that discussed 88 applications for this study. It compared the various technologies currently in use with hand-held portable devices and the critical issues raised by recent smartphone technology modifications in the healthcare sector. The utilization of cutting-edge technology minimally resource-intensive in the healthcare system was also recommended.

This research [73] has practical implications for expanding economic opportunities in health care on both sides of the border, expanding access to health care for at-risk populations, and improving public health and insurance services for folks in the border region through innovative health projects of international cooperation. Transnational medical consumers already use the opportunity to assist those not covered by the U.S. medical system by gaining access to resources at the border. In July-August 2002 and April-May 2005, this study was carried out in Los Algodones, Mexico, and on the border regions of Arizona and California that connect the United States and Mexico. The information comes from 33 semi-structured interviews, surveys, and participant observations with transnational medical consumers as they searched for health resources in Mexico. It took these interviews and surveys from opportunity and snowball samples. 36% were male, and 64 percent were female. Seventy percent were married, fifteen percent were single and had never been married, and the remaining fifteen percent were widowed or divorced. They had mostly graduated from high school or some college but didn't have a degree. The majority of interviewed said their annual income is between $15,000 and 25,000 dollars, or less than $65,000.

5.7. ACCOUNTABILITY

There will always be three components to an accountability system: an exact meaning of positive objectives or targets, the capacity to gauge and screen objective accomplishment, and a bunch of ramifications for suppliers or associations on the off chance that achievements regarding objectives or goals are not palatable. In healthcare, establishing goals and objectives is complex and contentious. Quality of care and patient experience is unaffected by quantitative targets for care volume. Improving a population's health and well-being may have only a tenuous or fragile connection to targets related to care delivery. If the goal is to provide providers of care and services with helpful feedback, monitoring the process or managing outcomes requires accurate, adequate, and timely information. The results of execution disappointment by suppliers are coercive. The definition of a clear mandate in the form of specific goals and objectives, the attribution of these mandates to skilled providers or organizations, and the design of incentives to support the accountability relationship and improvement present numerous challenges for accountability regimes in healthcare systems. The objectives are connected to the intricate function of production, and they will require a wide range of skills, knowledge, and abilities on the part of providers and governing bodies, as well as the capacity to work together to improve care and services. Fig. (**38**) represents IoT 4-Layer Architecture for HMS.

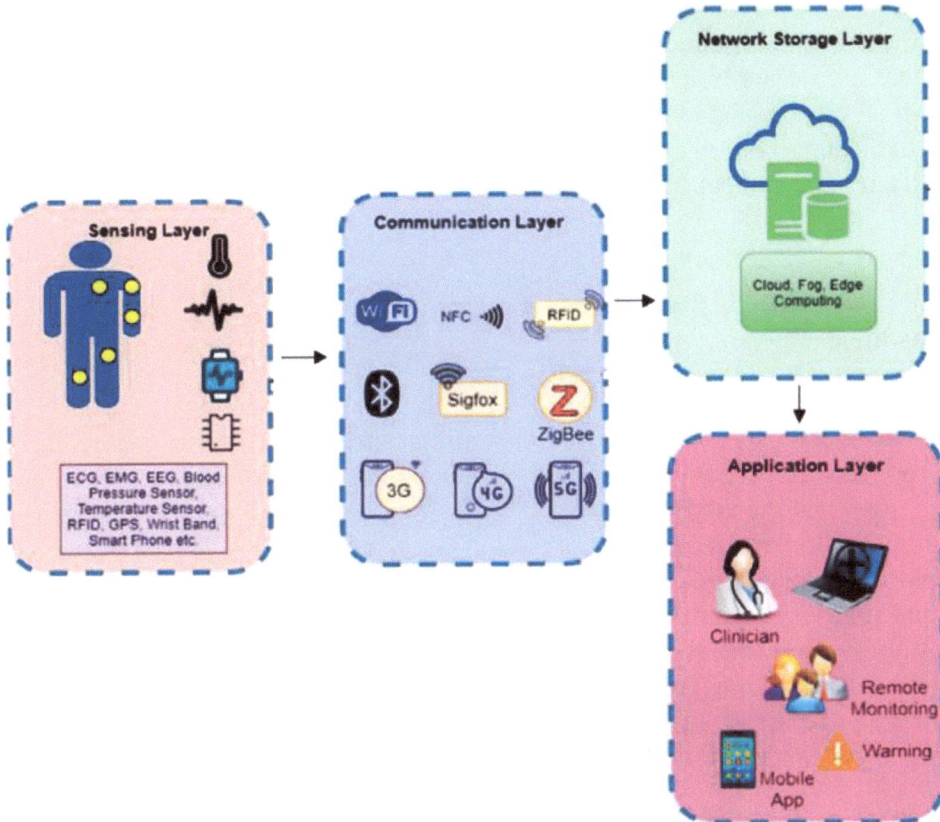

Fig. (38). IoT 4-Layer Architecture for HMS [74].

An IoT Security Risk Management Model [75] for Secured Practice in a Healthcare Environment, is proposed in the recommendation. Six processes are described. The primary focus of the planning stage is identifying the research questions or just conducting a case study based on its advantages and disadvantages. During the design phase, the unit of analysis will be described, categorize the underlying issues of the anticipated research, and develop procedures to maintain the quality of the case study. The Hospital Kuala Lumpur (HKL) is chosen as a case study because it is the largest government hospital in Malaysia and serves as a model for numerous pilot implementation projects, from medical health to technological infrastructure. There are 53 distinct departments at HKL. It includes the pharmaceutical department, clinical departments, clinical support services, and training and research. The hospital maintains its service standards by adhering to the Hospital Performance Indicator for Accountability (HPIA). The internal business process, customer focus, employee satisfaction, learning and development, financial and office management, and environmental support are the HPIA indicators. The preparation stage focuses on learning how to conduct a case study, create a protocol, conduct a pilot case, and get necessary approvals. It developed a case study protocol to guarantee the study's reliability, and the team comprises experienced researchers familiar with the case study approach. The collection stage includes:

- Following the case study's protocol.
- Gathering evidence from various sources.
- Creating a database.
- Keeping track of the evidence chain.

The work consisted of a series of semi-structured interviews with HKL's IT officers and healthcare professionals to obtain an overview of the company's operations and the current state of its IoT implementation. Analyze the stage that examines alternative explanations and interpretations of the findings using theoretical propositions and other strategies. Sharing the stage is where enough textual and visual materials are assembled to display the evidence necessary to draw the study's conclusion. The final product is presented as a Model of IoT Security Risk Management for Healthcare Practice. It incorporates the HPIA strategies and COBIT5 Framework for IoT Risk Management and the phases necessary to achieve it.

The work is a framework [76] for healthcare information security context. In addition to acting as a validator for evaluating the security of existing systems of interest, the proposed framework also serves as a security guideline for the system's design. It uses an identifier to define a resource's or information's security context (SC). The security context comprises an audit list of actions (Audit) and an access control list (ACL). An effort that it can perform on the piece of information is specified in an ACL. The previous actions carried out on the context-related data are listed in an audit list. The propagation context will involve the transmission or exchange of information among various components. It creates the audit list for the security context.

The task is to efficiently collect and process data using fog computing between cloud computing and sensors. There are three layers to the IoT/fog computing-based healthcare system architecture [77]. The layer of sensors or devices: is answerable for gathering medical services information from sensors and gadgets that communicate information through a WiFi or cell (4G/LTE) organization to the mist layer to process and execute undertakings. These sensors and devices are attached to them. Real-time data sensing and transmission are possible with these sensors and devices. The layer of fog computing: acts as a link between the cloud computing layer and IoT sensors, which receive health data from various medical IoT sensors and devices. It is used to process and analyze IoT healthcare data in real-time. It is responsible for notifying users in real-time whether they are in the "possibly infected or uninfected" category. Additionally, this layer is connected to the cloud for storing, analyzing, and compiling each patient's medical record. The fog layer's tasks that cannot be processed or executed are stored, processed, and carried out by the cloud computing layer. The patient's status and details are transferred from the fog layer to the cloud for any necessary future actions. It studies, analyzes, or predicts a patient's health history. The fog layer can access the cloud layer and retrieve the required data. The approach prioritizes scheduling IoT tasks according to their importance rather than length. Three classes are selected to group high, medium, and low-priority functions together. Class 1 only receives lessons of low reputation. Class 2 only receives tasks of medium stature. Class 3 only receives positions of high priority. Additionally, there are three subcategories in the VM List. Also, each category is only used for a particular kind of work. The first category includes virtual machines (VMs) with low capabilities and performance. These VMs are designed to perform low-priority tasks. The VMs in Category 2 are specifically designed to receive and serve missions of medium importance and have medium capability and performance. The VMs in Category 3h are explicitly intended to receive and perform high-importance tasks. They have increased capacity and performance.

With both in-band and stand-alone deployment, the work [78] aims to investigate the realistic performance of NBIoT in terms of effective throughput, patiently served per cell, and latency in healthcare monitoring systems. A minimum bandwidth of 180 kHz, equivalent to one physical resource block (PRB) in LTE transmission, is the foundation for NB-IoT. It can use NB-IoT in three different operational modes with a minimum spectrum requirement of 180 kHz:

- As a stand-alone dedicated carrier.
- In-band within an existing LTE carrier's PRB.
- Within a current LTE carrier's guard band.

In the time domain, the ten ms-long frame structure of the NB-IoT downlink is comparable to that of LTE. Each frame has ten one-millisecond-long subframes, each with two slots containing seven OFDM symbols. It has a single physical resource block (PRB) in the frequency domain, 12 subcarriers separated by 15 Khz, and a standard cyclic prefix (CP). A single resource element (RE), the smallest transmission unit, comprises one subcarrier and one symbol. NB-IoT supports both single-tone and multi-tone transmissions in the uplink. The same SC-FDMA scheme is used for multi-tone transmission, with a subcarrier spacing of 15 kHz. However, subcarrier spacings of 15 kHz and 3.75 kHz are supported by single-tone communication. The 15 kHz frequency has the same numerology as LTE. These wireless sensors send and receive data *via* a long-distance wireless link. With NB-IoT, you can use cellular base stations already in place to cover the entire facility and the people who live there. Even when powered by batteries, NB-IoT guarantees that the terminals used by end users will have a long lifespan.

The work [79] provides a novel platform for using blockchain-based smart contracts to monitor patient's vital signs. Hyperledger Fabric, an enterprise-distributed ledger framework for developing blockchain-based applications, is used in the design and development of the proposed system. The healthcare IoT blockchain platform that has been designed features a modular architecture in which each layer is decoupled from the others. Developers can add or remove any module without affecting the system as a whole. There are four layers to the developed system. Various healthcare devices with computing, data storage, and communication capabilities comprise the proposed IoT physical layer. Since there is no global internal protocol for physical healthcare sensing devices, the connectivity layer aims to provide routing management. The availability layer is likewise answerable for offering assistance, including security for the board, message intermediaries, and the organization of the executives. The DLT is an agreement of shared, synchronized, and reproduced computerized information disseminated across the whole blockchain network, where each member has a record duplicate. The big data module makes it possible for blockchain to store data online, making it more effective and dependable. Large amounts of transactional data from various parties are held in structured forms in ledgers in the blockchain, where they are further utilized in the analysis procedure. A single network has been granted to all parties in the blockchain, making it simple for the client to access these particulars. A piece of computer code that the external client application triggers to manage, access, and modify the ledger is known as the smart contract. An intelligent agreement is initiated and installed on each network peer. In the proposed system, event management sends a notification each time a new block is added to the ledger in response to a predefined condition being met. The developed services offered by the designed medical blockchain platform are made available through the application programming interface (API), which is how clients access the application and manage the blockchain network. Users can securely communicate with one another and share their resources and assets using blockchain technology. The blockchain relies on consensus algorithms, asymmetric ciphers, and a peer-to-peer network for communication. The top layer is the application layer, which is the final layer and serves as a user interface and is used to manage and control healthcare devices. The developed system comprises the technical infrastructure that provides a service to the blockchain for the smart contract and DL through a user service framework. To maintain the uniformity of the distributed ledger, the medical blockchain model has a reliable authorized peer in which each peer holds a copy of the register for the blockchain network. A data lake stores and maintains medical data related to healthcare sensors and network participation in the distributed ledger—a chain of blocks stores immutable transactions in the blocks. The blockchain network is utilized as exchange logs that record and keep up with every progression in the information lake. The following patient information is stored in the data lake as an off-chain ledger (database), including the most recent values for vital signs and information about healthcare devices, among other things. Data analytics and other healthcare services are two more applications for the off-chain database. Each member is expected to sign up for blockchain before presenting their exchange. The private key needed to sign the transaction is contained in the enrollment certificate. Reading and writing data from the distributed ledger is what is referred to as a transaction in the blockchain network. Through the healthcare IoT server, participants (patient, nurse, and doctor) can submit a transaction to either generate a new task or obtain a response from a current job. Subsequently, the medical care IoT server sends a solicitation to the blockchain organization to play out an errand as per the solicitation. Only authenticated users can use and access blockchain services after successful enrollment. Users use client applications to request vital sign information. With the request, the vital-sign data is sent to the server, which activates the transaction's smart contract. Subsequently, the agreement cycle is executed in the blockchain network, which attaches the exchange data to the blockchain and records the imperative sign data in the state data set. After the transaction is completed successfully, the client is informed about the ledger upgrade *via* email. Fig. (**39**) portrays the same.

A real-time health monitoring system [80] for elderly residents of geriatric residences is suggested. It made this system so caregivers could better control how they monitor their patient's health and communicate with their patient's families. Wearable technology, such as watches and Android-powered smartphones, are utilized in this project. The goal is to collect and analyze data from sensors attached to patients with medical conditions to detect or, ideally, anticipate episodes of conditions like bipolar disorder, seasonal affective disorder, and chronic obstructive pulmonary disease (COPD). Each day, smartphone users are required to complete a health-related questionnaire. After completing the questionnaire, patients are asked to blow into the microphone to determine their maximum expiratory flow. The day's data are transferred to a distant server for analysis. The wearable IoT device, which corresponds to the Hexiwear biometric bracelet, makes up the first layer. It has sensors that can measure heart rate, body temperature, and blood oxygenation and can function as an IoT node. A mobile application for smartphones is one of the components of the "WolkAbout IoT Platform," which supports the Hexiwear bracelet and stores all information generated by the bracelet's sensors in the cloud. This middleware utilized the help-situated figuring (SOC) worldview, which depends on administrations that uncover their usefulness through a web Programming interface. The subsystem that enables family members and caregivers to interact with the monitoring of patient's vital signs and medical information is the mobile application. React Native was used in the development of the Abuelómetro system. It used the Samsung Galaxy S7 for development and testing; this smartphone runs the Nougat 7.0 version of Android. For capacity data in the middleware, MongoDB was utilized, which is an instrument that permits us to foster data sets situated to records rather than relations. Fig. (**40**) portrays the same.

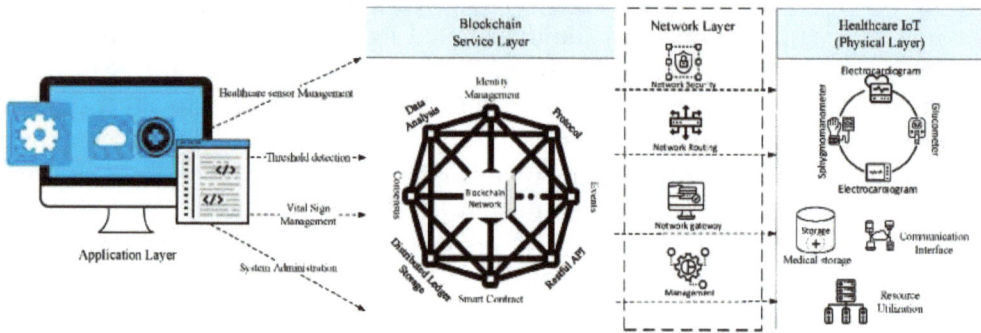

Fig. (39). Proposed layered-based healthcare IoT blockchain platform architecture for secure vital-sign monitoring [79].

The Common Recognition and Identification Platform (CRIP), a component of the CareStore project that aims to support caregivers and citizens in seamlessly managing health routines, is the subject of this study [81], which presents the design, development, implementation, and evaluation of the platform. In particular, the CRIP provides sensor-based assistance for seamless user and health device identification. The Normal Surrounding Helped Residing Home Stage is an open-source runtime execution stage for the execution of administrations, applications, gadget drivers, and a UI for staff and occupant's collaboration with the background. Using RFID and biometrics as identification technologies, the Common Recognition and Identification Platform is used to identify staff, residents, and devices. It is a shared online platform for uploading and storing healthcare and AAL drivers and applications that the CAALHP and CRIP can seamlessly download and install. An embedded Linux platform is used to integrate the hardware modules. This platform runs special software to handle all communications and interactions between the hardware and the CAALHP. The software was written in C++ as a Linux daemon for the chosen operating system, Linux, specifically the official Raspberry Pi distribution Raspbian. All classes that implement the CRIP's primary functions are contained in this module middleware. A biometric or NFC module's internal interrupt is started when a user interacts with the hardware and the hardware's data is read. The class CripHttpServer executes a more compelled HTTP server, in light of the libmicrohttpd library, to deal with the REST demands enrolled when the server begins. A URL is assigned to each registered method so it can be invoked when a REST request is received. It must use the interfaces ICripBluetooth, ICripBiometric, and ICripNfc abstract access to hardware peripherals such as Bluetooth, biometric, and NFC reader/writer, respectively, and a specified hardware factory by the interface ICripHardwareFactory to gain access to these devices. Fig. (**41**) represents the same.

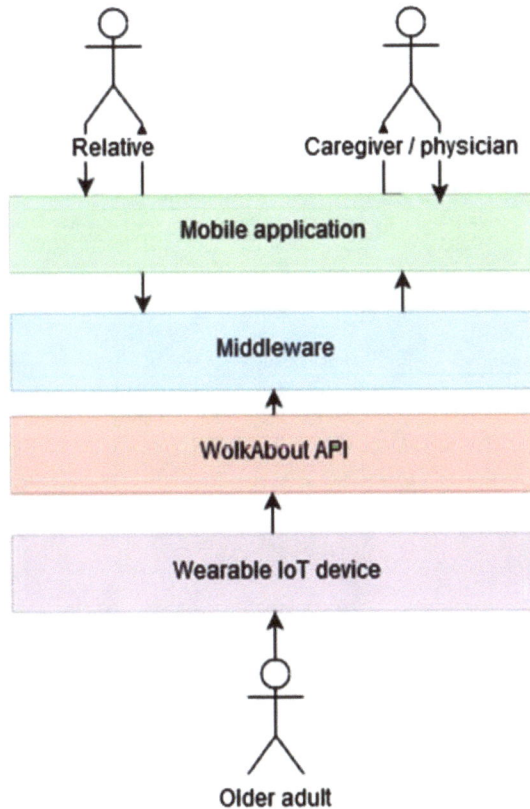

Fig. (40). System architecture of Abuelómetro [80].

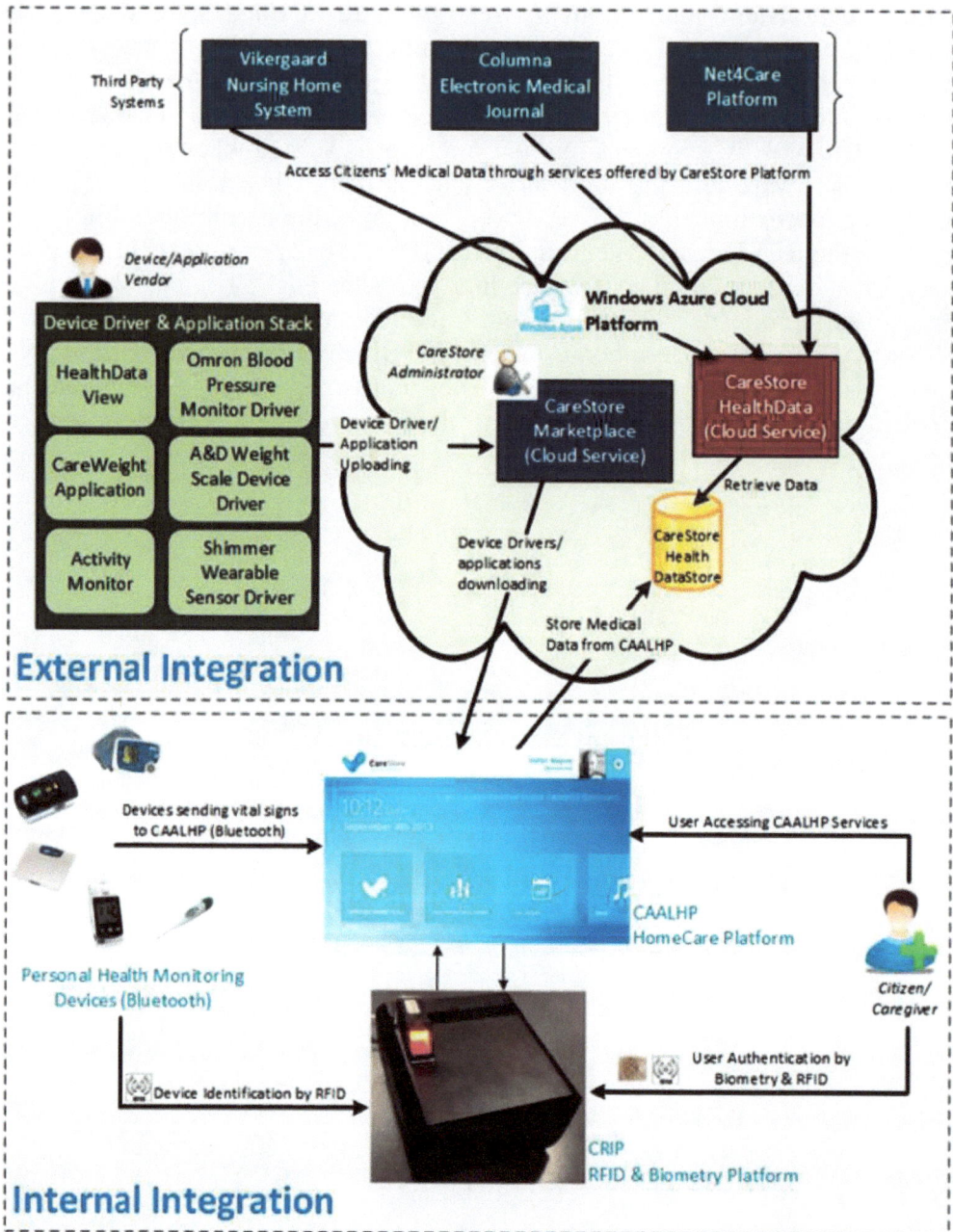

Fig. (41). Overview of the CareStore Platform, comprised by three main systems: the CAALHP, the CRIP and the Marketplace [81].

PISIoT [82] is built on a layered architecture that clearly defines and explains each module's activities and functions. It consists of five layers. There are various components in each layer, each of which has a particular role and relationship. Patients can view and track their biomedical variables, available IoT-based services, medical history, and recommendations through the presentation layer, which facilitates communication between the patient and the platform. It can manually enter water and food consumed throughout the day on the forum. When patients enter food or drinks consumed with an Internet-connected smartphone or computer, calories, carbohydrates, fat, and proteins are automatically retrieved from the device provider's database. The checking network layer comprises various IoT-based gadgets, for example, wearable and brilliant gadgets connected to telecom hardware, which have correspondence interfaces that work with data trading. Based on the activities performed throughout the day, these devices enable the collection of information on the patient's biomedical variables (heart rate, calories burned, sleep, minutes of physical activity, and weight). The incorporation layer comprises wearable and savvy gadget suppliers and gets the patient's information and interviews to produce the replies mentioned. It is responsible for the medical recommendations and critical variables identified by the data analysis layer. Linking, invoking, selecting, and confirming the availability of IoT-based services is the responsibility of the IoT-based services layer. The storage and backup of the patient's medical history and the data gathered by the utilized devices are the responsibility of the data management layer. Fig. (**42**) portrays the same.

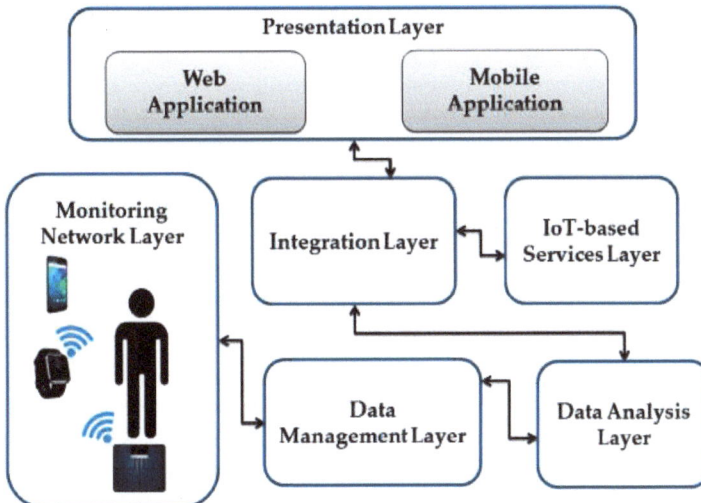

Fig. (42). Architecture of PISIoT [82].

The framework [83] uses two application-layered protocols—CoAP and HTTP—to provide end-to-end security. CoAP and HTTPs are two application layer protocols used to solve security and privacy issues in electronic healthcare systems. IP, REST, 6LowPAN, Bluetooth, Wi-Fi, ZigBee, and QoS are just a few of the many communication protocols in this layer. It is in charge of sending data across the network by using various routers and switches. Since sensors bring data into this layer, data transmission from the sensor layer to the IoT gateway's network layer is critical. It serves as a link between two distinct environments. It fosters doors ARM Corte-M3 and M4, which are the best choices in the IoT climate. Frames are created by packing data into packets with a header at the network layer. The structures or data of these patients move on to the application layer, where they are stored and analyzed to make decisions. The loss or delay of any packet can be dangerous because it must analyze healthcare data immediately. It uses a Cooja simulation environment and the Contiki operating system version 2.7 A Copper extension for Mozilla Firefox is used to support CoAP in Cooja. Fig. (**43**) represents the same.

The IoT layer [84] comprises a network of multiple sensors placed around the hospital beds to collect environmental and physiological data and send it to the MEC layer. The system selects 5G to connect the IoT directly to the MEC layer and transmit large amounts of IoT sensing data every second with high QoS. Authorized physicians can now acquire patient ECG data and analysis results from the MEC layer. Based on the diagnosis results generated by the proposed ECG diagnosis model, doctors can quickly decide whether or not to further evaluate the patient's condition with the assistance of artificial intelligence algorithms for automatic ECG diagnosis in the MEC layer. Besides, medical caretakers can screen the patient's state of being progressive through the observing terminal, associated with the MEC layer, so that they can react quickly in crises. The real-time acquisition of health-related statistical information and user environmental data, such as ECG, GPS, weather, and temperature data, is the responsibility of the IoT-based user subsystem. These data are obtained from human body-connected wireless sensing devices. The processing hardware and electrodes for the wearable sensor nodes are embedded in sportswear. Materials that are flexible and soft are used to make sportswear. The hardware module performs an ECG signal detection, digitization, and wireless data transmission, allowing for accurate ECG measurements. The cloud subsystem is in charge of storing various user data and the final ECG analysis result. There is a lot of storage space in it. It will keep the analysis results and share a summary of each user's medical information with authorized medical personnel, users, and hospitals. It can access medical records at any time and by authorized parties. The MEC layer will periodically send the information about the collected ECG data to the cloud system for permanent storage. It can likewise be received by some other server in the MEC layer. Similarly, the user's previous alarm messages regarding their cardiovascular health are also saved on the cloud server for experts to analyze further to provide emergency plans in the event of a crisis. The ECG dataset used in this study has 160,948 records and was used to train and test the proposed model. Fig. (**44**) represents the same.

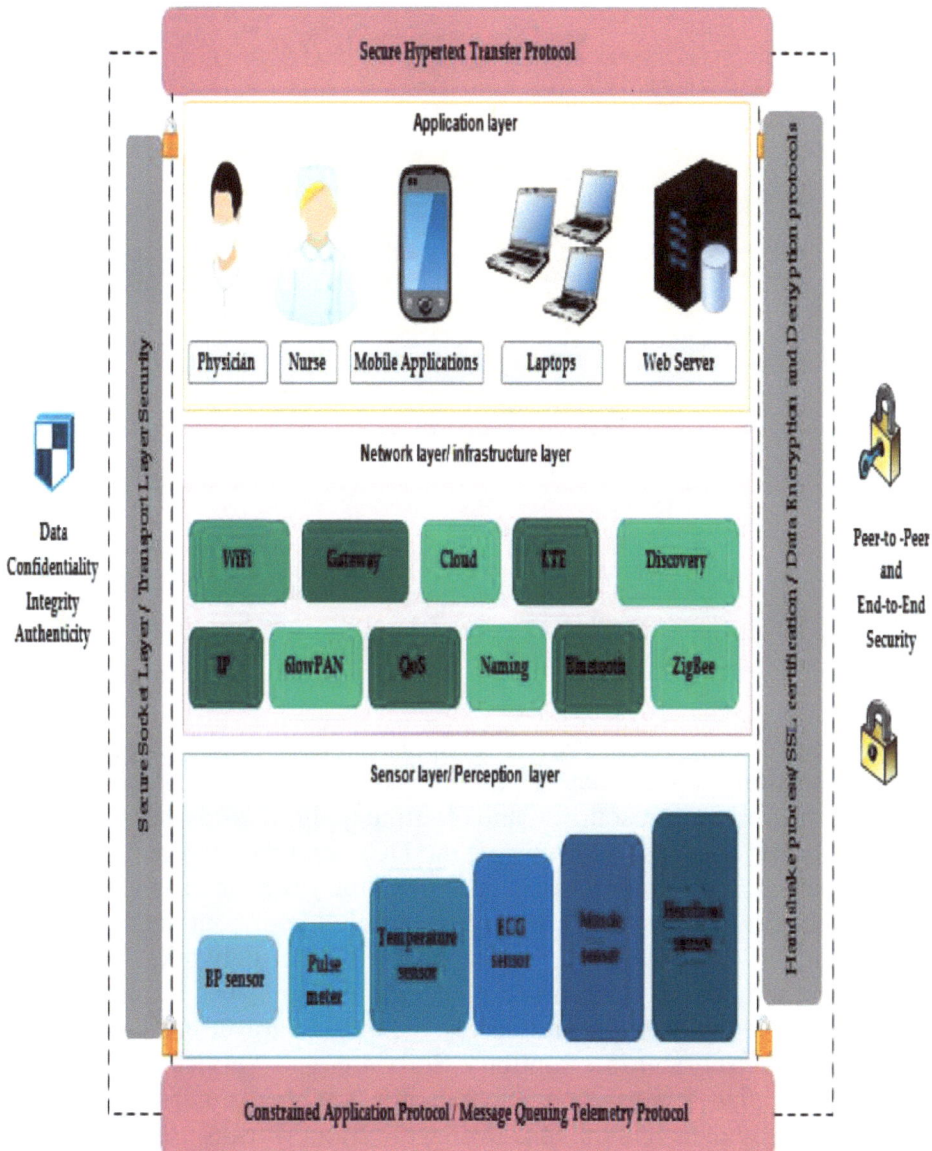

Fig. (43). Security framework for IoT-based real-time health application [83].

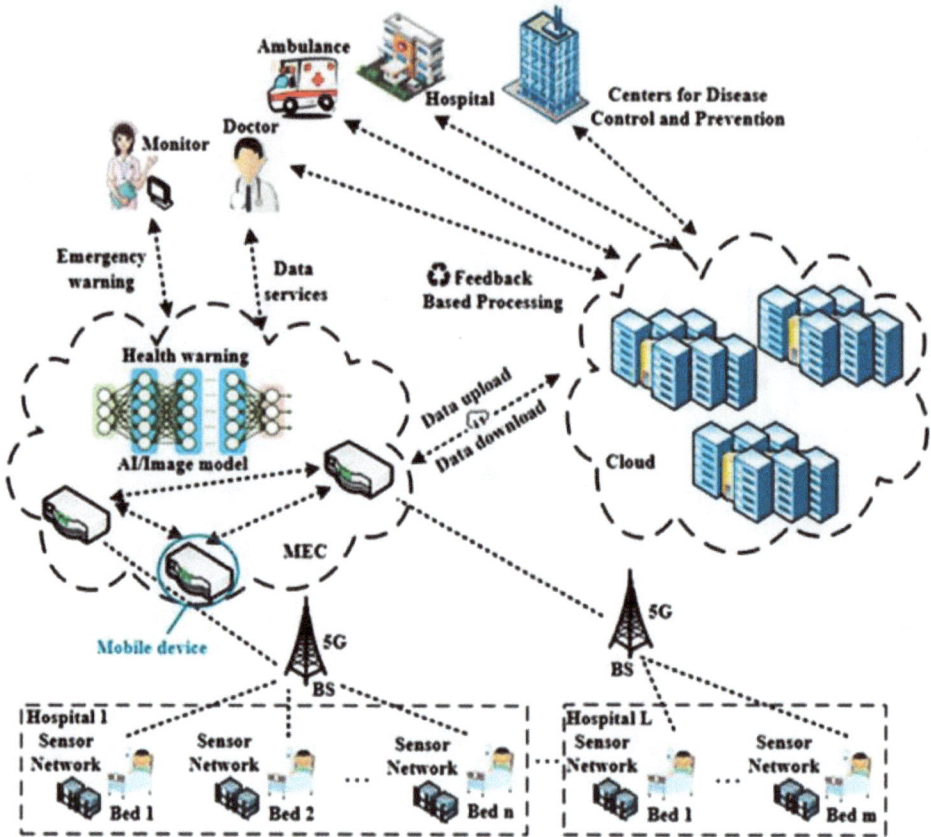

Fig. (44). System Framework [84].

These devices [85] are referred to as lightweight nodes. They can store and process a portion of the data on the blockchain because they have limited computing power and resources and continuously record the critical health parameters of the patients. As required, the DCs send data to the edge. The IPFS storage system stores complete transactions and the generated hash string is stored in the blockchain. Additionally, the proposed intelligent contract-based ePoW is used to authenticate the data transactions in the network. The proposed blockchain-based security and privacy scheme register all three nodes. At long last, the DL-based protection and security conspire are utilized to change and distinguish organizational interruptions. Software-as-a-Service (SaaS) is used to implement this plan at various network nodes, such as routers, gateways, edge servers, and Cloud data centers. In addition, the framework is used in a large-scale distributed network model or on a single host that successfully communicates, either in the edge-blockchain or cloud-blockchain layers. It also works together with other systems to detect cyberattacks. It considered a progression of emergency clinics as a contextual investigation, where a few ongoing wearable CPS, verification servers, and base stations are interconnected. There are several units in a hospital, including gastroenterology. Private rooms are provided for patient's convenience. These units, and wards are interconnected to survey, store, and send the patient's information. The web layer addresses the genuine client, where it can convey projects without limitation. IoMT devices are categorized according to their location and purpose. Fig. (45) represents the same.

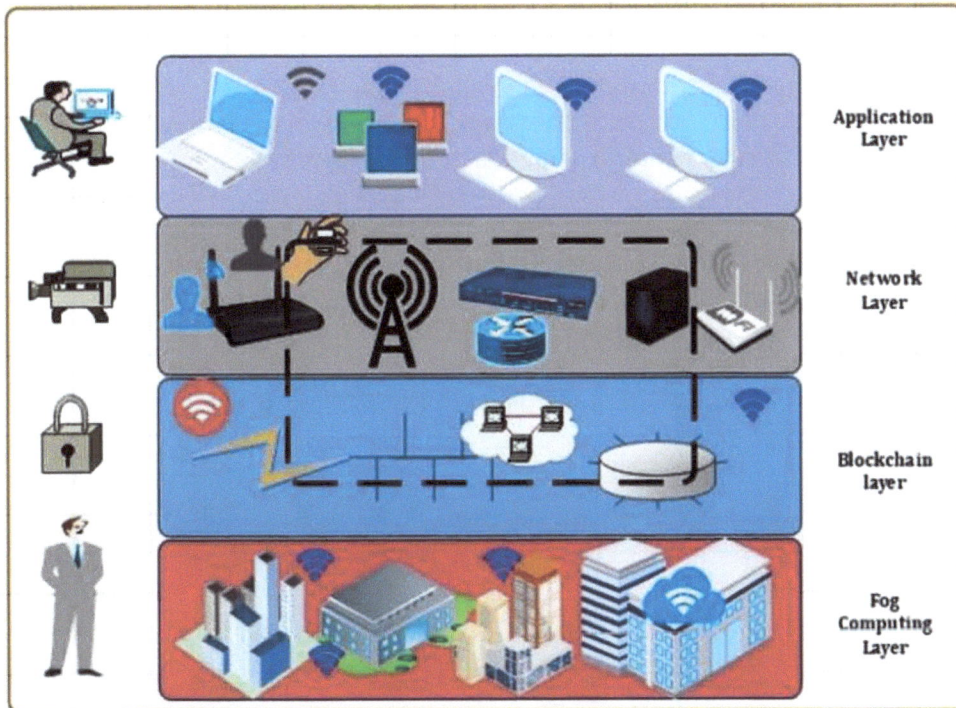

Fig. (45). Proposed Framework [85].

The data perception layer, the edge layer, the network layer, the data management (cloud layer), the application layer, and the business layer make up the proposed system architecture [86]. A federated multi-attack edge layer detection mechanism is the proposed system. The interruption discovery framework should have discussed the harming tackles issue while sending the loads for conglomeration to the server. ICU IoT devices with sensors are contained in the healthcare data perception layer. There are two types of case devices for the ICU: devices for monitoring the health and environment of the room and the patients. IoT gateways make up the blockchain layer that is edge-based. There are some healthcare sensing devices in each gateway. Physical healthcare sensors do not have a global internal protocol; As a result, the gateways could support a wide range of network access protocols. Detecting multiple attacks is the job of an Internet of Things gateway. It built a light IDS for the edge server (ES) to normalize their data and catch several ANN-based attacks. It protects the cloud or other resources in the event of a specific attack. The proposed module will be developed in FL mode and trained in the edge layer. It will do this by preventing data from its gateway. The closer the attack resources are, the shorter the intrusion's detection time will be. Because the FL model works with smaller data sets, there will also be less computing and processing power available. The weights of each local model will be transferred to a blockchain-distributed ledger and stored in chained blocks that link gateway nodes to server nodes in the subsequent cloud layer after the module learning process is finished. A further application for these chained blocks will be aggregation and averaging. Data transfers between lower and upper layers must be protected at the network layer. It is referred to as the connectivity layer because it manages the route. The cloud-based blockchain layer takes average weights from the ESs and updates the global ANN algorithm weights in the blockchain ledger. The application layer monitors vital healthcare signs. Based on the analyzed and received data from lower layers, the business layer assists the entire healthcare application service managers in creating executive reports, business models, and flowcharts. By creating a natural testbed environment in the Cyber Range Lab of UNSW, it is an IoT traffic-based dataset. The Canberra Testbed was set up with actual and simulated IoT regular and botnet attack traffic. The data is available in csv format and there are more than 73 million records with 46 features in each raw. Fig. (**46**) represents the same.

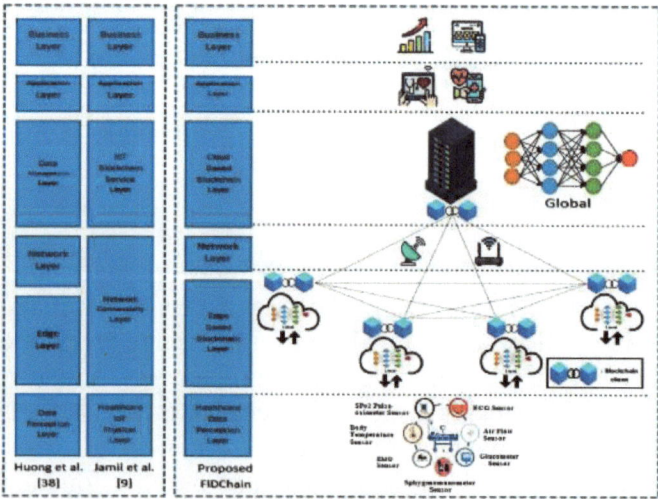

Fig. (46). Proposed System model [86].

5.8. DRAWBACKS

In the ongoing frameworks, wearable gadgets were utilized. Wearable devices ought to be embedded in the body to give data. If patients with SARS-CoV-2 need to be monitored, this condition can cause anxiety and risks because the virus may be transmitted through wearable devices. In addition, wearable devices require battery charge and must be removed from the wearer's body to charge. The cultural stigma associated with using medical devices that are physically in touch with the body may need to be confronted in the context of home-based monitoring.

Additionally, the absence of feature selection models for covid 19 detection in the current work raises the possibility of time complexity. Wearable device concerns can be avoided with noncontact healthcare technology. Noncontact technology does not require physical contact to monitor a patient's condition. Even though wearable gadgets can be productively used for observing the SARS-CoV-2 contaminated patients, they come to the detriment of plausible constriction of the infection. When they connect, change, or take off wearable devices, healthcare workers, especially nurses, risk contracting a disease. If medical professionals take every possible precaution, such as covering their hands with gloves or masks, the risk of contracting the virus will be reduced; However, employing noncontact technology will, without a doubt, eliminate all potential routes of virus transmission. Likewise, a superior advancement-based highlight choice is used for the discovery of Coronavirus, which relies upon upgraded profound learning.

5.9. FUTURE DIRECTIONS

5.9.1. Edge Architecture in H-IOT

A subset of a broader IoT system is the H-IoT. A recent trend is the application of IoT in healthcare. The market data show that the use of fitness trackers or wearables has increased significantly over the past few years, and this trend is expected to continue in the future. IoThNet is a healthcare-focused system developed due to the evolution of smart health monitoring devices and enhanced connectivity to the Internet of Things communication infrastructure. The patients associated with the organization can be followed to adjust their well-being boundaries like vital signs and biometric data for better analysis and the nature of conveyed clinical consideration. It raises a requirement to improve a normalized design to work with data trading between the different partaking substances. It would significantly facilitate the widespread adoption of H-IoT by establishing a standard or reference architecture. Numerous commercial organizations and consortiums are working to develop a variety of standard architectures to put various IoT applications into action. Fig. (**47**) portrays Wearable smart log patch with Internet of Things (IoT) sensor in edge computing environment.

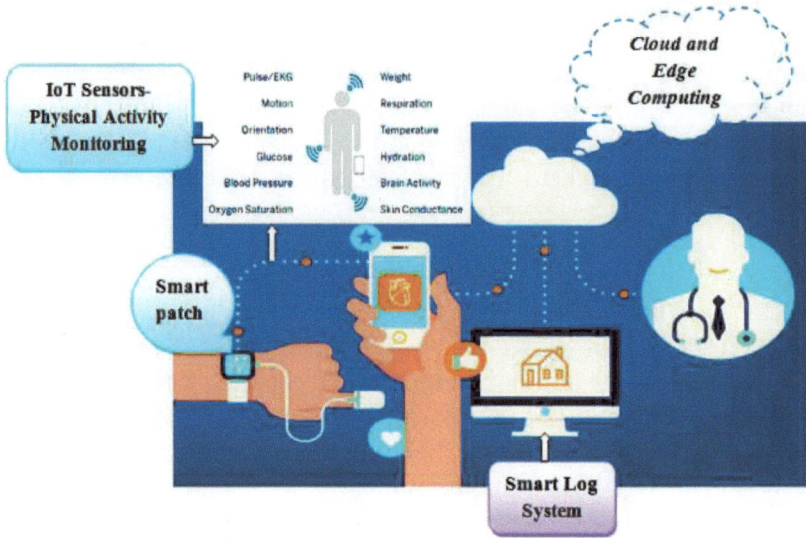

Fig. (47). Wearable smart log patch with Internet of Things (IoT) sensor in edge computing environment [87].

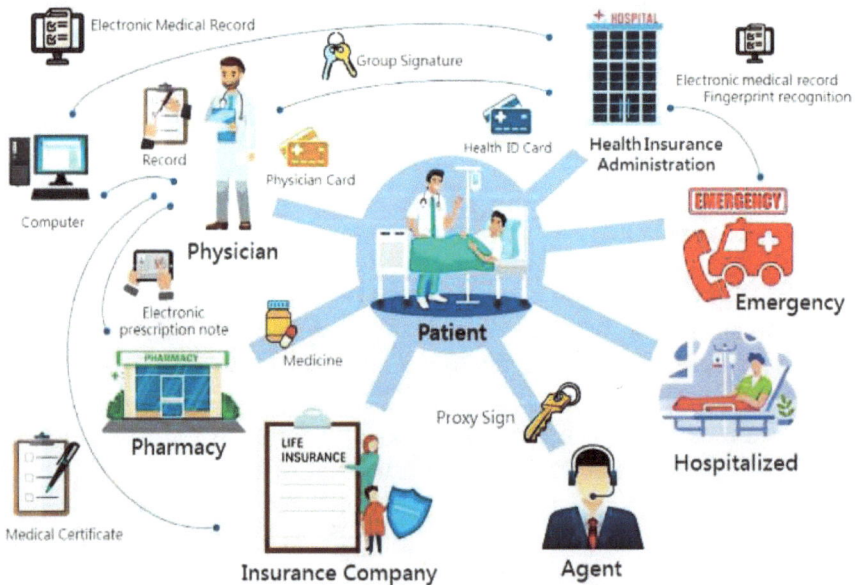

Fig. (48). The Integrated Medical Information System (IMIS) process [88].

5.9.2. Cryptography with Computing in H-IOT

The internet of things, or IoT, is making rapid inroads into daily life. It is one of the new technologies that is attracting a lot of academic researchers as well as businesses in the industrial sector. It aims to combine digital and physical worlds into a single, intelligent system that can perform a specific task without human intervention, such as transport manufacturing, healthcare, smart homes, intelligent buildings, smart cities, and smart grids. The issues with internet security are distinct from those with IoT security. Privacy, authorization, verification, access control, system configuration, information storage, and management are all aspects of IoT security. Recent trends include blockchain, lightweight cryptography, lightweight authentication, secure architecture for smart cities, and data privacy preservation. Fig. (**48**) represents integrated medical information system (IMIS) process.

5.9.3. Blockchain Based H-IOT

Blockchain offers numerous advantages for individuals, healthcare providers, and medical researchers. It will investigate and adapt medicine to establish a single saved location for all health information, keep track of adapt details simultaneously, and provide granular access authorizations for a group of data. Health researchers require comprehensive datasets for various diseases, accelerated biomedical detection, and rapid drug development to develop individual treatment devices based on genetics, lifecycle, and environment. Blockchain's allocated information method will produce many datasets by incorporating patients from various ethnic and socioeconomic backgrounds and geographic locations. Because Blockchain collects health information throughout a person's lifetime, it provides accurate data for longitudinal studies. The group of people currently underserved by the medical community or not typically included in science would see their health information gathered by the healthcare blockchain expanded. Blockchain's distributed information environment makes it simple to engage audiences and the general public to produce outcomes more reflective. The healthcare blockchain might aid the development of novel varieties of "smart" healthcare provider apps that will circumvent the most recent medical research and develop individualized treatment methods. Fig. (**49**) depicts workflow of blockchain-based healthcare applications.

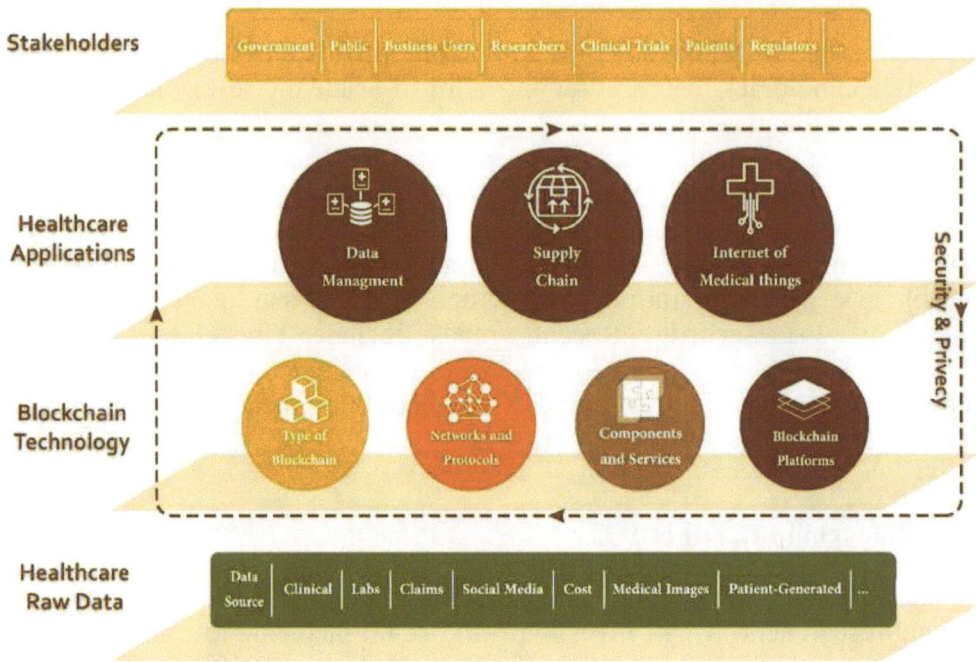

Fig. (49). workflow of blockchain-based healthcare applications [89].

5.9.4. Machine Learning in H-IOT

The development of medical technologies, drugs, and rehabilitation protocols to diagnose, treat, and manage critical illnesses like cancer, heart disease, and neurological disorders, as well as to improve healthcare and life expectancy, has resulted from synergistic collaborations in pharmaceutical research. A lack of cross-disciplinary interaction between the academic and federal investigation, industry, regulatory, and clinical communities has limited the traditional synergies between technology development and research. A collaborative paradigm is necessary to treat patients and assist them in maintaining their health [90]. It must actively partner with all stakeholder groups—researchers and technology developers, healthcare providers, patients, regulatory sectors, and payors—to meet the global challenge of providing quality healthcare with preventive, personalized, and precision medicine at an affordable cost. It could develop the synergy and foundation needed for developing and implementing future point-o--care technologies in various clinical or semi-clinical settings on a global collaborative platform involving researchers with active participation from clinicians and industry in a data-rich environment with patient-centred information databases. It would ensure high-quality global healthcare. Molecular, cellular, microfluidic, acoustics-based tests, noncommunicable disease screening technologies, and biosensor-based monitoring are at the forefront of POC technology development trends. The information assortment and informatics for continuous information investigation are primary for opportune POC diagnostics, alarms, and preventive, customized, and précised medical services. With reliable diagnostics and data analytics, it can use POC technologies to screen and monitor high-risk patients for meaningful clinical use. The clinical management, treatment, and therapeutic intervention made possible by the expressive use of secure, accurate, and dependable data can contribute to providing high-quality healthcare. It can reach patients *via* ICT and POC technologies to encourage adherence to preventive medicine and healthy living. It suggested that workflows be altered to test and treat patients in one visit to improve efficiency. Fig. (**50**) represents the Heart disease risk prediction system.

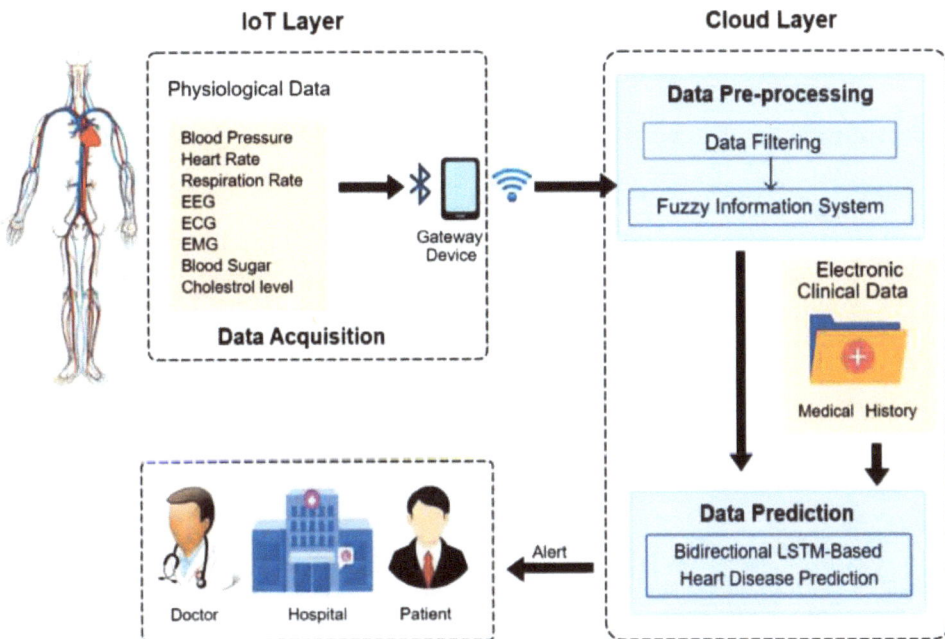

Fig. (50). Heart disease risk prediction system [91].

5.9.5. Digital Twin in H-IOT

The healthcare industry is being transformed by digital twins, making healthcare more individualized, intelligent, and proactive. For individuals to provide the appropriate kind of care at the proper time and in the right manner, a significant need exists to represent a virtual replica with the development of individualized healthcare. A digital representation of healthcare data, including electronic medical data, hospital environments, human physiology, operational staff, and laboratory results, is built with DTs in the healthcare industry. They use the virtual replicas of their clients, which are provided by DT technologies, to keep an eye on their health and provide care services tailored to each client's specific requirements. Specifically, the medical services industry utilizes individual's data separate from their PDTs. The PDT-based, high-quality health data about each patient is then analyzed to predict potential risks and monitor progress over time. It can make decisions and recommendations. Healthcare providers are eager to have personalized client data. Fig. (**51**) represents the Composition of a digital twin.

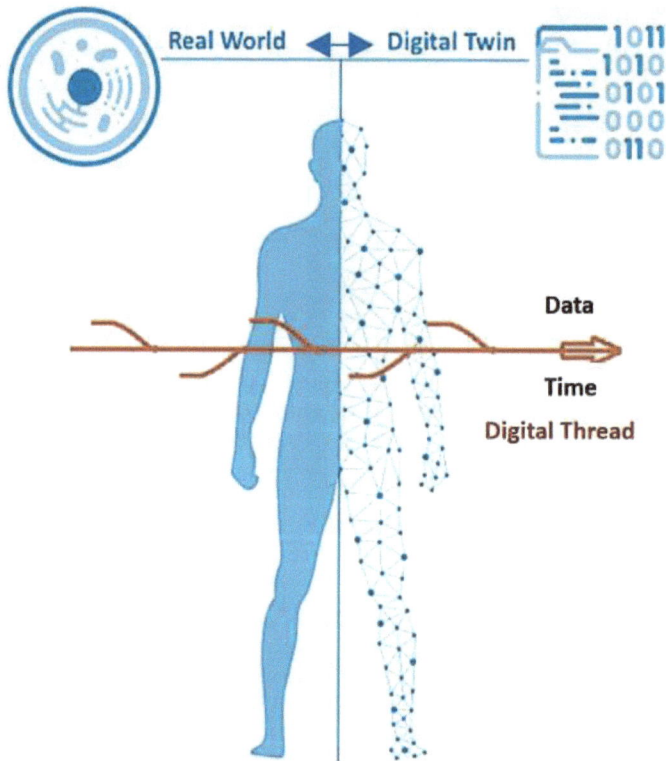

Fig. (51). Composition of a digital twin [92].

5.9.6. Unified Network Integration Framework

All aspects of human-machine interaction are experiencing a paradigm shift due to the rise of the Internet of Things in recent years. From the assembling business to medical care, from administration to finding the board, and from buyer administrations to guard, IoT has seen enormous reception in a couple of years. The fourth industrial revolution, or Industry 4.0, has begun by incorporating IoT into the consumer goods and manufacturing industries. In contrast, the integration of IoT into the healthcare industry is referred to as "Medicine 4.0" and "Health 2.0." Wellbeing 2.0 follows the age of dramatic reception of demonstrative apparatuses in the medical care areas. Implementing proactive treatment plans and detecting disorders are more accessible thanks to Health 2.0's shift toward ubiquitous patient monitoring. It could beneficially incorporate this method into existing techniques because it significantly contributes to measuring integration about a perceived optimal integration target. Both quantitative and qualitative measurements are required. Since all the processes require a lot of resources, researchers should concentrate on simplifying the existing methods. The validity of the currently available measures requires additional research. Fig. (**52**) represents the same.

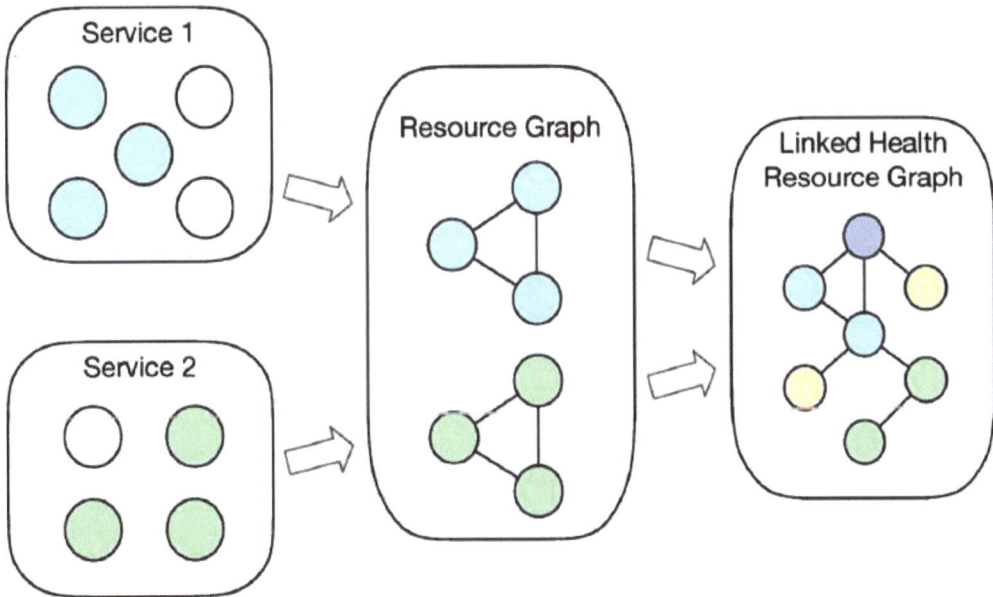

Fig. (52). Integration Process [93].

5.9.7. Context Aware Accessibility

Most chronic disease-related morbidity and mortality, also known as health risk behaviors or unhealthy, modifiable behaviors, are caused by health risk behaviors. The cost and prevalence of chronic diseases resulting from these modifiable behaviors significantly strain available healthcare resources. A social-ecological approach to public health considers that people are part of the society and environments in which they live. Digital behavior change interventions (DBCIs) that are more individualized are being created using new approaches incorporating various intelligent technologies better to support health improvement goals across the care continuum. From primary prevention initiatives to the efficient management of chronic diseases, context-aware DBCIs have the potential to enhance population health management. DBCIs that are context-aware can tailor aspects of the intervention based on dynamic contextual factors that could influence the user's behavior. Fig. (**53**) represents the same.

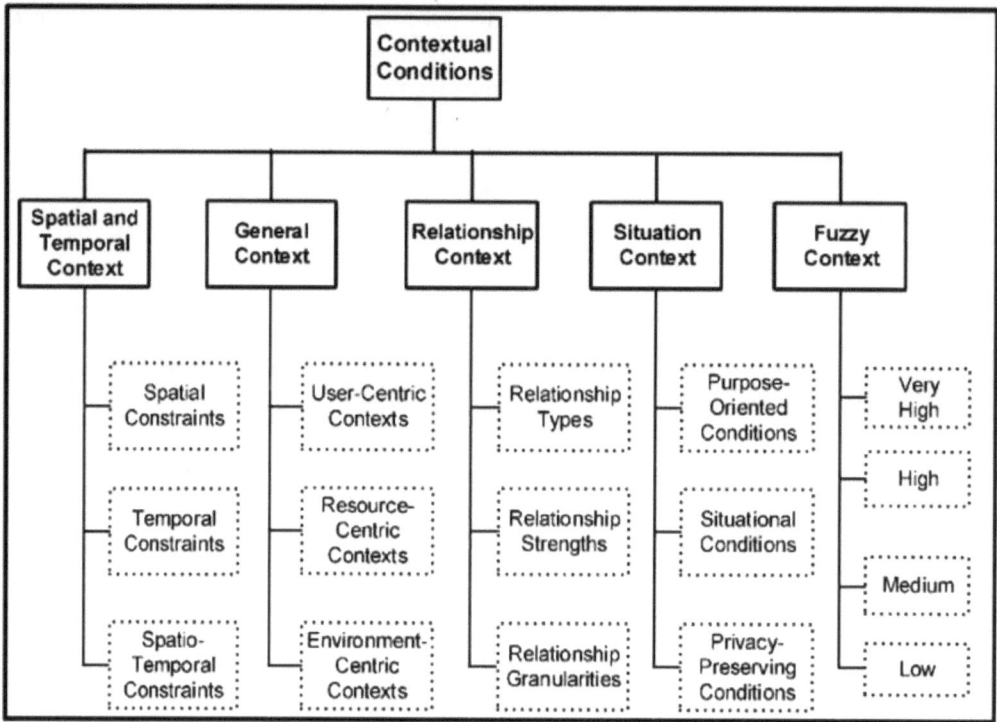

Fig. (53). A taxonomy of contextual conditions [94].

5.9.8. Edge and Fog Computing

Through cutting-edge technology known as the "Internet of Things," the upcoming technological developments and research have shifted the center of medical sciences not only for analysis but also for how to prevent diseases with incomplete recognition and appropriate and precise health information. The focus of the Internet of Things is the physical objects, such as appliances, electronics, and devices that are constantly developing around the world and can feature internet connectivity within an IP address using unique identities. It makes it possible for the various objects to interact with one another and act accordingly. Application-oriented operations are computed by the network components between the cloud and devices, as shown by the architectural framework of fog and edge computing. Because the fog layer dynamically accepts a large amount of aural data from the sensor network system in a short period, its primary focus is to control the incoming data so that the system can respond quickly to the number of users and the conditions required. Due to the potential for patients to suffer irreparable harm due to decision delays and anxiety, this task gains importance in healthcare settings. Fig. (**54**) represents the modelling phase.

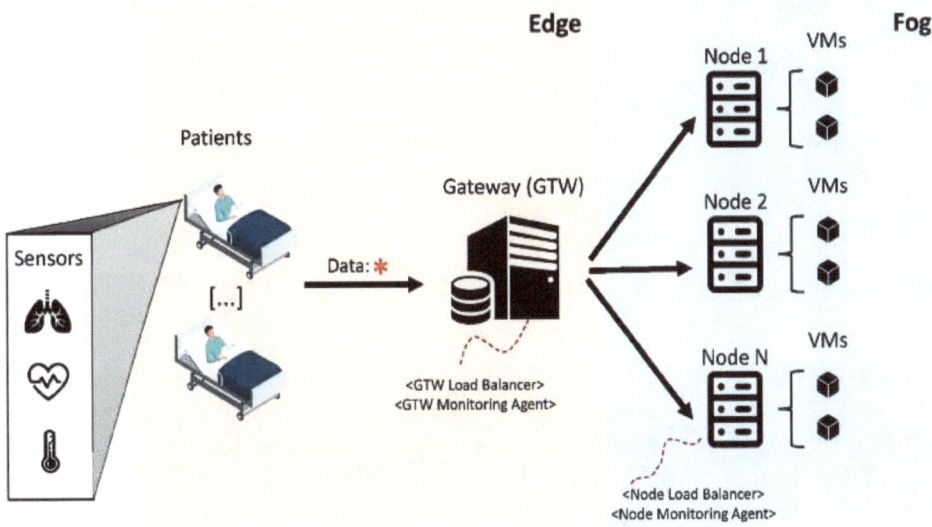

Fig. (54). Overview of Modelling Phase [95].

5.9.9. Sensors and Actuator Integration in H-IOT

There are numerous applications for wireless sensor network technologies in entertainment, travel, retail, industry, medicine, dependent person care, emergency management, and many other fields that have the potential to alter our way of life. Pervasive healthcare systems provide rich contextual information and alerting mechanisms against abnormal conditions with continuous monitoring. Artificial intelligence research, wireless sensors and sensor networks, and pervasive computing have combined to create the interdisciplinary concept of ambient intelligence. To realize the broad vision of intelligent healthcare, researchers in the medical, computer and networking fields collaborate. Fig. (**55**) represents the same.

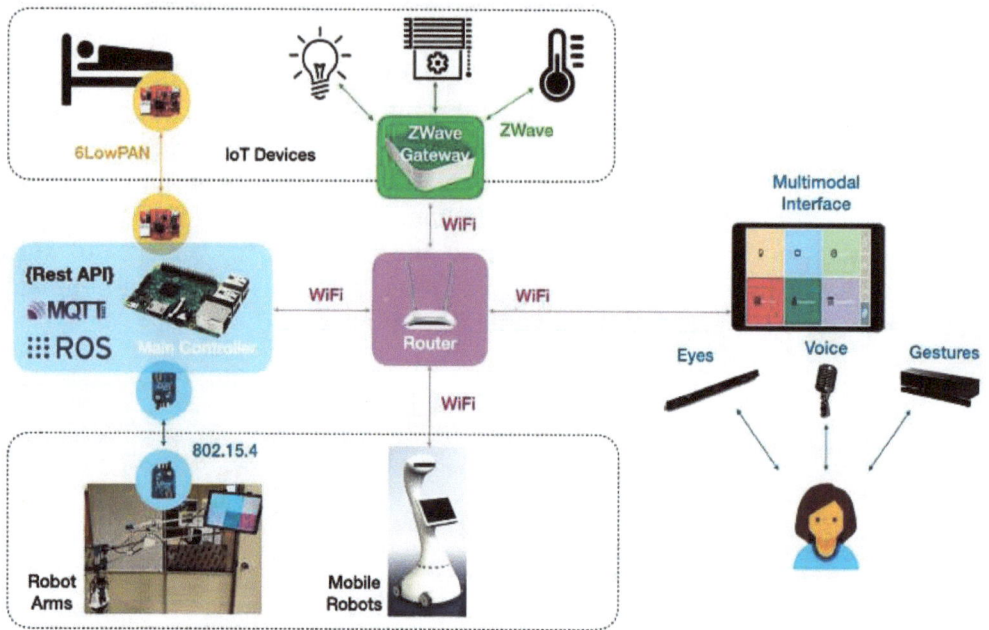

Fig. (55). Network Architecture [96].

CONCLUSION

Given that the millennial generation has only experienced the post-globalization period of the human timeline, the Internet of Things (IoT) today represents a significant milestone in technological advancement. It is especially true for millennial. To monitor a patient's recovery in the healthcare monitoring department, manual inspection in the presence of a doctor or other qualified medical assistants was unquestionably necessary. It held up the outcomes of medical tests for days before being used to make a diagnosis. Machines with artificial intelligence that use continuous monitoring to aid in disease detection have been introduced with the advent of IoT devices. These machines alert healthcare providers or physicians *via* an alert system. The shift of tasks from a manual, hectic, and time-consuming method to a smarter, automated, and time-efficient one was a significant benefit of this transformation. Utilizing these algorithms has resulted in the development of numerous novel architectures. These algorithms serve as the foundation for successful and highly accurate prediction models.

REFERENCES

[1]   N. Ambika, Enhancing security in iot instruments using artificial intelligence. *IoT and Cloud Computing for Societal Good* Springer International Publishing, 2022.
[http://dx.doi.org/10.1007/978-3-030-73885-3_16]

[2]   C. González García, B.C. Pelayo G-Bustelo, J. Pascual Espada, and G. Cueva-Fernandez, "Midgar: Generation of heterogeneous objects interconnecting applications. A domain specific language proposal for internet of things scenarios", *Comput. Netw.,* vol. 64, pp. 143-158, 2014.
[http://dx.doi.org/10.1016/j.comnet.2014.02.010]

[3]   Y.B. Zikria, R. Ali, M.K. Afzal, and S.W. Kim, "Next-Generation internet of things (IoT): Opportunities, challenges, and solutions", *Sensors,* vol. 21, no. 4, p. 1174, 2021.
[http://dx.doi.org/10.3390/s21041174] [PMID: 33562343]

[4]   S. Li, L.D. Xu, and S. Zhao, "The internet of things: A survey", *Inf. Syst. Front.,* vol. 17, no. 2, pp. 243-259, 2015.
[http://dx.doi.org/10.1007/s10796-014-9492-7]

[5]   L.D. Xu, W. He, and S. Li, "Internet of things in industries: A survey", *IEEE Trans. Industr. Inform.,* vol. 10, no. 4, pp. 2233-2243, 2014.
[http://dx.doi.org/10.1109/TII.2014.2300753]

[6]   N. Ambika, An Economical Machine Learning Approach for Anomaly Detection in IoT Environment.*Bioinformatics and Medical Applications: Big Data Using Deep Learning Algorithms,* A. Suresh, S. Vimal, Y. Harold Robinson, Dhinesh Kumar Ramaswami, R. Udendhran, Eds., wiley publications: Hoboken, New Jersey, 2022, pp. 215-234.
[http://dx.doi.org/10.1002/9781119792673.ch11]

[7]   M. Lombardi, F. Pascale, and D. Santaniello, "Internet of Things: A general overview between architectures, protocols and applications", *Info.,* vol. 12, no. 2, p. 87, 2021.
[http://dx.doi.org/10.3390/info12020087]

[8]   G. Marques, and R. Pitarma, "An indoor monitoring system for ambient assisted living based on internet of things architecture", *Int. J. Environ. Res. Public Health,* vol. 13, no. 11, p. 1152, 2016.
[http://dx.doi.org/10.3390/ijerph13111152] [PMID: 27869682]

[9]   B. Jo, R. Khan, and Y.S. Lee, "Hybrid blockchain and internet-of-things network for underground structure health monitoring", *Sensors,* vol. 18, no. 12, p. 4268, 2018.
[http://dx.doi.org/10.3390/s18124268] [PMID: 30518124]

[10]   F. Wu, T. Wu, and M. Yuce, "An Internet-of-things (IoT) network system for connected safety and health monitoring applications", *Sensors,* vol. 19, no. 1, p. 21, 2018.
[http://dx.doi.org/10.3390/s19010021] [PMID: 30577646]

[11]   G. Gardašević, K. Katzis, D. Bajić, and L. Berbakov, "Emerging wireless sensor networks and internet of things technologies—foundations of smart healthcare", *Sensors,* vol. 20, no. 13, p. 3619, 2020.
[http://dx.doi.org/10.3390/s20133619] [PMID: 32605071]

[12]   G. Marques, and R. Pitarma, "mHealth: Indoor environmental quality measuring system for enhanced health and well-being based on internet of things", *J. Sens. Actuator Netw.,* vol. 8, no. 3, p. 43, 2019.
[http://dx.doi.org/10.3390/jsan8030043]

[13]   G. Marques, I.M. Pires, N. Miranda, and R. Pitarma, "Air quality monitoring using assistive robots for ambient assisted living and enhanced living environments through internet of things", *Electronics,* vol. 8, no. 12, p. 1375, 2019.
[http://dx.doi.org/10.3390/electronics8121375]

[14]   A.A. Al-Atawi, F. Khan, and C.G. Kim, "Application and challenges of iot healthcare system in COVID-19", *Sensors,* vol. 22, no. 19, p. 7304, 2022.
[http://dx.doi.org/10.3390/s22197304] [PMID: 36236404]

[15]   S. Zaim, J.H. Chong, V. Sankaranarayanan, and A. Harky, "COVID-19 and multiorgan response", *Curr. Probl. Cardiol.,* vol. 45, no. 8, p. 100618, 2020.
[http://dx.doi.org/10.1016/j.cpcardiol.2020.100618] [PMID: 32439197]

[16]   A.M.U.D. Khanday, B. Bhushan, R.H. Jhaveri, Q.R. Khan, R. Raut, and S.T. Rabani, "NNPCov19: Artificial neural network-based propaganda identification on social media in COVID-19 Era", *Mob. Inf. Syst.,* vol. 2022, pp. 1-10, 2022.
[http://dx.doi.org/10.1155/2022/3412992]

[17]   R. Brindha, A. Kavitha, and B. Bhushan, "A systematic review literature on computer-aided detection methods for COVID-19 detection in x-ray and ct image modalities", *9th International Conference on Innovations in Electronics and Communication Engineering,* vol. 355, 2022pp. 227-233 Ibrahimpatanam, Hyderabad
[http://dx.doi.org/10.1007/978-981-16-8512-5_25]

[18]   M. Yousif, C. Hewage, and L. Nawaf, "IoT technologies during and beyond COVID-19: A comprehensive review", *Future Internet,* vol. 13, no. 5, p. 105, 2021.
[http://dx.doi.org/10.3390/fi13050105]

[19]   R.K. Chandana Mani, B. Bhushan, V. Rajyalakshmi, J. Nagaraj, and T. Ramathulasi, "A pilot study on detection and classification of COVID Images: A deep learning approach", *9th International Conference on Innovations in Electronics and Communication Engineering (ICIECE-2021)* Ibrahimpatanam, Hyderabad, 29-31, 2022.
[http://dx.doi.org/10.1007/978-981-16-8512-5_21]

[20]   T. Yang, M. Gentile, C.F. Shen, and C.M. Cheng, "Combining point-of-care diagnostics and internet of medical things (IoMT) to combat the COVID-19 pandemic", *Diagnostics,* vol. 10, no. 4, p. 224, 2020.
[http://dx.doi.org/10.3390/diagnostics10040224] [PMID: 32316113]

[21]   D. Shome, T. Kar, S. Mohanty, P. Tiwari, K. Muhammad, A. AlTameem, Y. Zhang, and A. Saudagar, "COVID-Transformer: Interpretable COVID-19 detection using vision transformer for healthcare", *Int. J. Environ. Res. Public Health,* vol. 18, no. 21, p. 11086, 2021.
[http://dx.doi.org/10.3390/ijerph182111086] [PMID: 34769600]

[22]   A. Aljumah, "Assessment of machine learning techniques in iot-based architecture for the monitoring and prediction of COVID-19", *Electronics,* vol. 10, no. 15, p. 1834, 2021.
[http://dx.doi.org/10.3390/electronics10151834]

[23]   P. Di Marco, P. Park, M. Pratesi, and F. Santucci, "A bluetooth-based architecture for contact tracing in healthcare facilities", *J. Sens. Actuator Netw.,* vol. 10, no. 1, p. 2, 2020.
[http://dx.doi.org/10.3390/jsan10010002]

[24]   M. Ayadi, A. Ksibi, A. Al-Rasheed, and B.O. Soufiene, "COVID-AleXception: A deep learning model based on a deep feature concatenation approach for the detection of COVID-19 from chest x-ray images", *Healthcare,* vol. 10, no. 10, p. 2072, 2022.
[http://dx.doi.org/10.3390/healthcare10102072] [PMID: 36292519]

[25]   A. Suleiman, I. Bsisu, H. Guzu, A. Santarisi, M. Alsatari, A. Abbad, A. Jaber, T. Harb, A. Abuhejleh, N. Nadi, A. Aloweidi, and M. Almustafa, "Preparedness of frontline doctors in jordan healthcare facilities to COVID-19 outbreak", *Int. J. Environ. Res. Public Health,* vol. 17, no. 9, p. 3181, 2020.
[http://dx.doi.org/10.3390/ijerph17093181] [PMID: 32370275]

[26]   R.K. Shinde, M.S. Alam, S.G. Park, S.M. Park, and N. Kim, "Intelligent IoT (IIoT) device to identifying suspected COVID-19 infections using sensor fusion algorithm and real-time mask detection based on the enhanced mobilenetv2 model", *Healthcare,* vol. 10, no. 3, p. 454, 2022.
[http://dx.doi.org/10.3390/healthcare10030454] [PMID: 35326932]

[27]   M. Loey, F. Smarandache, and N.M. Khalifa, "Within the lack of chest COVID-19 X-ray Dataset: A novel detection model based on GAN and deep transfer learning", *Symmetry,* vol. 12, no. 4, p. 651, 2020.

[http://dx.doi.org/10.3390/sym12040651]

[28]   H. Mukhtar, S. Rubaiee, M. Krichen, and R. Alroobaea, "An IoT framework for screening of covid-19 using real-time data from wearable sensors", *Int. J. Environ. Res. Public Health,* vol. 18, no. 8, p. 4022, 2021.
[http://dx.doi.org/10.3390/ijerph18084022] [PMID: 33921223]

[29]   S. Hussain, Y. Yu, M. Ayoub, A. Khan, R. Rehman, J.A. Wahid, and W. Hou, "IoT and deep learning based approach for rapid screening and face mask detection for infection spread control of COVID-19", *Appl. Sci.,* vol. 11, no. 8, p. 3495, 2021.
[http://dx.doi.org/10.3390/app11083495]

[30]   H.S. Munawar, H. Inam, F. Ullah, S. Qayyum, A.Z. Kouzani, and M.A.P. Mahmud, "Towards smart healthcare: UAV-based optimized path planning for delivering COVID-19 self-testing kits using cutting edge technologies", *Sustainability,* vol. 13, no. 18, p. 10426, 2021.
[http://dx.doi.org/10.3390/su131810426]

[31]   M.L. Hoang, M. Carratù, V. Paciello, and A. Pietrosanto, "Body temperature—indoor condition monitor and activity recognition by MEMS accelerometer based on IoT-Alert System for people in quarantine due to COVID-19", *Sensors,* vol. 21, no. 7, p. 2313, 2021.
[http://dx.doi.org/10.3390/s21072313] [PMID: 33810301]

[32]   N. El-Rashidy, S. El-Sappagh, S.M.R. Islam, H.M. El-Bakry, and S. Abdelrazek, "End-To-End deep learning framework for coronavirus (COVID-19) detection and monitoring", *Electronics,* vol. 9, no. 9, p. 1439, 2020.
[http://dx.doi.org/10.3390/electronics9091439]

[33]   M. Umair, M.A. Cheema, O. Cheema, H. Li, and H. Lu, "Impact of COVID-19 on IoT adoption in healthcare, smart homes, smart buildings, smart cities transportation and industrial IoT", *Sensors.,* vol. 21, no. 11, p. 3838, 2021.
[http://dx.doi.org/10.3390/s21113838] [PMID: 34206120]

[34]   T.A. Kumar, R. Rajmohan, M. Pavithra, S.A. Ajagbe, R. Hodhod, and T. Gaber, "Automatic face mask detection system in public transportation in smart cities using IoT and deep learning", *Electronics,* vol. 11, no. 6, p. 904, 2022.
[http://dx.doi.org/10.3390/electronics11060904]

[35]   I. Politis, G. Georgiadis, A. Kopsacheilis, A. Nikolaidou, and P. Papaioannou, "Capturing twitter negativity Pre-vs. mid-COVID-19 pandemic: An LDA application on london public transport system", *Sustainability,* vol. 13, no. 23, p. 13356, 2021.
[http://dx.doi.org/10.3390/su132313356]

[36]   S. Ahmad, F. Mehmood, F. Khan, and T.K. Whangbo, "Architecting intelligent smart serious games for healthcare applications: A technical perspective", *Sensors,* vol. 22, no. 3, p. 810, 2022.
[http://dx.doi.org/10.3390/s22030810] [PMID: 35161556]

[37]   J. Končar, A. Grubor, R. Marić, S. Vučenović, and G. Vukmirović, "Setbacks to IoT implementation in the function of FMCG supply chain sustainability during COVID-19 pandemic", *Sustainability,* vol. 12, no. 18, p. 7391, 2020.
[http://dx.doi.org/10.3390/su12187391]

[38]   S. Habib, and N.N. Hamadneh, "Impact of perceived risk on consumers technology acceptance in online grocery adoption amid COVID-19 pandemic", *Sustainability,* vol. 13, no. 18, p. 10221, 2021.
[http://dx.doi.org/10.3390/su131810221]

[39]   L. Meng, "Using iot in supply chain risk management, to enable collaboration between business, community, and government", *Smart Cities,* vol. 4, no. 3, pp. 995-1003, 2021.
[http://dx.doi.org/10.3390/smartcities4030052]

[40]   J. Končar, R. Marić, G. Vukmirović, and S. Vučenović, "Sustainability of food placement in retailing during the COVID-19 pandemic", *Sustainability,* vol. 13, no. 11, p. 5956, 2021.
[http://dx.doi.org/10.3390/su13115956]

[41]   R. Carrasco-Navarro, L.F. Luque-Vega, J.A. Nava-Pintor, H.A. Guerrero-Osuna, M.A. Carlos-Mancilla, and C.L. Castañeda-Miranda, "MEIoT 2D-CACSET: IoT two-dimensional cartesian coordinate system educational toolkit align with educational mechatronics framework", *Sensors,* vol. 22, no. 13, p. 4802, 2022.
[http://dx.doi.org/10.3390/s22134802] [PMID: 35808304]

[42]   H. Susanto, F.Y. Leu, W. Caesarendra, F. Ibrahim, P. Haghi, U. Khusni, and A. Glowacz, "Managing cloud intelligent systems over digital ecosystems: Revealing emerging app technology in the time of the COVID19 pandemic", *Applied System Innovation,* vol. 3, no. 3, p. 37, 2020.
[http://dx.doi.org/10.3390/asi3030037]

[43]   M. Gong, L. Liu, X. Sun, Y. Yang, S. Wang, and H. Zhu, "Cloud-based system for effective surveillance and control of COVID-19: useful experiences from Hubei, China", *J. Med. Internet Res.,* vol. 22, no. 4, p. e18948, 2020.
[http://dx.doi.org/10.2196/18948] [PMID: 32287040]

[44]   S. Tuli, S. Tuli, R. Tuli, and S.S. Gill, "Predicting the growth and trend of COVID-19 pandemic using machine learning and cloud computing", *Internet of things,* vol. 11, p. 100222, 2020.
[http://dx.doi.org/10.1016/j.iot.2020.100222]

[45]   R. Singh, "Cloud computing and COVID-19", *3rd International Conference on Signal Processing and Communication (ICPSC),* 2021 Coimbatore, India
[http://dx.doi.org/10.1109/ICSPC51351.2021.9451792]

[46]   Z. Nuryana, A. Pangarso, and F.M. Zain, "Factor of zoom cloud meetings: Technology adoption in the pandemic of COVID-19", *Int. J. Eval. Res. Educ.,* vol. 10, no. 3, pp. 816-825, 2021.
[http://dx.doi.org/10.11591/ijere.v10i3.21726]

[47]   V. Naumov, E. Putin, S. Pushkov, E. Kozlova, K. Romantsov, A. Kalashnikov, F. Galkin, N. Tihonova, A. Shneyderman, E. Galkin, A. Zinkevich, S.M. Cope, R. Sethuraman, T.I. Oprea, A.T. Pearson, S. Tay, N. Agrawal, A. Dubovenko, Q. Vanhaelen, I. Ozerov, A. Aliper, E. Izumchenko, and A. Zhavoronkov, "COVIDomic: A multi-modal cloud-based platform for identification of risk factors associated with COVID-19 severity", *PLOS Comput. Biol.,* vol. 17, no. 7, p. e1009183, 2021.
[http://dx.doi.org/10.1371/journal.pcbi.1009183] [PMID: 34260589]

[48]   R. Mukherjee, A. Kundu, I. Mukherjee, D. Gupta, P. Tiwari, A. Khanna, and M. Shorfuzzaman, "IoT-cloud based healthcare model for COVID-19 detection: An enhanced k-nearest neighbour classifier based approach", *Comput.,* vol. 105, no. 4, pp. 849-869, 2021.
[http://dx.doi.org/10.1007/s00607-021-00951-9]

[49]   C. González García, E.R. Núñez Valdéz, V. García Díaz, B.C. Pelayo García-Bustelo, and J.M. Cueva Lovelle, "A review of artificial intelligence in the internet of things", In: *Int. J. Of Interactive Multimedia And Artif. Intell.* vol. Vol. 5. , 2019, no. 4, p. 1.
[http://dx.doi.org/10.9781/ijimai.2018.03.004]

[50]   M. Mittal, G. Battineni, L.M. Goyal, B. Chhetri, S.V. Oberoi, N. Chintalapudi, and F. Amenta, "Cloud-based framework to mitigate the impact of COVID-19 on seafarers' mental health", *Int. Marit. Health,* vol. 71, no. 3, pp. 213-214, 2020.
[http://dx.doi.org/10.5603/IMH.2020.0038] [PMID: 33001435]

[51]   A.T. Shumba, T. Montanaro, I. Sergi, L. Fachechi, M. De Vittorio, and L. Patrono, "Leveraging IoT-Aware technologies and ai techniques for real-time critical healthcare applications", *Sensors,* vol. 22, no. 19, p. 7675, 2022.
[http://dx.doi.org/10.3390/s22197675] [PMID: 36236773]

[52]   C. Perera, A. Zaslavsky, P. Christen, and D. Georgakopoulos, "Context aware computing for the internet of things: A survey", *IEEE Commun. Surv. Tutor.,* vol. 16, no. 1, pp. 414-454, 2014.
[http://dx.doi.org/10.1109/SURV.2013.042313.00197]

[53]   L. Catarinucci, D. de Donno, L. Mainetti, L. Palano, L. Patrono, M.L. Stefanizzi, and L. Tarricone, "An IoT-aware architecture for smart healthcare systems", *IEEE Internet Things J.,* vol. 2, no. 6, pp.

515-526, 2015.
[http://dx.doi.org/10.1109/JIOT.2015.2417684]

[54] C. González García, V. García-Díaz, B. García-Bustelo, and Juan Manuel Cueva Lovelle, *Protocols and Applications for the Industrial Internet of Things* IGI Global: US, 2018, p. 356.

[55] A.I. Maarala, X. Su, and J. Riekki, "Semantic reasoning for context-aware internet of things applications", *IEEE Internet Things J.,* vol. 4, no. 2, pp. 461-473, 2017.
[http://dx.doi.org/10.1109/JIOT.2016.2587060]

[56] A. Ahad, M. Tahir, M.A. Sheikh, K.I. Ahmed, and A. Mughees, "An intelligent clustering-based routing protocol (CRP-GR) for 5G-Based smart healthcare using game theory and reinforcement learning", *Appl. Sci.,* vol. 11, no. 21, p. 9993, 2021.
[http://dx.doi.org/10.3390/app11219993]

[57] S. Alletto, R. Cucchiara, G. Del Fiore, L. Mainetti, V. Mighali, L. Patrono, and G. Serra, "An indoor location-aware system for an IoT-based smart museum", *IEEE Internet Things J.,* vol. 3, no. 2, pp. 244-253, 2016.
[http://dx.doi.org/10.1109/JIOT.2015.2506258]

[58] C. Perera, A. Zaslavsky, P. Christen, and D. Georgakopoulos, "Ca4iot: Context awareness for internet of things", In: *IEEE International Conference on Green Computing and Communications* Besancon: France, 2012.
[http://dx.doi.org/10.1109/GreenCom.2012.128]

[59] F. Jimenez, and R. Torres, "Building an IoT-aware healthcare monitoring system", In: *2015 34th International Conference of the Chilean Computer Science Society (SCCC)* Santiago: Chile, 2015.
[http://dx.doi.org/10.1109/SCCC.2015.7416592]

[60] H. Elayan, M. Aloqaily, and M. Guizani, "Digital twin for intelligent context-aware IoT healthcare systems", *IEEE Internet Things J.,* vol. 8, no. 23, pp. 16749-16757, 2021.
[http://dx.doi.org/10.1109/JIOT.2021.3051158]

[61] M. Min, X. Wan, L. Xiao, Y. Chen, M. Xia, D. Wu, and H. Dai, "Learning-based privacy-aware offloading for healthcare IoT with energy harvesting", *IEEE Internet Things J.,* vol. 6, no. 3, pp. 4307-4316, 2019.
[http://dx.doi.org/10.1109/JIOT.2018.2875926]

[62] U. Satija, B. Ramkumar, and M. Sabarimalai Manikandan, "Real-time signal quality-aware ECG telemetry system for IoT-based health care monitoring", *IEEE Internet Things J.,* vol. 4, no. 3, pp. 815-823, 2017.
[http://dx.doi.org/10.1109/JIOT.2017.2670022]

[63] P. Bai, S. Kumar, G. Aggarwal, M. Mahmud, O. Kaiwartya, and J. Lloret, "Self-sovereignty identity management model for smart healthcare system", *Sensors,* vol. 22, no. 13, p. 4714, 2022.
[http://dx.doi.org/10.3390/s22134714] [PMID: 35808211]

[64] P. Cabrera-Barona, T. Blaschke, and S. Kienberger, "Explaining accessibility and satisfaction related to healthcare: a mixed-methods approach", *Soc. Indic. Res.,* vol. 133, no. 2, pp. 719-739, 2017.
[http://dx.doi.org/10.1007/s11205-016-1371-9] [PMID: 28890596]

[65] T. Graham-Steed, E. Uchio, C.K. Wells, M. Aslan, J. Ko, and J. Concato, "Race and prostate cancer mortality in equal-access healthcare systems", *Am. J. Med.,* vol. 126, no. 12, pp. 1084-1088, 2013.
[http://dx.doi.org/10.1016/j.amjmed.2013.08.012] [PMID: 24262722]

[66] L. Mao, and D. Nekorchuk, "Measuring spatial accessibility to healthcare for populations with multiple transportation modes", *Health Place,* vol. 24, pp. 115-122, 2013.
[http://dx.doi.org/10.1016/j.healthplace.2013.08.008] [PMID: 24077335]

[67] J. Sanchez, G. Byfield, T.T. Brown, K. LaFavor, D. Murphy, and P. Laud, "Perceived accessibility versus actual physical accessibility of healthcare facilities", *Rehabil. Nurs.,* vol. 25, no. 1, pp. 6-9, 2000.

[http://dx.doi.org/10.1002/j.2048-7940.2000.tb01849.x] [PMID: 10754921]

[68]   A. Ghanemi, M. Yoshioka, and J. St-Amand, "Post-coronavirus disease-2019 (COVID-19): toward a severe multi-level health crisis?", *Med. Sci.,* vol. 9, no. 4, p. 68, 2021.
[http://dx.doi.org/10.3390/medsci9040068] [PMID: 34842764]

[69]   H.Y. Lee, M.N. Oh, Y.S. Park, C. Chu, and T.J. Son, "Public health crisis preparedness and response in Korea", *Osong Public Health Res. Perspect.,* vol. 4, no. 5, pp. 278-284, 2013.
[http://dx.doi.org/10.1016/j.phrp.2013.09.008] [PMID: 24298444]

[70]   D. Ngoc Su, D. Luc Tra, H.M. Thi Huynh, H.H.T. Nguyen, and B. O'Mahony, "Enhancing resilience in the Covid-19 crisis: Lessons from human resource management practices in Vietnam", *Curr. Issues Tour.,* vol. 24, no. 22, pp. 3189-3205, 2021.
[http://dx.doi.org/10.1080/13683500.2020.1863930]

[71]   D. Zavras, "Studying healthcare affordability during an economic recession: The case of Greece", *Int. J. Environ. Res. Public Health,* vol. 17, no. 21, p. 7790, 2020.
[http://dx.doi.org/10.3390/ijerph17217790] [PMID: 33114353]

[72]   Y.K. Talwar, S. Karthikeyan, N. Bindra, and B. Medhi, "Smartphone-a user-friendly device to deliver affordable healthcare-a practical paradigm", *J. Health Med. Inform.,* vol. 7, no. 7, p. 3, 2016.
[http://dx.doi.org/10.4172/2157-7420.1000232]

[73]   J. Miller-Thayer, "Health migration: crossing borders for affordable health care", *j. of field actions.,* vol. 2010, no. 2, 2010.

[74]   S.B. Junaid, A.A. Imam, A.O. Balogun, L.C. De Silva, Y.A. Surakat, G. Kumar, M. Abdulkarim, A.N. Shuaibu, A. Garba, Y. Sahalu, A. Mohammed, T.Y. Mohammed, B.A. Abdulkadir, A.A. Abba, N.A.I. Kakumi, and S. Mahamad, "Recent advancements in emerging technologies for healthcare management systems: A survey", *Healthcare,* vol. 10, no. 10, p. 1940, 2022.
[http://dx.doi.org/10.3390/healthcare10101940] [PMID: 36292387]

[75]   H. Zakaria, N.A.A. Bakar, N.H. Hassan, and S. Yaacob, "IoT security risk management model for secured practice in healthcare environment", *Procedia Comput. Sci.,* vol. 161, pp. 1241-1248, 2019.
[http://dx.doi.org/10.1016/j.procs.2019.11.238]

[76]   O. Sangpetch, and A. Sangpetch, "Security context framework for distributed healthcare IoT platform", In: *International conference on IoT technologies for healthcare* Västerås: Sweden, 2016.
[http://dx.doi.org/10.1007/978-3-319-51234-1_11]

[77]   T. Aladwani, "Scheduling IoT healthcare tasks in fog computing based on their importance", *Procedia Comput. Sci.,* vol. 163, pp. 560-569, 2019.
[http://dx.doi.org/10.1016/j.procs.2019.12.138]

[78]   H. Malik, M.M. Alam, Y. Le Moullec, and A. Kuusik, "NarrowBand-IoT performance analysis for healthcare applications", *Procedia Comput. Sci.,* vol. 130, pp. 1077-1083, 2018.
[http://dx.doi.org/10.1016/j.procs.2018.04.156]

[79]   F. Jamil, S. Ahmad, N. Iqbal, and D.H. Kim, "Towards a remote monitoring of patient vital signs based on iot-based blockchain integrity management platforms in smart hospitals", *Sensors,* vol. 20, no. 8, p. 2195, 2020.
[http://dx.doi.org/10.3390/s20082195] [PMID: 32294989]

[80]   L.A. Durán-Vega, P.C. Santana-Mancilla, R. Buenrostro-Mariscal, J. Contreras-Castillo, L.E. Anido-Rifón, M.A. García-Ruiz, O.A. Montesinos-López, and F. Estrada-González, "An IoT system for remote health monitoring in elderly adults through a wearable device and mobile application", *Geriatrics,* vol. 4, no. 2, p. 34, 2019.
[http://dx.doi.org/10.3390/geriatrics4020034] [PMID: 31067819]

[81]   J. Miranda, J. Cabral, S. Wagner, C. Fischer Pedersen, B. Ravelo, M. Memon, and M. Mathiesen, "An open platform for seamless sensor support in healthcare for the internet of things", *Sensors,* vol. 16, no. 12, p. 2089, 2016.

[http://dx.doi.org/10.3390/s16122089] [PMID: 27941656]

[82]   I. Machorro-Cano, G. Alor-Hernández, M.A. Paredes-Valverde, U. Ramos-Deonati, J.L. Sánchez-Cervantes, and L. Rodríguez-Mazahua, "PISIoT: A machine learning and iot-based smart health platform for overweight and obesity control", *Appl. Sci.,* vol. 9, no. 15, p. 3037, 2019.
[http://dx.doi.org/10.3390/app9153037]

[83]   A. Hussain, T. Ali, F. Althobiani, U. Draz, M. Irfan, S. Yasin, S. Shafiq, Z. Safdar, A. Glowacz, G. Nowakowski, M.S. Khan, and S. Alqhtani, "Security framework for iot based real-time health applications", *Electronics,* vol. 10, no. 6, p. 719, 2021.
[http://dx.doi.org/10.3390/electronics10060719]

[84]   Y. Zhang, G. Chen, H. Du, X. Yuan, M. Kadoch, and M. Cheriet, "Real-time remote health monitoring system driven by 5G MEC-IoT", *Electronics,* vol. 9, no. 11, p. 1753, 2020.
[http://dx.doi.org/10.3390/electronics9111753]

[85]   M.A. Almaiah, F. Hajjej, A. Ali, M.F. Pasha, and O. Almomani, "A novel hybrid trustworthy decentralized authentication and data preservation model for digital healthcare IoT based CPS", *Sensors,* vol. 22, no. 4, p. 1448, 2022.
[http://dx.doi.org/10.3390/s22041448] [PMID: 35214350]

[86]   E. Ashraf, N.F.F. Areed, H. Salem, E.H. Abdelhay, and A. Farouk, "FIDChain: Federated intrusion detection system for blockchain-enabled iot healthcare applications", *Healthcare,* vol. 10, no. 6, p. 1110, 2022.
[http://dx.doi.org/10.3390/healthcare10061110] [PMID: 35742161]

[87]   G. Manogaran, P. Shakeel, H. Fouad, Y. Nam, S. Baskar, N. Chilamkurti, and R. Sundarasekar, "Wearable IoT smart-log patch: An edge computing-based bayesian deep learning network system for multi access physical monitoring system", *Sensors,* vol. 19, no. 13, p. 3030, 2019.
[http://dx.doi.org/10.3390/s19133030] [PMID: 31324070]

[88]   H.Y. Chen, Z.Y. Wu, T.L. Chen, Y.M. Huang, and C.H. Liu, "Security privacy and policy for cryptographic based electronic medical information system", *Sensors,* vol. 21, no. 3, p. 713, 2021.
[http://dx.doi.org/10.3390/s21030713] [PMID: 33494288]

[89]   S. Khezr, M. Moniruzzaman, A. Yassine, and R. Benlamri, "Blockchain technology in healthcare: A comprehensive review and directions for future research", *Appl. Sci.,* vol. 9, no. 9, p. 1736, 2019.
[http://dx.doi.org/10.3390/app9091736]

[90]   N.A. Mahoto, A. Shaikh, M.S. Al Reshan, M.A. Memon, and A. Sulaiman, "Knowledge discovery from healthcare electronic records for sustainable environment", *Sustainability,* vol. 13, no. 16, p. 8900, 2021.
[http://dx.doi.org/10.3390/su13168900]

[91]   A.A. Nancy, D. Ravindran, P.M.D. Raj Vincent, K. Srinivasan, and D. Gutierrez Reina, IoT-Cloud-based smart healthcare monitoring system for heart disease prediction *via* deep learning, *Electronics,* vol. 11, no. 15, p. 2292, 2022.
[http://dx.doi.org/10.3390/electronics11152292]

[92]   M.N. Kamel Boulos, and P. Zhang, "Digital twins: From personalised medicine to precision public health", *J. Pers. Med.,* vol. 11, no. 8, p. 745, 2021.
[http://dx.doi.org/10.3390/jpm11080745] [PMID: 34442389]

[93]   C. Peng, and P. Goswami, "Meaningful integration of data from heterogeneous health services and home environment based on ontology", *Sensors,* vol. 19, no. 8, p. 1747, 2019.
[http://dx.doi.org/10.3390/s19081747] [PMID: 31013678]

[94]   A.S.M. Kayes, R. Kalaria, I.H. Sarker, M.S. Islam, P.A. Watters, A. Ng, M. Hammoudeh, S. Badsha, and I. Kumara, "A survey of context-aware access control mechanisms for cloud and fog networks: Taxonomy and open research issues", *Sensors,* vol. 20, no. 9, p. 2464, 2020.
[http://dx.doi.org/10.3390/s20092464] [PMID: 32349242]

[95]   T.A. Nguyen, I. Fe, C. Brito, V.K. Kaliappan, E. Choi, D. Min, J.W. Lee, and F.A. Silva, "Performability evaluation of load balancing and fail-over strategies for medical information systems with edge/fog computing using stochastic reward nets", *Sensors,* vol. 21, no. 18, p. 6253, 2021.
[http://dx.doi.org/10.3390/s21186253] [PMID: 34577460]

[96]   A. Brunete, E. Gambao, M. Hernando, and R. Cedazo, "Smart assistive architecture for the integration of iot devices, robotic systems, and multimodal interfaces in healthcare environments", *Sensors,* vol. 21, no. 6, p. 2212, 2021.
[http://dx.doi.org/10.3390/s21062212] [PMID: 33809884]

SUBJECT INDEX

A

Acute 112, 179
   coronary syndrome 112
   respiratory syndrome 179
Adaptive neuro-fuzzy inference system
   (ANFIS) 83
AI-based decision support system 48
Application(s) 10, 14, 23, 40, 63, 68, 85, 132,
   135, 138, 164, 166, 167, 169, 185, 186,
   187, 195, 196
  computer-based 40
  machine-learning 63
  programming interface (API) 10, 135, 138,
   185
Automobiles 146, 155, 177
  autonomous 146
Autonomous solutions 163

B

Bipolar disorder 186
Blockchain 185, 186
   network 185, 186
   technology 185
Bluetooth 52, 174
   connection 52
   sensor 174
Breast cancer 43, 62, 79
   prognosis 43
   screening 79

C

Cancer 85, 176
  lung 85
  prostate 176
Cardiac dysrhythmia 101
Cardiovascular disease risk 34
CARLA outcome measure 47
Centroids 121, 177

census block 177
computed 121
Characteristics, sociodemographic 99
Chronic obstructive pulmonary disease
   (COPD) 169, 186
Cloud 9, 10, 15, 16, 61, 83, 135, 148, 152,
   153, 164, 165, 166, 167, 169, 174, 183,
   184, 187
  and artificial intelligence 169
  based hardware 166
  computing 61, 183
  computing layer 184
  database 16, 174
  execution 167
  miner 83
  public 165
Cluster(s) 84, 123
  activity 84
  formation 123
Clustering algorithm 121
Common recognition and identification
platform (CRIP) 187, 188, 189
Computer 25, 39, 156
  algorithm 25
  program 39
  vision 156
Computing power 130
Conditions 15, 32, 37, 61, 67, 91, 133, 138,
   186, 196, 204
  heart 67
  neuropsychiatric 15
  respiratory 138
Consumption, fuel 163
Convolutional 29, 30, 81, 82, 120, 147, 151,
   156, 167
  neural network (CNN) 29, 30, 82, 151, 156,
   167
  pathways 29
Coronary atherosclerosis 101
Coronavirus, acute respiratory syndrome 1,
   129

Smart 173, 158, 168, 185
  contracts, blockchain-based 185
  gateway, wearable 173
  home services 158
  PLS Version 168
Smartphone 14, 53, 118, 150, 169
  app 150, 169
  based depressed mood prediction system 14
  device's sensor streams 118
  stores 14
  transmits data 53
Social 7, 10, 137, 157
  isolation 10
  media platforms 7, 157
  networks 137
Software, smartphone-based 180
Solar corona 19
Somatization 91
SparkFun sensor 146
Speech recognition process 25
Statistical package for social science (SPSS)
    9, 87, 102, 161
Storage 14, 61, 129, 133, 135, 173, 190
  business 129
  devices 61
Support vector machine (SVM) 25, 34, 79, 88
System 25, 59, 169, 181, 196
  eGAP 59
  healthcare-focused 196
  learning-based 25
  medical 181
  microelectronics 169

T

Techniques 37, 43, 59, 63, 68, 77, 85, 86, 118,
    125, 156
  applied data mining 125
  boosting 63
  computer vision 156
  deep-stacked autoencoder 118
  effective clustering 59
  mining 77
Technologies, wireless sensor network 204
Thrombolysis 47, 90
  therapy 47
Transportation 129, 155, 156, 163
  public 155
Transportation 166, 177
  network 177

restrictions 166

U

UCI 38, 39, 67, 82
  repository 38, 39, 67
  standards 82
  web portal 67

V

Video frames 173
Virtual 141, 167, 184
  climate 141
  machines (VMs) 167, 184
Virus1, 146, 196
  single-stranded RNA 1
  transmission 146, 196
Vision transformer 141
Visual analysis system 115

W

Web of Science databases 6
Wi-Fi 13, 53, 61, 117, 136, 137, 152, 164, 191
  application 61
  certified product 117
  network 137
Wireless 16, 61, 132, 134, 151, 169, 170, 185,
    191, 204
  body area network (WBAN) 134, 169
  communications 61, 132
  connection 16
  data transmission 191
  human body-connected 191
  sensors 185, 204
Wisconsin breast cancer 67

Z

ZigBee 132, 142
  networking protocol 132
  protocol 142
Zoom cloud meeting 168

* 9 7 8 9 8 1 5 1 7 9 4 7 7 *